Physical Therapy Management
An Integrated Science

Physical Therapy Management

An Integrated Science

JANE WALTER, P.T., Ed.D.

Associate Professor and Program Director
Department of Physical Therapy
School of Allied Health Sciences
Oakland University
Rochester, Michigan

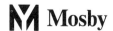 **Mosby**

St. Louis Baltimore Boston Chicago London Philadelphia Sydney Toronto

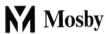

Copyright © 1993 by Mosby-Year Book, Inc.
A C.V. Mosby imprint of Mosby-Year Book, Inc.

Mosby-Year Book, Inc.
11830 Westline Industrial Drive
St. Louis, MO 63416

1 2 3 4 5 6 7 8 9 0 CL MV 97 96 95 94 93

Library of Congress Cataloging-in-Publication Data
Walter, Jane, 1945-
    Physical therapy management : an integrated science / Jane Walter.
        p.   cm.
    Includes bibliographical references and index.
    ISBN 0-8016-6416-0
    1. Physical therapy services—Administration.   I. Title.
    [DNLM: 1. Physical Therapy—methods. 2. Physical Therapy—
    organization & administration—United States.   WB 460 W232p]
    RA975.5.P6W35   1992
    362.1′786—dc20
    DNLM/DLC   92-48211
    for Library of Congress   CIP

Sponsoring Editors: David K. Marshall/Martha Sasser
Associate Managing Editor, Manuscript Services: Deborah Thorp
Production Supervisor: Carol A. Reynolds
Proofroom Manager: Barbara M. Kelly

. . . .

To my parents, Donald and Lorine Walter, for their support, patience, and work ethic.

. . . .

Contributors

Cheryl Cooper, M.A., P.T.
Clinical Coordinator
Physical Therapy
Nova-Care, Inc.
Baltimore, Maryland

Samuel B. Feitelberg, M.A., P.T.
Professor and Chairman
Department of Physical Therapy
University of Vermont
Burlington, Vermont

Jan Gwyer, Ph.D., P.T.
Director of the Physical Therapy Graduate Program
Duke University
Durham, North Carolina

Donald E. Jackson, M.S., P.T.
Executive Vice President
National Easter Seal Society
Chicago, Illinois

Colleen Kigin, M.P.A., P.T.
Director, Physical Therapy Services
Massachusetts General Hospital
Boston, Massachusetts

Kathleen Jakubiak Kovacek, P.T.
Administrator for Rehabilitation Services
Cottage Hospital and Henry Ford Rehabilitation
Grosse Pointe Farms, Michigan

Peter R. Kovacek, M.S.A., P.T.
President
Kovacek Physical Therapy
Harper Woods, Michigan

Jane Walter, P.T., Ed.D.
Associate Professor and Program Director
Department of Physical Therapy
School of Allied Health Sciences
Oakland University
Rochester, Michigan

··········

Foreword

··········

In this book on physical therapy management, Jane Walter, Ed.D., P.T., breaks new ground. This is the first textbook of its kind solely devoted to physical therapy practice. I have known Dr. Walter for many years, both through our work as physical therapists and our work on behalf of the American Physical Therapy Association, and it is with great pleasure that I write this foreword for an exciting new book.

As those of us in the profession know and understand, physical therapy is a specialized field that cannot be readily interpreted by the usual management theories and practices. The profession has developed into a hybrid organization because of the special relationship physical therapists have with the patient and the institutions that deliver the service and because of the changing health care environment's current emphasis on cost savings and regulation.

Physical therapy is a relatively new profession. Nevertheless, it has evolved rapidly in the latter part of this century into one of the more crucial health care delivery systems. Not only is physical therapy concerned with serving the injured or handicapped patient, but it also helps the older individual to maintain a desired quality of life and provides outreach to corporate and industrial employees and employers to help prevent injuries and maintain a safe and secure workplace. This changing mission, coupled with the variety of health care settings in which physical therapists work, and the intricacies of health insurance coverage and reimbursement make physical therapy management a complex operation. It is imperative to have effective management in today's changing health care environment.

This book speaks directly to the issues concerning the physical therapy manager in this climate. It gives the reader an in-depth overview of health care systems and how physical therapy fits into the "big picture." Dr. Walter's synthesis and analysis of management systems, planning strategies, and marketing keys directly into what is happening in physical therapy today, making the book a state-of-the-art guide to managing a practice. Her attention to laws and regulations, reimbursement, and fiscal management makes it indispensable reading for the physical therapy manager.

Dr. Walter's book is a genuine accomplishment: a comprehensive presentation of what it takes to manage a practice today. Her sound insights and her acute knowledge of the physical therapy field and health care in general are communicated with a special sensibility. It is well researched and documented, and the case studies and examples make the material readily understandable. This book is what the physical therapy industry has needed for a long time. Before we relied on networking with other professionals, sharing accomplishments and failures. Now we have a book that pulls all that knowledge and expertise together. Dr. Walter has created a book that is "must" reading for anyone setting up or continuing in private practice, in a hospital, or clinic.

Ernest A. Burch, Jr., P.T.

Preface

Physical therapy practice is not a belt factory in which known raw materials are manipulated in specific ways to produce known and measurable finished products. This is not a textbook of management theory but a textbook of applied management within a physical therapy environment. This text is based on theories that emphasize the relationship of structure and function and the organization as a system. In addition, references are made to classical concepts of organizational structure and behavioral concepts of group dynamics and human relations within the organization.

The product of the physical therapy service is difficult to measure both at the beginning and at the end of the process. For many, the service that occurs at the time of production should be the focus of our management and our understanding. As a profession that focuses on functional and dysfunctional human movement, physical therapy offers many challenges to the manager who must make sense out of the product, the service, and the productivity of the professional involved, while understanding the relationship of the service to the mission of the institution and the community in which the service is provided. Like the plant manager is Studs Terkel's *Working,* physical therapy managers are "human engineers"* who must master the art of understanding human nature and help the individual to maximize his/her potential for the good of the organization.

Health care is a constantly evolving, extremely complex system. As health care continues to evolve in the United States, systems that were once hierarchical and closed are flattening the organizational structure, and managers are finding new ways to scan the environment and adapt to changing needs and regulations. Alternative physical therapy services are developing where traditional structures and functions no longer meet the needs of the community of interest or organizational mission. Entrepreneurial ventures are evolving in physical therapy with a variety of coalition structures, and physical therapy is joining collectivities of professionals to offer contractual services to community and institutional groups.

Health care is in a constant state of change. A 1984 study predicted that "(1) 90% of health care will be delivered by contract arrangements; (2) 90% of hospitals will be part of a multihospital system; (3) 40% of all physicians will be employed by health care organizations; (4) nontherapeutic services will account for 25% of hospital revenue; (5) national debate will govern health care rationing; (6) trustees will be more involved in hospital management; [and] (7) a two-tiered delivery system will continue to exist."†

Although a follow-up study has not been done to track these changes, contract arrangements are increasing for all health care providers as independent and group

---

*Terkel S: *Working.* New York, Ballantine Books, 1974, p. 248.

†From Staff: *Hospitals.* Excerpts from meeting of American Association for Hospital Planning, Houston, July, 1983 in Colachis SC: New directions in health care. *Arch Phys Med Rehabil,* June 1984, vol 65, p. 294.

contractors, and major services such as laundry, purchasing, and food services are being contracted from outside vendors. Many community-based hospitals are finding it to their benefit to join other hospitals in a variety of arrangements to share services, and an increasing number of multihospital systems are being formed locally, regionally, and nationwide. We are also in the midst of a national debate on health care financing, with over 20 national health care plans introduced to Congress. Health care rationing in terms of identifying what will be paid for by national plans is a major component of most of these proposals. The changes in the health care system continue to increase costs with few effective cost-containment measures.

A physical therapy manager is a person who bridges the gap between administration and the worker; between the patient and the reimbursement agency; between the worker (client) and the employer; between the marketplace and the practice. It is critical that this person understand the organization, the market, the community, the practice, the outcome of the service, and the myriad of other components of a successful operation, while grounding practices in current management theories.

Three skill areas that are critical to the manager are (1) human resource skills to develop and maintain teams; resolve conflict; train, coach, and counsel staff; and negotiate; (2) management science skills including measurement and forecasting skills to measure productivity, plan, monitor programs, develop budgets and programs, and make accurate projections; and (3) service delivery skills to assess markets and profitability, utilize resources effectively and efficiently, assure quality care, recognize and reduce risks, develop new approaches to care, and take responsibility to explore the ethical dilemmas encountered in the provision of services.

Many skills are developed and honed in clinical practice that will enhance the effectiveness of the physical therapy manager. These include, but are not limited to, communication skills, knowledge of scheduling issues, time management skills, knowledge of health care from the perspective of the clinician, and skills related to managing subordinates. It has been common practice in many health professions, including physical therapy, to promote industrious physical therapists who are effective clinicians to management positions. As health care continues to expand and become more complex, the management of components of the system is also becoming more complex. Physical therapy managers today must be as well prepared as possible to assume this critical leadership position within the profession. In addition to being "mentored" on the job, it is important to develop the new skills needed by today's manager through formal education, networking, and continuing self-study.

The role of the manager in health care is a critical one for the effective and efficient operation of the system and to develop and manage creative changes, which are necessary to bring the cost of health care under control. The manager promotes the profession of physical therapy within the organizational components of the health care system and assures the continuing viability of the services, which are needed by the collective communities of interest including patients (consumers, clients, citizens), referral sources, human service agencies, and community service groups.

Organizations—as do many systems—tend toward entropy. That is, left unattended or improperly managed, organizations that are not aware of the environment will eventually fail because the environment in which they exist is constantly changing and the product that they produce may be less and less valued by society. This is especially true of a health care organization today.

Among the many challenges facing the physical therapy manager is that of managing in a time of limited resources: manpower, money, time, and space. That challenge requires a keen understanding of the principles of management and the ability to manage scarce resources optimally and fairly.

. . . .
ORGANIZATION OF THE BOOK

Chapter 1 introduces the concept of systems and how health care organizations function as systems from an organizational and functional perspective.

Chapter 2 focuses on community-based physical therapy systems and the degree to which these systems are responsive to the needs of the community.

Complex physical therapy environments such as multihospital settings and managed-care environments are discussed in Chapter 3. These highly complex systems are the focus of the development of alternative structures to meet the needs of the customer and to reduce the complex hierarchical structure of the institution.

One of the most complex approaches to flattening the organizational structure in complex organizations is the concept of service/product line management. This concept is presented in detail by Samuel Feitelberg, P.T., M.A., a guest contributor to Chapter 4.

Common filters in a system include the roles and rules by which the participants are defined in the system. Chapter 5 presents the laws and regulations that define the delivery of physical therapy services in a variety of settings.

Complex organizations must develop complex systems to manage the information generated by the institution. As society moves toward a more technologically sophisticated system of information management, health care institutions will find more and more opportunities to streamline the management of patient, regulatory, reimbursement, and organizational information through computerized systems. Chapter 6 focuses on this area of information management.

Mangement theories have evolved from an intuitive and trial and error approaches of the industrial era to modern contingency approaches. The breadth of management theories are presented in Chapter 7.

Chapter 8 focuses on the manner in which individuals behave within an organization. This behavior is a result of what the individual brings to the organization and reactions to the organizational environment. Managers must understand human development, the changing physical therapy environment, and theories of managing people within the organizational environment in order to appropriately manage people within the organization.

Chapter 9 presents the mechanisms most often used by managers to control organizational behavior through institutional policies and procedures.

There are several overlapping areas of responsibility in an organization. When some individuals representing one aspect of the organization have rights, other individuals have certain obligations. Chapter 10 discusses these rights and obligations and other ethical aspects of physical therapy management.

A critical aspect of management is the planning of facilities, new programs, and budgets. There are a variety of planning techniques and schemas that managers use in conducting both short-term and long-term planning. Planning strategies are presented in Chapter 11.

The key to space designs in physical therapy departments and practices is flexibility. Chapter 12 presents guiding principles for planning space from laws such as the Americans with Disabilities Act and general principles related to space decisions.

The marketing of physical therapy services within the institution, to communities of interest and to the general public is critical as the profession moves toward greater autonomy. Chapter 13 discusses marketing principles related to physical therapy.

Quality assurance and measures of productivity have always been critical facets of physical therapy practice. As business and health care delivery systems embrace the concepts of total quality management and continuous quality improvement, physical therapy managers must respond to the shift toward greater incorporation of quality improvement in organizations. Chapter 14 explores the relationships between quality and productivity in physical therapy management.

The increased bureaucratization of health care reimbursement has led to a very complex system of fiscal management in physical therapy. In addition, soaring health care costs have lead most health care organizations to adopt cost-saving and cost-cutting measures as a means of controlling costs. Chapter 15 presents the complexities of reimbursement and its effect on the practice of physical therapy, as well as the principles of fiscal management of a physical therapy practice.

In Chapter 16 the author speculates on the future of physical therapy management in a changing physical therapy and health care environment.

Jane Walter, Ed.D., P.T.

Acknowledgments

Foremost, I would like to thank David Marshall and Martha Sasser, my editors, and Julie Tryboski and Barbara Menczer for their guidance and encouragement. They have made the process of writing this book a pleasant and rewarding experience.

I also wish to recognize the many hospital administrators who were so supportive during my tenure at Mary Hitchcock Memorial Hospital in Lebanon, New Hampshire. They include William Wilson, William Donaldson, William Richwagen, Eugenia Monroe Hamilton, and Paul Gardent. These last two individuals facilitated my involvement in many administrative projects and led me to pursue doctoral education in administration.

In addition, special recognition belongs to Dr. Otto Goldkamp, who generously gave his time and talent to help me and many other physical therapists to develop as autonomous professionals, and Dr. Robert Krout, who gave me the opportunity to assume my first management position. Dr. Edward D. Harris, Jr., and Dr. Ronald Olson provided the freedom to apply innovative and creative solutions to management problems and instilled confidence through their constructive and continuing feedback.

A special thank you to all of the professionals and staff who worked in Rehabilitation Medicine at Mary Hitchcock Memorial Hospital: Kathy Cepeda, Alison Corpieri, Liz Hewitt, Margaret Rahn, David Robator, Debbie VanArman, Mike Emery, Stuart Binder-MacLeod, Ron Renz, Ginny Hunt, Cheryl Cooper, Bonnie Sussman, Cyndi Stabenow, Beth Wolf, Polly Bingham, and Yvonne Martin.

Several professors at the University of Vermont greatly influenced this work including my doctoral advisor, Dr. Robert Carlson, and Drs. Robert Larson, Robert Nash, and Edward Ducharme. The influences of these scholars appear throughout the text.

A very special thank you to Samuel Feitelberg, who is one of the finest physical therapy administrators I know. His contributions to physical therapy management have been countless and he continues to lecture on the subject widely. A particular thank you goes to Mr. Feitelberg for his support during the creation and writing of this book; he wrote Chapter 4, which is an adaptation of his many lectures on service line management. I wish to also thank three outstanding Michigan-based physical therapy managers, administrators and teachers: Kathleen Jakubiak Kovacek, P.T.; Peter R. Kovacek, M.S.A., P.T.; and Kristine Thompson, M.Ph., P.T. Their untiring efforts in reading early drafts provided insightful feedback and helped to refine concepts.

This text is a management text that truly reflects the challenges of the physical therapy manager in the health care system. Many of the concepts presented in this text were refined and clarified through many discussions with staff of the American Physical Therapy Association. Special appreciation is extended to Frank Mallon, Esq.; R. Charles Harker, Esq.; Brian Rasmussen; Bob Mansell; and Phyllis Quinn and staff members in their respective departments for their timely and expert assistance. The depth of these individuals' understanding of the issues and the systems in which physical therapy must exist is outstanding and was invaluable in discussing many of the concepts in this text.

My appreciation also to the faculty and staff of the Program in Physical Therapy, and Ronald Olson (Dean) and Arthur Griggs (Assistant to the Dean) of the School of Health Sciences at Oakland University for their support over the past year. Special thanks to Linda Berlinski, a second-year physical therapy student, who retrieved many of the articles used in this text. Her dependability and perseverance were critical to completion of the project.

Jane Walter, Ed.D., P.T.

Contents

CHAPTER 16
· · · · · · · · · · ·
THE FUTURE OF PHYSICAL THERAPY MANAGEMENT 271

Health Care Systems

I. **Organizational systems**

II. **Systems**

III. **Organizational structure**
   A. Building pyramids as an organizational structure
   B. Hierarchical health care organizational structures
   C. Small systems structure in physical therapy

IV. **Definitions**

V. **Appendix**
   Creating an organizational chart

ORGANIZATIONAL SYSTEMS

Organizations are commonly referred to as rational, natural, or open systems. A system is a set of elements that are so related that a change in any element causes changes in other elements within the system. Systems are made up of sets of components that work together for the overall objective of the whole.

A rational system is described as "a collectivity oriented to the pursuit of relatively specific goals and exhibiting a relatively highly formalized social structure."[2(p21)] Rational systems (e.g., General Motors, IBM) represent most of the organizations that we deal with in our society and have also been referred to as closed systems operating more independent of the environment.

A natural system is defined as "a collectivity whose participants are little affected by the formal structure or official goals but who share a common interest in the survival of the system and who engage in collective activities, informally structured, to secure this end."[2(p22)] Natural systems are usually seen as agreements among individuals in organizations like buying cooperatives, in which individuals give some tangible service to the organization in order to secure a mutual goal such as specific types of foods bought at a reasonable price.

An open system is defined as "a coalition of shifting interest groups that develop goals by negotiation; the structure of the coalition, its activities, and its outcomes are strongly influenced by environmental factors."[2(p23)] Open systems are seen in organizations such as day care or alternative schooling systems in which the individuals define the nature of the organization according to their specific interests or philosophies. Such a system may change as the community changes.

For the most part, physical therapy services are found in rational, closed organizations. However, most administrators have recognized that a closed system will not be a healthy organization and have developed some of the characteristics of an open system, such as environmental scanning. Such scanning functions are now seen in vice presidential–level positions in the organization where the individual is responsible for assessing the needs of the community of interest and making short- and long-term plans to bring about adjustments in the mission and function of the organization. These efforts even extend into individual departments where individuals are designated to devote part of their efforts to marketing or community outreach projects. There are a few unique physical therapy practices that can be characterized as truly open systems, and they will be discussed later.

SYSTEMS

A system is represented by an input, throughput, output, and feedback loop set within a specific environment (Fig 1–1).

In a health care organization and from a patient care perspective, input may be characterized by the ill person who enters the system; throughput represents the clinical environment, the tests, the hospital stay, and the professional consultations that are used to diagnose and treat the person; output is either a well person or a person who remains ill, but whose condition is being controlled medically or managed in terms of therapies; and the feedback loop is made up of quality assessment and improvement activities that assess the degree to which ill persons are treated and the degree to which they get well and stay well. The environment may be represented by the community if this is a community hospital, by the state or region if the organization is a tertiary care center, or by a larger world view if the facility offers unique services not found in other locations (Fig 1–2).

ORGANIZATIONAL STRUCTURE

In looking at or building any organization, it is important to understand that the structure of the organization is driven by activities, decisions, and relationships.[3(p194)] The functions of an organization should determine their structure; however, that is not always the manner in which individuals build an organization. The mechanical structure of an organization cannot dictate relationships of individuals in a meaningful way. There must first be a need for individuals to interact. The organizational structure, then, depicts or frames that interaction.

Organizational structures are depicted by organizational trees that show levels of responsibility, span of control, reporting relationships, and functional relationships.

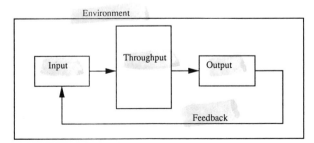

FIG 1–1.
System design.

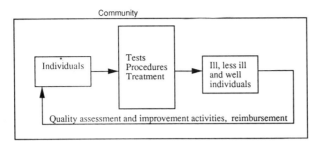

FIG 1–2.
System design of a community hospital.

Building Pyramids as an Organizational Structure

During the time of the Pharaohs, let us imagine that the pyramid builders had to have a very formal structure in order to complete the task of building the pyramids. In this example, the builder is the final authority in this system. His span of control extends to the stone movers who, according to this chart, have responsibility (span of control) for the team leaders who move the stones as well as for the stone masons who cut and shape the stones. This organizational chart depicts four levels of responsibility commonly described and built from the bottom up. The slaves are responsible to the team leaders, who are responsible to the stone mover, who is responsible to the builder. The vertical lines depict lines of authority, whereas the horizontal lines depict span of control. In some organizations, horizontal lines may also depict lines of communication and staff positions. Communication horizontal lines are drawn between boxes rather than on the top of the boxes, as depicted in this example. In this example the slaves depicted horizontally to the pyramid builder would be responsible only to him for functions such as his personal well-being and would be considered staff to the pyramid builder (Fig 1–3).

The organizational chart depicts not only the relationship of each member of

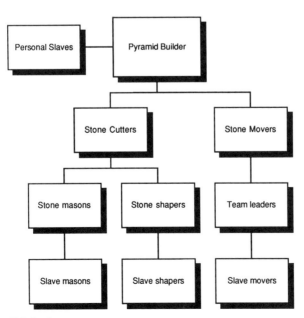

FIG 1–3.
Organizational structure: pyramid builders.

the system, but the activities that must be performed. Given that all functions are represented in this organizational chart, there is a clear line of authority in the performance of the activities. It can be assumed that these functions were being carried out in the oppressive environment of Egypt in 1300 B.C., and, therefore, there is little doubt that communications only flowed one way—from the top down. That perception of unidirectional communications is one of the weaknesses of the hierarchical organization. However, given the environment in which the builder worked and the grave consequences of dissatisfaction with his work, it was critical to build a system that reliably responded to commands.

Hierarchical Health Care Organizational Structures

The first hospitals were seen as workshops for the physician—facilities in which patients could be gathered and cared for under the physician's direction. The social structure was determined by the decisions that were made in relation to the care of the patient. Such a system called for a highly structured organization in which the physician was clearly at the top of the decision-making hierarchy (Fig 1–4). These structures are referred to as hierarchical pyramids. The hierarchy refers to the levels in which the organization is divided. Each level suggests a specific reporting relationship, degree of independence, and level of responsibility. The pyramidal structure is created by the diminishing number of positions in the higher levels of authority. Although the system may be depicted as a single pyramid, it is most accurate to represent the multiple pyramids within a system to understand the complex and highly structured nature of the organization (Fig 1–5).

In highly structured systems, power and authority often come from the positional power of formal position and title. The more structured and hierarchical the system, the more authority those at the top of the pyramid have over the levels below them. As these systems become more flattened, the professionals serving in these authority levels must "learn to operate without the might of the hierarchy behind them. The crutch of authority must be thrown away and replaced by their own personal ability to make relationships, use influence, and work with others to

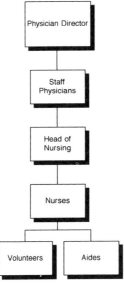

FIG 1–4.
Organizational structure: early hospitals.

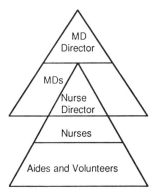

FIG 1–5.
Pyramidal structure: early hospitals.

achieve results."[4(p361)] This move away from traditional systems and the changing role of physical therapy managers will be discussed in greater detail later. Organizational systems may also be depicted in prose (Fig 1–6).

It was in this kind of formalized structure that organized physical therapy was first developed as a component of the army hospital and then as a component of the acute care and rehabilitation hospitals during the early polio epidemics.[5]

Small Systems Structure in Physical Therapy

Physical therapy departments, practices, and joint ventures are built according to the output (product) of the system. A typical organizational chart of a small private practice is represented in Figure 1–7, in which the owner determines the clientele to be served and the relative volume of the work.

By keeping the organization relatively flat and simple, the owner can predict outcomes with some certainty, and the system is stable. Given that the secretary, bookkeeper, and physical therapists report directly to the owner (owner's span of control), it is easy to make adjustments when, for example, the secretary reports a significant increase in appointments for the following week, the bookkeeper reports that there will be a 3-month delay in medicare payments, or one of the physical therapists is pregnant and will be on maternity leave in 6 months. The owner, as the primary decision maker in this system, has built a system that can be easily monitored in which changes can be made relatively quickly to cover all contingencies.

Let's take the same system and add the fact that the owner has decided to keep the practice open 14 hours a day (7 A.M. to 9 P.M.) 6½ days a week. Given that adjustments might have to be made in this system quickly in order to accommodate environmental stressors, it would be unrealistic for the owner to presume that she can

```
1.0   Physician  Director
    1.1  Staff  Physicians
       1.1.1 Director of Nursing
          1.1.1.1 Staff Nurses
             1.1.1.1.1. Aides
             1.1.1.1.2. Volunteers
```

FIG 1–6.
Prose depiction of organizational system.

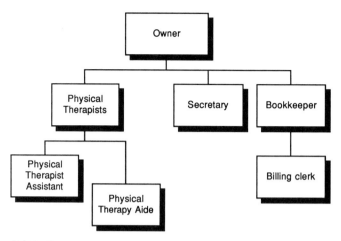

FIG 1–7.
Organizational structure: small physical therapy practice.

be available at all hours to make decisions. Therefore, she creates a senior physical therapist position, or junior partner position, and places that person directly in her line in a one-on-one position (Fig 1–8). "The one-on-one concept reflects a desire to have one person in authority at all times who can deal with emergencies that can arise at any time in an organization that must operate continuously around the clock."[6(p407)]

This assistant-level position gives this person all the authority of the owner in her absence, as evidenced by her span of control to monitor activities of the secretary line, the bookkeeper line, and the physical therapist line.

Although the lines of authority do not now place the physical therapists, physical therapist assistants, or aides in a direct line with the owner, it is critical that the lines of communication remain open in the system. In order for the system to remain sta-

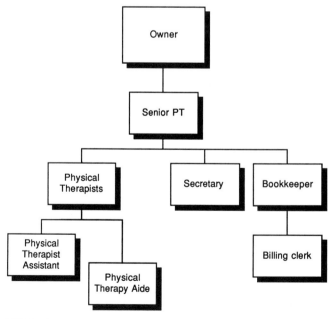

FIG 1–8.
Depiction of one-on-one organizational concept. *PT* = physical therapist.

ble and respond in a timely fashion, communications must move up as well as down the organizational structure. More complex organizational structures will be dealt with in other chapters in discussions of multihospital systems.

DEFINITIONS

Boundary: Defined by the constraints of the system and occurring between the system and the environment. The limitations imposed by the system limiting growth or change. In analysis, consider the rigidity or looseness of the boundaries.

Closed system: Any other set of elements that can be classified as a system but does not possess the characteristics of an open system; self-contained—moving toward entropy (i.e., nuclear fission, some primitive societies).

Entrepreneurial: Related to establishing and running an independent business operation.

Entropy: Universal law of nature in which all forms of organization move toward disorganization or death. Entropic process asserts itself in all biological systems as well as in closed physical systems.

Environment: The larger context in which a system operates, from which it receives its purposes and resources, and to which it is responsible for the use of resources and for the adequacy of its output. In an organization, society is an environment.

Equifinality: A system can reach the same final state from differing initial conditions and a variety of paths (i.e., regionalization of services).

Feedback: A process built into a system by which output performance is compared with criterion performance and by which the information about the adequacy of the performance of the system and about the adequacy of its output is communicated to the designer and manager of the system.

Inputs: Consists of those elements that are transformed by the system; whatever becomes subject to the system, or the material upon which the system operates. Raw materials used in a process to achieve a product or output.

Negentropy: Importation of more energy from the environment than is expended. Energy is stored (i.e., bringing in new technology before the population is defined or ready to use it).

Open system: Characteristics of an open system are as follows: (1) Importation of energy (energy derived from the environment). (2) Throughput (transformation of energy). (3) Output (export product). (4) Cycle of events. (5) Possess negative entropy. (6) Information input, negative feedback, and coding process. (7) Steady-state and dynamic homeostasis. (8) Differentiation and elaboration. (9) Equifinality.

Output: Embody the purposes for which the system functions. Identification and determination of outputs represent the preferred first step of analysis. The end of an organization, agency, or agent that may or may not positively affect an outcome. The product of a system; the result or outcome of processes employed by the system.

Steady state: The point at which input equals output and no reserves are available. This is not a static situation. There is a continuous inflow of energy from the external environment and a continuous export of products from the system.

Subsystem: A part of a system, comprised of two or more components, with a purpose of its own and designed to interact with its peer subsystems in order to attain the overall purpose of the system.

Suprasystem: A larger entity, designed for a specific purpose, that is comprised of two or more systems.

System: Set of elements so related that a change in the state of any element induces changes in the state of other elements. Made up of sets of components that work together for the overall objective of the whole.

References

1. Staff: Hospitals, Excerpts from the meeting of the American Association for Hospital Planning, Houston, Tex, July 1983, in Colachis SC: New directions in health care. *Arch Phys Med Rehabil* 1984; 65:291–294
2. Scott WR: *Organizations: Rational, Natural, and Open Systems.* Englewood Cliffs, NJ, Prentice Hall, Inc, 1981.
3. Drucker PF: *The Practice of Management.* New York, NY, Perennial Library, 1986.
4. Kanter RM: *When Giants Learn to Dance.* New York, NY, Simon and Schuster Inc, 1989.
5. Pinkston D: Evolution of the practice of physical therapy in the United States, in Scully R and Barnes ML: *Physical Therapy.* Philadelphia, Pa, JB Lippincott Co, 1989.
6. Webber RA: *Management: Basic Elements of Managing Organizations.* Homewood, Ill, Richard D Irwin, Inc, 1979.

APPENDIX 1.1

Creating an Organizational Chart

1. Identify the FUNCTIONS of the positions and levels by naming job functions, not people.

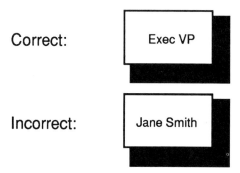

Correct: Exec VP

Incorrect: Jane Smith

2. For those positions that represent a function (personal secretary) which supports another position (executive vice president for finance), use a horizontal line between the two functions.

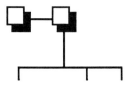

3. **For those positions that represent a function which is subordinate to another function, use a vertical line.**

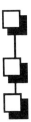

4. **When more than one position represents functions that are subordinate to another function, use a combination of vertical and horizontal lines or vertical lines.**

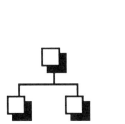 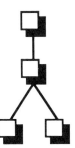

5. **When functions within the organizational chart are equal, place them on the same organizational level.**

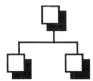

6. **When a function is not equal to others on the same level, but not subordinate to another function on that level, place that function below the other functions.**

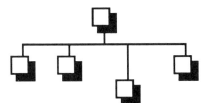

7. **Organizational charts may be represented vertically. When represented vertically, the levels descend from left to right.**

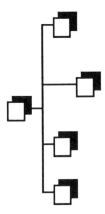

8. **One form of organizational chart shorthand may be employed using a wider and longer box to suggest a number of individuals within one category (staff, supervisors, aides, etc).**

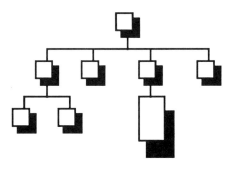

CHAPTER 2

Community-Based Physical Therapy Systems

I. **Community health care systems**

II. **Assessment of community demands for physical therapy**
A. Step 1: Determine the demand for the program
B. Step 2: Determine the roles and rules governing the proposed program
C. Step 3: Develop the concept
D. Step 4: Fieldtest the concept
E. Step 5: Assess the impact of the program

III. **Physical therapy human resource needs in the community**

IV. **Community-based practice settings**
A. The community hospital
B. Home health care

V. **Cases**
A. Practice Privileges: Case 2.1
B. Practice Privileges: Case 2.2

VI. **Definitions**

COMMUNITY HEALTH CARE SYSTEMS

The role of the physical therapist in the community health care system is often as a consultant and health care contractor who works with human service and community service organizations. From a management perspective, the physical therapy manager must be competent enough in health systems research to make an assessment of community physical therapy demands and needs. Skills needed by the manager include the ability to assess the morbidity and mortality statistics of the community as they apply to physical therapy, determine the physical therapy demands of a targeted population, plan an appropriate intervention, conduct a feasibility study of the projected intervention, assess the outcomes of the intervention, and develop a business plan to implement successful interventions.

In the tenth Mary McMillan Lecture, Helen Hislop dreamed that "physical therapy shall achieve greatness as a profession."[1(p1069)] She emphasized the need to elevate our practice to reflect the values of society and meet criteria set by the public that the profession have scientific, humanistic, and social merit.[1(p1077)] That challenge must be taken up by physical therapy managers to promote clinical and community research, to deal with the dilemma of high touch vs. high tech as exercise equipment invades the clinical and community-based health care environments, and to assess the social impact of the physical therapy services provided within the clinic and community. Taking part in community health care systems provides the ideal opportunity to follow up on patients and assess the impact of physical therapy on the individual and the community.

The community health care system focuses on the community hospital and uses human service agencies and community service agencies as extensions of the health care providers. Human service agencies include agencies such as visiting nurse associations, Women, Infant and Children programs, United Way, hospice, Alcoholics Anonymous (AA), senior centers, organizations devoted to helping the homeless, and the Red Cross. Many of these agencies receive federal, state, and local support to carry out community-based programs. Community service agencies are those clubs or organizations that have a commitment to assisting the community members with medical care and other kinds of support. They include women's clubs, which often provide transportation and other services to shut-ins; Lions Clubs, which have a commitment to aiding the blind; Rotary, which often provides business-related assistance; Elks, which may be willing to devote fund-raising activities to specific community health care projects; Shriners, who support crippled and burned children through a variety of services, including free hospital and clinic services; and Daughters of the American Revolution, which supports scholarships for health care–related study. These groups either raise money from members or hold auctions, raffles, fairs, and other community events to raise money for worthy causes, many of which are health care related.

· · · · · · · · · · ·
ASSESSMENT OF COMMUNITY DEMANDS FOR PHYSICAL THERAPY

Many millions of dollars are spent by public health researchers and the federal government in assessing the needs of a community for various health care services. This chapter is concerned with the concept of community demand as it relates to physical therapy. "The *demand* for health care is an economic concept, while the *need* for health care refers to the amount of services that should be made available regardless of economic considerations."[2(p2)] Although health care need is often a driving force that intuitively causes the health care provider or the community to seek services, the economic, sociological, and cultural aspects of the population must be considered in determining the true demand for the service.

As an example, let's assume that you are the manager of a large physical therapy department in an academic health center in an urban setting. At a management meeting you heard that the homeless located around the hospital use the emergency room for assessment of musculoskeletal injuries and other pathologic conditions, and the administration would like to find a way to reduce the high cost of providing emergency room care for problems that may be able to be handled in other ways. You have decided to assess your community homeless population to see if it is feasible to launch a physical therapy program for the homeless to assess and treat musculoskeletal problems before they become severe enough to require emergency room care.

Step 1: Determine the Demand for the Program

"Of greatest importance is the establishment of a population denominator (i.e., the total number of individuals with whom one is dealing). A denominator permits the calculation of specific incidence and prevalence rates (i.e., new occurrences of conditions and all existing conditions regardless of time of onset)."[3(p28)] Census data are oftentimes used with mortality and morbidity reports to determine the population to be studied. The problems in this case are the probable inaccuracies of these reports, especially of the actual number of homeless, cause of death and birth defects, as well as comorbidities.

In this case, actual emergency room records should be retrospectively reviewed as to the diagnoses and treatments administered to the homeless in the past 6 months to establish morbidity rates. Included in that investigation is an assessment of all medical problems for each homeless person seen in the emergency room, the reason for the emergency room visit, the number of times the same person was treated and the primary complaint at each visit, the intervention, and the impressions of those treating the patient. This will result in a profile of the possible clients that will be served by physical therapy intervention. This information will also provide a data base from which to begin the assessment of the proposed program. The total population may have to be estimated if census figures are not available from city, county, or state health statistic resources.

There may be a great need to provide physical therapy services to the homeless in a large urban center, but a manager will find it very difficult to find reliable statistics regarding the homeless since they are not accurately counted by most agencies. In addition to whatever statistics may be available through state and county resources, the physical therapy manager must consider the availability of federal, state, local, and institutional financial support for physical therapy; the demographics of the homeless, including the transitory nature and average length of time a homeless person remains homeless; and the degree to which the homeless seek medical help.

Step 2: Determine the Roles and Rules Governing the Proposed Program

Federal guidelines exist for fundable medical services for the homeless. In addition, there may be state and local guidelines related to this population. All of these guidelines must be gathered and an assessment made regarding the scope of services available now and the potential role of physical therapy in these services.

Roles of various health care workers must be determined in caring for this population and the role physical therapy will play. For example, physical therapists practicing in states that allow evaluation without referral could play a triage role with this population to sort out and refer musculoskeletal, prosthetic/orthotic, and cardiopulmonary symptoms (to name only a few possible areas of triage). This triage function is often performed by social workers and nurses and could be supplemented by physical therapists.

The emphasis of the program as preventive or curative must be determined, and the scope of services needed to provide each of these approaches must be assessed. This is a critical step in physical therapy. It is common to assume that physical therapists will treat any problem that is determined to be present and treatable by physical therapy measures. It may be that the focus of the proposed program will be to prevent musculoskeletal injuries and refer any other major rehabilitation problems, but not to engage in treatment beyond the protocol established for the program. This is a decision that must be made early in order to shape the program.

Step 3: Develop the Concept

The assessment process at this point will suggest a preliminary approach, in this case a possible demand for minor prosthetic and orthotic adjustments for homeless people who are amputees or have severe arthritis.

The preliminary approach is shared with colleagues and interested parties to determine the degree of interest and acceptance. In this case, the concept is for the orthotist in your department to accompany the county nurse on street rounds once a week with a small portable workbench in the nurse's van to make minor adjustments and referrals to the county hospital for major prosthetic and orthotic services. The orthotist will seek a referral for new orthotics from the physician covering the homeless program and will proceed to fabricate those splints. The project has been discussed with the county hospital administration, and they are willing to pilot test the concept for 1 month if all parties are willing to assist in finding funding if the program is to continue.

Step 4: Fieldtest the Concept

Triage guidelines, a demographic survey to determine exactly who takes part in the service, and a follow-up questionnaire to determine if the person who receives treatment continues to use the service, returns to the emergency room, improves function, or decreases pain are developed to monitor the program and assess the results.

The plan is now ready to be presented to the county nursing department responsible for the homeless program and the medical staff covering the clinics.

A physical therapist who is interested in research is chosen to accompany the orthotist to conduct the interviews of the clients and to do the follow-up.

The fieldtest is set up for a 1-month period, with another month to assess the absence of the service. The orthotist will also be on call for the emergency room to triage orthotic problems for the targeted population.

Step 5: Assess the Impact of the Program

The primary goal of the assessment is to determine if the program served its purpose (reduce use of the emergency room) while also assessing unexpected results (new referrals).

From a management perspective, it is also critical to perform a feasibility analysis. The primary goal of this analysis is to assess if the return from the program will be sufficient to justify the resources needed to carry it out. This analysis should be presented as a projected income and expense statement for 1 to 5 years. In the case of this project, income may be in the form of federal, state, and local dollars, grant dollars, reduced use of emergency room facilities, and good will. Expense should project realistic levels of service and resources utilizing existing systems such as county nursing vehicles, hospital buildings, and donated materials. This is the kind of project that community service agencies will be very supportive of and their in-kind contributions should be considered in projecting expenses and income (Table 2–1).

TABLE 2–1. Assessing the Demand for Physical Therapy Services in a Community

Step 1	Determine the demand for the program
Step 2	Determine the roles and rules governing the proposed program
Step 3	Develop the concept
Step 4	Fieldtest the concept
Step 5	Assess the impact of the program

· ·
BOX 2–1 MAJOR COMPONENTS OF HUMAN RESOURCE SHORTAGE ISSUES

- Shortage of physical therapists
- No. of physical therapists/10,000 is increasing

· · · · · · · · · · ·
PHYSICAL THERAPY HUMAN RESOURCE NEEDS IN THE COMMUNITY

In 1952 there were 5,000 physical therapists in the United States, which represented approximately 0.3 therapists per 10,000 population. At that time there was an estimated annual deficit of approximately 2,000 physical therapists. In 1991, there were approximately 66,000 physical therapists in the work force,* representing 2.87 therapists per 10,000 population and an estimated annual deficit of 1,351 physical therapists. Approximately 4,200 new licensees are added to the supply of physical therapists per year, with an estimated 2.4% attrition rate (1,585). This results in a total gain of approximately 2,615 physical therapists. Therefore, first, there is a deficit of physical therapists in the United States. Second, the number of physical therapists per 10,000 population is increasing. The Bureau of Labor Statistics has projected that positions for physical therapists will increase by between 48% and 62% by the year 2000 (Box 2–1).

Currently the demand for physical therapists is 1 for every 44 hospital beds, 1 for every 93 skilled nursing facility beds, and 1 for every 10 rehabilitation beds. These facilities, in addition to schools and home health agencies, are experiencing the greatest shortages of physical therapists.

The increased demand for physical therapy in these settings has been influenced by the move of physical therapists into private practice settings, specialized centers, sports physical therapy, industrial settings, and public schools. In addition, the demand of the public for timely rehabilitation to their premorbid state has placed greater emphasis on outpatient care and private clinics.

Physical therapists work in a multitude of systems including community-based organizations such as community hospitals and home health agencies, in private practices, school systems, large hospital systems, managed health care environments such as health maintenance organizations and multihospital systems (Table 2–2).

Many of the regulatory changes in health care have dramatically affected the human resource needs for physical therapists. Diagnosis related groups (DRGs) emerged from cost-containment legislation and cover 467 principal diagnoses in which fixed payments are determined for medicare reimbursement. This prospective payment system has decreased hospital stay, increased the number of admissions to nursing homes that require skilled nursing, influenced the role of the nursing home as a step-down level of care from the hospital, and, therefore, increased the demand for rapid turnover of the patient in the acute care setting and more acute physical therapy services in the skilled nursing facility. This shift of patients has increased the need for physical therapists in nursing homes and home health agencies.

The demand for physical therapy services in public schools has grown dramati-

---

*In 1991 there were approximately 71,000 licensed physical therapists in the United States. Of this number 70% (49,700) were full time, 23% (16,330) were part time; and 7% (4,970) were retired or not working.

TABLE 2–2. Type of Facility or Institution in Which (or for Which) Respondents Practice*

Facility	1978	1983	1990
Hospital	47.1	41.9	29.6
Private office	9.9		
Physical therapy office		14.6	24.9
M.D. office		2.7	2.2
Rehabilitation center	9.2	9.1	10.8
Nursing home	8.2	6.0	5.5
Home health agency	5.8	8.3	7.0
School system	5.7	4.7	5.1
Academic institution	5.2	4.3	4.0
Prepaid health care organization	0.4	0.9	1.2

*Adapted from Staff: *1990 Active Membership Profile Report.* Alexandria, Va, American Physical Therapy Association, 1990.

cally. Both public law (PL) 94–142 and PL 99–457* assured the public that children with disabilities would be provided with physical therapy services and other rehabilitation services to improve or correct conditions that interfered with the child's ability to take part in the educational experience. Those laws have significantly increased the demand for physical therapists.

As can be seen from the examples above, the demand for physical therapists comes from a variety of sources. In 1952, when the number of therapists per 10,000 population was 0.3, the primary practice site of the physical therapist was the hospital setting. Rarely did physical therapists work in alternative sites. Today, the need for physical therapists from DRGs and PL 94–142 and PL 99–457 alone place staggering demands on the supply of physical therapists.

The impact of these shortages in physical therapy has included increased salaries, increased resources being used for recruitment and retention, increased burnout for physical therapists trying to fill the void, and encroachment by other professions such as occupational therapists, athletic trainers, and exercise physiologists.

· · · · · · · · · · ·
COMMUNITY-BASED PRACTICE SETTINGS

A variety of service delivery systems exist within the community, and physical therapists work in many of them, including community hospitals, home health settings, nursing homes, private practices, and managed care settings. Of these practice settings, the physical therapy services within the community hospital and the home health agency are most connected to the success of the community. Although private practices, nursing homes, and managed care services exist as successful delivery systems in the community, they are often focused on a specific market or target within the community. The mission of community hospitals and home health agencies is to maintain and enhance the health of the citizens and the integrity of the community.

---

*PL 94–142 was originally called the Education for All Handicapped Children law but was renamed in 1991 to the Individuals With Disabilities Education Act. The law guaranteed that all public schools would provide special education and rehabiliation (physical therapy, occupational therapy, and speech) for all children from the age of 3 years with disabilities that interfered with the child's ability to take part in the educational process. PL 99–457 extended the rights of the child to receive special educational services and rehabilitation to the 0- to 3-year-old population.

Community hospitals are a source of community pride, just like the church and schools, and the home health agency is an extension of that community hospital system.

The Community Hospital

The Board of Trustees of the community hospital is often comprised of both community leaders and physicians. Some board bylaws will even specify the percentage of board members who will be physicians and the pool from which they will be drawn. This is understandable given the history of the development of hospital administration by physicians. However, conflict of interest questions arose regarding physician ownership or control of the environment (hospital) in which they practiced medicine. Another factor that lead to decreased dominance of the physician as trustee and administrator was the bureaucracy of regulations governing hospitals, which made it increasingly apparent that those individuals responsible for the administration of the hospital had to have special training in health care regulation and management. The burden of administration made it increasingly impossible for the physician-administrator to practice medicine, and the physician eventually turned to the experts to manage the increasingly complex health care environment of the hospital.

As you can see in the organizational structure for the community hospital (Fig 2–1), however, it is clear that the physician groups still have a significant voice in the administration of the community hospital. The director of the medical staff holds a position parallel to the president of the hospital and reports directly to the Board of Trustees. Usually both the president and the director of the medical staff sit at Board of Trustee meetings to deal with organizational and medical issues.

The majority of community hospitals have a flattened organization—there are relatively few layers of administrators or middle managers between the worker and the president of the hospital. The span of control of the president is usually divided between vice president–level administrators who are responsible for the operations of the major departments of the hospital, the financial status of the organization, and the management of the human resources of the institution.

At one time having a hospital within the community, like a church or school, was a source of community pride. It was health care being delivered and administrated by neighbors who understood the community's needs and relationships. The Board of Trustees of the hospital was comprised of strong community leaders who brought the values of the community to the local hospital providing services that met the need of the citizens. In many rural areas, however, few community hospitals can survive the high cost of providing health care without forming stronger and more formal relationships with larger hospital systems. With these mergers comes a loss of a sense of community as boards and medical staffs merge and the focus of the community hospital shifts to provide outreach for the larger system. These hospitals often focus their services on maternity care, ambulatory surgery, geriatric day hospitals, patient education centers, alcohol and drug rehabilitation, or physical rehabilitation services, and in the process lose some of their emphasis on general medical care.

As the community hospital has changed its focus, the physical therapy needs have changed significantly. Traditionally, the small community hospital would staff a small physical therapy service with one or two full-time or part-time physical therapists. Now, as the community hospital becomes more focused, the physical therapy needs change according to the focus of the facility. For example, the physical therapy manpower needs of a hospital that focuses on maternity care and ambulatory ser-

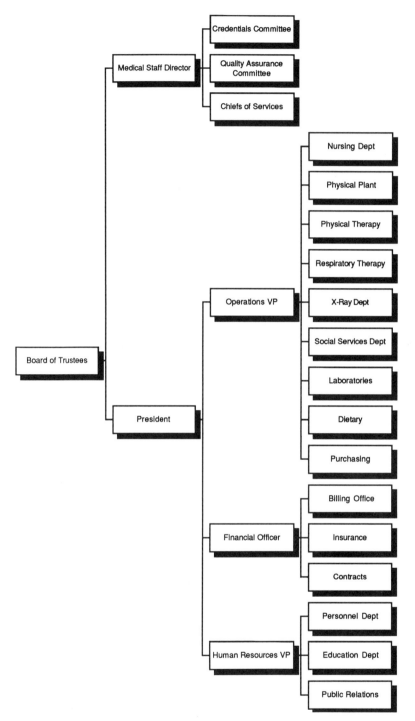

FIG 2–1.
Organizational chart for a community hospital. *VP* = vice president.

vices, where patient stay is short and rehabilitation is primarily carried out in an out-patient setting, is quite different from a community hospital that serves as a geriatric day hospital and a rehabilitation center.

The community hospital that has remained relatively simple in its organizational complexity has become a focal point for physical therapists in the area of practice privileges.* In 1983, Louise Yurko, P.T., sued for clinical privileges at Carterett General Hospital in Morehead City, NC. "The 4th US District Court of Appeals decided that: The courts have ruled that medical staff privileges granted to the physician constitute a property interest entitled to due process protection. The clinical privileges held by the physical therapist are sufficiently analogous to those of the physician's medical staff privileges to make a claim to a property interest under the due process clause of the 14th amendment."[5]

The granting of practice privileges within a community hospital that does not have a physical therapy department and in which there is little competition for physical therapy services has been seen as very positive by physical therapists involved in these settings. Look at the organizational chart again for a community hospital (see Fig 2–1). As you can see, physical therapists are traditionally responsible to the administrative lines of the organization. Although in many states and by the bylaws of the institution, within many institutions, physical therapists work under the prescription of a physician, there is no direct reporting relationship and no functional relationship in the organization. By being granted staff privileges, physical therapists in community hospitals are given the right to sit on credentials committees and quality assurance committees to represent themselves in these bodies. They are often put in a communication loop with the physician. As persons with privileges, they are asked their opinions about the policies and directions of the institution that they would otherwise not be privy to in an administrative line position. Practice privileges in these environments can be seen as positive and powerful in moving the physical therapist from a technician to a professional in the eyes of colleagues within the community hospital setting.

The community hospital is clearly related to the tertiary† center that serves as a referral center for the community for services which cannot be provided within the community. In some instances that relationship is implicit and depends on the referral relationships of the health care professionals using the services. In other in-

---

*The Joint Commission on the Accreditation of Healthcare Organizations (JCAHO) defines practice privileges as the authorization by the governing body to provide specific patient care and treatment services in the organization within well-defined limits based on an individual's license, education, training, experience, competence, and judgment. In December 1983, JCAHO revised the accreditation standards for hospital staff to say that an institution should establish procedures that would open staff membership to nonphysicians and dentists. The standards offered an avenue for the inclusion of licensed individuals who are permitted by law and by the institution independently in that institution. In accordance with these standards, clinical privileges were delineated to allow the applicant to provide patient care services independently within his or her legally defined scope of practice. All members are subject to medical staff and departmental bylaws, rules, and regulations and are subject to review as part of the hospital quality assurance program. In the granting of such privileges, the institution is encouraged to take into consideration local, state, and federal licensing laws, accreditation standards, and the particular health care needs of the institution patient population. The JCAHO considers the medical staff qualified to evaluate the applicant's professional competence and to make recommendations to the institution's governing board, which is ultimately responsible for granting privileges. Any licensed individual permitted by law to provide patient care may apply for hospital practice privilege.

In 1991 the American Physical Therapy Association (APTA) Task Force on Practice Privileges adopted the JCAHO definition of practice privileges and added the following: "The privileges may encompass the full scope of physical therapy practice as defined by state law or be limited to a specific clinic service or patient population." From APTA Task Force on Practice Privileges Report to the House of Delegates, June 1991.

†A tertiary center is a center to which patients are referred for services that are not commonly available in the primary care setting. Primary care is wholistic care that is often provided by one health care provider or health care center. Your family physician is a primary caregiver. He or she is the entry point into the health care system and takes care of minor and major disturbances within his/her scope of practice or within the resources available in the primary care setting. When special tests or special care is needed, the primary care provider makes a referral to the tertiary center, expecting that you will return after the special problem has been resolved to continue to receive primary care in your community. Physical therapists are also primary care providers, and as referral practices evolve with direct access, physical therapists are expected to use the physical therapy or rehabilitation services of a tertiary care center to supplement the primary care provided to the patient.

stances the referral relationship is reinforced by housing a community health clinic of the tertiary center in the community, by giving referring practitioners practice privileges at the tertiary center, or by forming an organizational relationship with the institution. Some large multihospital systems have holding companies that either have sole or partial ownership of a variety of community-based clinics.

Home Health Care

Care of the patient in the home is provided through a number of different organizational structures. In some communities there are hospital-based home health agencies, whereas the majority of communities have their own free-standing home health agency. The most common agency structure is one that is headed by a Board of Directors which hires the head of the agency. Although physical therapists have moved into agency director positions, these positions are most often held by nursing or social work professionals. Large agencies are sometimes managed by professionals with advanced degrees in business or public health.

Typically, the organization is characterized as an open system and could be referred to as a loosely coupled system; that is, the majority of the professionals involved in the organization are independent contractors with a high level of professional autonomy. The director of the agency must maintain professional autonomy and at the same time be able to expect a certain degree of organizational cooperation and impose some controls. Those controls come in the form of documentation requirements, billing regulations, and quality assurance activities. Physical therapists are one of the autonomous professional groups represented in most home health agencies where a second skilled service qualifies the agency to receive medicare reimbursement.

Each agency deals with professionals differently. Oftentimes the agency has staff nurses who are salaried. This salaried relationship represents an implied contract and a master-servant relationship in which the "employee is employed on terms whereby the employer has the right, whether exercised or not, to control the work done and the way in which it is done by the employee."[6] The conditions of this contract are contained in personnel policies of the agency and specify items such as vacation and holiday allotments, work hours, termination, orientation, and benefits.

The agency usually contracts for specialized nursing personnel, occupational therapy, physical therapy, and respiratory therapy as independent contractors. The primary characteristics of the independent contractor relate to the degree of control of the agency over the work. The contracts are frequently generated by the agency, but are negotiable. They outline the roles and responsibilities as well as the liabilities of the two parties and detail the manner in which services will be delivered and payment will be made for those services. Like all contracts, these contracts should be carefully constructed, and advice from a lawyer should be sought. "The following points illustrate some considerations for careful construction of contracts:

1. Language of the contract is controlling in the absence of ambiguity or fundamental mistakes.

2. In interpreting contracts, utilize the ordinary meaning of terms.

3. Failure by one party to specify what it later claims was intended cannot alter the contract.

4. A contract clause that is clear and unambiguous will be interpreted in strict accordance with the written terms.

5. Contract terms must be accorded their first and customary meaning.

6. The written contract is presumed to be absolute.

7. Failure to include a term is proof that it was intended to be omitted.

8. Practices consistent with the agreement remain effective unless the contract expressly provides otherwise."[5]

The physical therapy manager who attempts to construct contracts without the assistance of the appropriate legal specialist will do a disservice to the institution in which the physical therapy practice is housed and to the parties with whom the con-

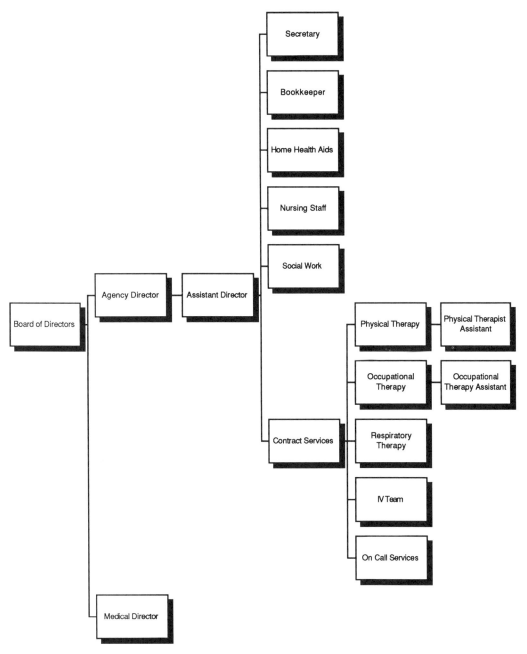

FIG 2–2.
Home health agency organizational chart. *IV* = intravenous.

tract is being written. Contract law is complex and specialized to the point that the manager should seek a lawyer with experience in health care, reimbursement, Internal Revenue Service, and employment practices.

From an organizational structure perspective, secretarial and billing services are usually a part of the organization and under the supervision of the director of the agency (Fig 2–2). As agencies have grown and provided more intense and around-the-clock services for more critically ill patients at home, there has been a need for a one-on-one administrative level (assistant director) so that decisions can be made expeditiously during the continuous coverage of the agency.

Each agency has a carefully monitored and expedited quality assurance program requiring a specific number of records to be reviewed each month. The quality assurance committee either employs professionals not affiliated with the agency or uses volunteer professionals to review the records and report to the quality assurance committee. That committee then reports to the agency director and the Board of Directors on the status of the services provided by the agency as a result of the review. The reports are shared with the professionals involved and action plans are developed to resolve any deficiencies noted in the review process.

Most agencies have complex bylaws and policies that detail the relationship of the agency to the community and the state. In some communities, the home health agency is an agency of the town/city and receives funding directly through the municipal budget process. In other communities, home health services are provided by a for-profit or nonprofit independent agency that applies to the town/city government for support for some services provided to welfare recipients and for some health screening and public health functions such as immunizations.

The role of the physical therapist assistant varies in home health agencies according to state laws and the structure of the agency. In states that clearly define the practice of the physical therapist assistant as occurring with on-site supervision, it is not economical or professionally reasonable to involve a physical therapist assistant in home health care unless the care calls for two individuals. However, in those states where the laws allow, many home health therapists and physical therapist assistants have found a rewarding experience in home health care for the physical therapist assistant, especially with the more chronically ill population. By using cellular telephones, the physical therapist and the physical therapist assistant are in constant contact as well as being in contact with the agency. The use of laptop computers greatly aids the transfer of orders, evaluation results, program plans, and progress notes, which are then easily exchanged by disk between the physical therapist and the physical therapist assistant and ultimately to the secretarial and billing personnel. Although the physical therapist assistant can be effectively utilized in any geographical setting, it is perhaps most advantageous in highly populated areas where the physical therapist and physical therapist assistant can plan their schedules so they are working in the same neighborhood. In that way, the physical therapist assistant will have the consultative services of the physical therapist available very quickly should the need arise. Other issues related to supervision will be discussed further in Chapter six.

CASE 2.1:

Practice Privileges

Colleen Kigin, P.T., M.S., M.P.A.

Jan Gwyer, P.T., Ph.D.

Jane Smith, P.T., M.S.,* was a therapist in private practice in a medium-size city in California. Her practice was situated across the street from a community hospital of 330 beds. The physicians consisted of private practitioners who had practice privileges at the hospital.

She had been treating a 45-year-old man with a bilateral knee replacement who had an underlying diagnosis of arthritis for over 2 years. The patient was a certified public accountant and owned his own business. He was in a car accident and was admitted to the community hospital.

The car accident occurred as a dumpster backed into the patient's Mercedes, during which he slammed on his brakes and fractured his hip. His right knee motion went from 70° to 25°. He was treated and returned to work. He then tripped over a plastic chair mat at work, again breaking his hip.

The above events were followed by a trail of lawsuits, including the dumpster company suing for injury of the garbage man hurt in the initial accident.

The patient called Ms. Smith from the hospital and stated that his physical therapy was not going well and that he needed her to treat him. Ms. Smith stated that she could only treat him if his physician agreed and arranged it. She acknowledged to herself, however, that she would have no idea how to bill this but she would consider that later.

At the same time, Ms. Smith was also negotiating with the very hospital the patient was in to take over the hospital physical therapy practice. The former director had been inadequate and had been dismissed. A group of orthopedic surgeons had a physical therapy and outpatient service nearby and were also anxious to have their therapists treat the patients that were in the hospital.

The patient's physician was not anxious to pursue this issue, and he was not seen by the therapist until he was discharged home.

Consider the practice privilege issues in this case. Does the patient have the right to ask for a specific health care provider? Why does the physician delay in pursuing this issue? What issues would this case pose for existing physical therapy services in the institution? What legal issues might arise from this case?

---

*All names of case study subjects in this book are fictitious.

······ CASE 2.2:
······

Practice Privileges

Colleen Kigin, P.T., M.S., M.P.A.

Jan Gwyer, P.T., Ph.D.

John Smith was a physical therapist who had contracted for cardiac rehabilitation services at a small community hospital. He did so through a flat fee as part of his physical therapy private practice. This contract for cardiac rehabilitation services came under the direction of the director of the physical therapy department. In 1980 he decided to leave the community hospital (in conjunction with partners in his practice) because he felt that this hospital was not offering enough compensation for the services offered. The hospital administration had been approached regarding this issue and had chosen not to pay the increased rate, and consequently the relationship ended.

Upon leaving the institution, Mr. Smith wrote the hospital administrator a letter requesting access to records of patients prior to discharge from the community hospital. This request was made because he still provided outpatient cardiac rehabilitation services to the community, which included patients who had been seen at this community hospital. In his letter requesting to see records, he told the hospital that having access to inpatient records was necessary for continuity of care.

The hospital administrator granted his request to have access to these records, but only if the physician signed the request. Mr. Smith was also allowed to review records in the medical records department as well as on the patient floors. The right to review records on the floors of present patients had actually not been requested by Mr. Smith, but it was something that was helpful to him in his practice. The criteria that the hospital administrator established for this process was that Mr. Smith would present a letter to the head nurse allowing the release of information. The head nurse then reviewed the document and allowed access to the records.

The therapist was restricted to only seeing records of patients being referred for cardiac rehabilitation. Even though Mr. Smith's practice was broader than cardiac rehabilitation in the private setting, he was not allowed access to records of any patients other than those with the diagnosis of cardiac dysfunction.

After receiving this initial letter, Mr. Smith began reviewing the records of patients. Subsequently, he received a follow-up letter from the hospital administrator which stated he had found evidence that Mr. Smith had exceeded the original intent of the agreement and that he was in fact observed treating patients. The administrator asked Mr. Smith to stop this activity if it was indeed happening. Mr. Smith had in fact accessed records in the hospital and had gone into each room to meet and talk to the patients. He talked with patients about risk factors and other topics, and, in fact, he had gotten one patient out of bed and ambulated with him.

After receiving the letter from the hospital administrator, Mr. Smith discontinued ambulation of patients. At this time he also requested the opportunity to consult with the patient prior to discharge. This letter was cosigned by six physicians who used Mr. Smith's services for cardiac rehabilitation. This time the hospital administrator denied his request because there was already a program in place that provided consultation to inpatients. The administrator did allow Mr. Smith to introduce himself to the patient so that the patient could meet him and establish a sense of ease about who would initiate the outpatient care. Only this level of contact was allowed by the administrator.

In 1983, Mr. Smith was contacted by a physician group that was affiliated with the hospital but separate from the actual organization of the hospital. This clinic saw a number of out-of-town patients for cardiac care and wanted a team to see the patients before discharging them from the hospital. They wanted the team to offer patient consultation regarding diet risk factors and activity levels. Dieticians from this particular clinic had been allowed into the community hospital to provide such care. With the perspective that if dieticians could be allowed to go into this hospital and provide this level of care then a consulting physical therapist should have the same rights, Mr. Smith again requested to be allowed to provide consultative services to this patient population. The hospital administrator responded in writing that he would allow the therapist to work with the patients from this particular clinic only if the consultation included home instruction.

In 1984 DRGs greatly affected the community hospital. The administrative staff was trying to decrease costs on its general fund ledger. The hospital administrators scrutinized marginal programs and particularly scrutinized those programs that were a financial drain to the institution. The cardiac rehabilitation program that had been started by Mr. Smith years ago was presently being directed by a therapist employed by the physical therapy department of the hospital. In fact, much of the work was done by an exercise physiologist who worked through the physical therapy department. It was unclear from those interviewed as to how the exercise physiologist billed for services, but it was a possibility that the billing was done under the auspices of a fellow therapist. This fellow therapist had contact with the cardiac rehabilitation program. The hospital decided to close down this service.

Mr. Smith was aware of the plan to close the cardiac rehabilitation service and wrote a letter requesting practice privileges in the hospital to provide cardiac rehabilitation. He had a great deal of support for this proposal now that the hospital could no longer provide this particular service. In fact, Mr. Smith had talked to an assistant administrator of the hospital, who said that he felt that the institution as a whole would welcome an application from him at this time. In the letter Mr. Smith requested practice privileges to evaluate and treat patients with cardiac disease. Even with plans to close the service under way, Mr. Smith was not authorized practice privileges immediately. He needed to further delineate what he wanted to do as a clinician. He added an addendum letter that relied heavily on the cardiopulmonary competencies which were prepared for the specialist certification process. He outlined what the advanced clinician in cardiac rehabilitation would and should do in caring for a patient.

Consequently, Mr. Smith did get practice privileges as an allied health care practitioner. However, it is unclear how much the physical therapy department participated in this decision, if at all. In fact, it is unclear if the physical therapy department was even aware that this process was being pursued. The paper trail shows that those who did participate in the decision included the internal medicine committee, which made the appointment of Mr. Smith to the medical staff of the department of internal medicine of the hospital as an allied health professional. This appointment was passed through nursing administration and the Board of Trustees of the hospital. On September 17, 1984, practice privileges were granted to the physical therapist. Nowhere in the documentation of this process did Mr. Smith have any tie or communication with the physical therapy department. There was no indication in the documentation that he needed to maintain any of the standards or policies of the department of physical therapy in terms of continuing education, quality assurance, or practice policies. There was also no indication that he was to have his privileges renewed or reviewed on any systematic basis.

Mr. Smith also requested, since he was unable to bill for medicare patients while they were inpatients, that the hospital bill for these services and reimburse him. The hospital administrator stated clearly that the hospital did not want any role in reimbursing or offering subsequent compensation to him, and his request was denied. This status remained as of 1990, and consequently Mr. Smith did not get paid if he chose to see a medicare patient.

Mr. Smith did bill for patients who had insurance company coverage for his services. The hospital, in choosing not to participate in any billing, does not send any bills for Mr. Smith's services. His private practice sends the bill accompanied by a letter from the administrator of the hospital stating that the patient has been seen while an inpatient at the hospital by the therapist and that the accompanying bill was for those services.

As the situation progressed, Mr. Smith realized that at times it would be necessary to use hospital rehabilitation equipment to treat various patients. He requested that the hospital allow him to use the equipment, which was denied, and the issue has never been resolved. Once again, it appears that this communication was with the hospital administration directly and that there was some minor communication, but no negotiation, with the physical therapy department.

It is of interest that the director of physical therapy is the same director who Mr. Smith originally worked under when he contracted for cardiac rehabilitation services directly through physical therapy. The relationship between Mr. Smith and the director of the department is cordial and communicative, but certainly not collegial or one in which Mr. Smith is considered part of the physical therapy department.

The hospital administration also realized that there could be a potential malpractice issue with granting practice privileges to nonphysicians. At this point, they changed or solidified the policy for the granting of practice privileges to a number of clinicians who now have practice privileges, including nurses and dieticians.

Another point of interest is that Mr. Smith was requesting practice privileges simultaneously at a second community hospital in the area, and received them. Mr. Smith presently does not see patients at the second community hospital nor has he seen patients there for the last 3 years. He does have close communication with physicians who work at this hospital and does see a number of their patients in his outpatient clinic. This particular hospital has a much tighter policy of granting practice privileges; Mr. Smith's privileges are reviewed every year by physicians on staff and he must show evidence of continuing education and undergo a tuberculosis test. The physicians know Mr. Smith well from the outpatient setting and feel very confident and comfortable giving him an excellent review, and his practice privileges are almost routinely renewed.

Consider the practice privilege issues in this case. What problems does this case pose for the existing physical therapy services in the institution? What rights and obligations are pointed out in the case? Which of these rights and obligations did the consulting physical therapist violate? Which did the administrator violate? Are there legal issues involved here?

References

1. Hislop HJ: The not-so-impossible dream. *Phys Ther* 1975;55:1069–1080.
2. Cordes SM: Assessing health care needs: Elements and processes, in *Community Assessment.* Rockville, Md, Aspen Systems Corp, 1978.
3. Gentry JT: *Introduction to Health Services and Community Health Systems.* Berkeley, Calif, McCutchon, 1978.
4. Staff: *Task Force on Practice Privileges Report to the House of Delegates.* Alexandria, Va, American Physical Therapy Association, 1991.
5. Yurko L: *Alternative Physical Therapy Services* [audio tape presentation]. Orlando, Fla, Combined Sections Meeting, American Physical Therapy Association, 1991.
6. Feitelberg SB: Principles and concepts in contractual arrangements for physical therapy services. *Phys Ther* 1970;50: .

CHAPTER 3

Physical Therapy in Complex Systems

Although many physical therapists still work for hospitals, the percentage has declined. New alternatives to the physician's office and the hospital have developed in most communities, and with that development new practice arenas for physical therapists have been developed. The degree to which insurance companies have played a role in the development of health care environments can be seen even in the categories of health care settings described as fee-for-service and managed health care settings.

FEE-FOR-SERVICE SETTINGS

In a fee-for-service model there is a free market. The insured person is free to seek the provider of choice. This is the model under which health care was originally established. During the first wave of economic development in the United States (up to 1900), there was no insurance, and although the individual was free to choose a health care provider, that choice was usually limited to the one physician in the community (or the area) and a dentist who covered several communities.[1] Payment was often made in terms of services or products rather than money, but payment was made directly to the professional (Fig 3–1).

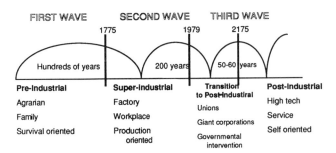

FIG 3–1.
Three waves of economic development in the United States. (Adapted from Toffler A: *The Third Wave.* New York, NY, William Morrow and Co, Inc, 1980.)

During the second wave of economic development (industrial revolution), factory owners began to realize that the best way to keep the worker on the job was to provide injury-related health care in the facility and offer this health care as a benefit to the worker. This movement brought about the company physician and nurse and, later, the occupational therapist,* who were paid by the industry to provide care within the factory. Although factories were sites of high incidences of injuries, there was often not enough business to keep the physician busy, so physicians moved out of the factories and still tried to serve those clients.

As it became obvious to the factory owner that maintaining increasingly complex (X-ray machines, surgical suites) health care facilities in the factory could become increasingly expensive, organized labor began to demand health care coverage that extended beyond the traditional on-the-job injury. Industrial leaders banned together to seek a third party to whom they could pay for health care for employees in anticipation of claims. Payments of claims would be negotiated and made by the third parties after the worker had paid a certain amount of health care (deductible). In these early days, the third parties (insurance companies) made no stipulation about the choice of the practitioner and would pay for the service as long as it was covered in the worker's plan.

During the third wave (transition to the post–industrial phase), health care organizations have grown to giant corporation size, and the field is dominated by government regulations and the growing probability of government intervention in the form of national health insurance. With the growth of the corporations, changing technology, governmental regulations, a changing US economy, and increasing costs, health organizations have developed new organizational structures and functions to meet the needs of the consumers and the insurance companies. Among these new functional units are the managed care systems.

Although the original physical therapists began the practice of physical therapy in physician offices as early as 1917 (Table 3–1), there is no documentation about how those services were reimbursed. It is probable that the physical therapist was paid a salary or hourly wage similar to the office nurse and was not considered as a professional who could receive direct payment for health care services provided. Since the physical therapist worked for the physician, it is assumed that the physician

---

*Occupational therapy (OT) had its beginnings in the early 1800s in the mental health field. Dr. Rufus Wyman was the first physician in the United States to supervise an OT program at McLean Asylum in Boston in 1818. The title OT was coined in 1917 by George E. Barton, an architect who helped to organize Consolation House at Clifton Springs, NY. This was an institution where, by means of occupation, people could be retrained or readjusted to enable gainful living. In 1923, hospitals treating industrial accident patients were required to include OT. Although OT continues to be closely affiliated with mental health care, there was a shift to industrial medicine during the 1930s. Occupational therapists now specialize in developmental OT, hand OT, psych OT, physical disabilities, and industrial OT.

TABLE 3–1. Timeline of the Development of the Profession of Physical Therapy*

1914	1916	1917
Polio epidemics; Wilhelmine Wright, Janet Merrill, Alice Lou Plastridge trained by Dr. Lovett in massage, muscle training, and corrective exercise	Janet Merrill first public health physical therapist	Division of Special Hospitals and Physical Reconstruction created in Surgeon General's Office

1918	1918	1921
Mary McMillan recognized as first Reconstruction Aide	Polio epidemic, World War I; large number of disabled Americans in need of rehabilitation; Reconstruction Aide Training Program established at Reed College, Eugene, Ore	American Women's Physical Therapeutic Association (precursor of APTA) founded

1922	1925	1926
Emma Vogel established first postwar course for physical therapists at Walter Reed Hospital	AMA created Council on Physical Therapy to define educational standards	Conversion to 4-year curriculum

1941–1945	1945	1950s	1965
World War II produced large number of Americans in need of services over a short period of time	Twenty-one PT schools to meet wartime needs; only a few awarded BS degrees; 3% of PTs were men	Polio epidemic	PT included in medicare provisions; 33% of PTs were men

1970s	1979	1980s	1992
APTA studies and promotes professional autonomy including practice independent of physician referral; APTA becomes sole accrediting body for PT and PTA educational programs	APTA set post–baccalaureate degree entry level as professional goal	ABPTS establishes mechanism for board certification of physical therapy specialties; APTA continues to promote autonomy, practice without referral, the elimination of physician-owned PT, and legislation supporting PT	Forty-two states allow evaluation without physician referral; 27 states allow evaluation and treatment without physician referral; 40% of physical therapy academic programs are at the post–baccalaureate degree level

*APTA = American Physical Therapy Association; *ABPTS* =American Board of Physical Therapy Specialties; *AMA* = American Medical Association; *PT* = physical therapy or therapist; *BS* = bachelor of science; *PTA* = physical therapist assistant.

billed for the service provided as an adjunct to the medical care provided and was paid by the procedure or service regardless of the person providing the service.

As the profession of physical therapy grew, physical therapists increasingly moved to rehabilitation centers, hospitals, and clinics as their practice settings. As in the physician's office, the physical therapist's services were not considered directly reimbursable services, but physical therapy was considered an ancillary service—ancillary to medical care. In that role, the physical therapist received payment for services based on hours worked rather than the service provided.

The first true public recognition of physical therapy as a fee-for-service profession occurred in 1965 with the passage of medicare legislation. During the time period that this legislation was under consideration, the American Physical Therapy Association (APTA), under the direction of the Executive Director of the APTA, Royce Noland, and the Director of Governmental Affairs, Robert Teckmeyer, made important strides in gaining recognition for physical therapy as a service to receive direct reimbursement under the medicare program. The inclusion of physical therapy in medicare legislation was one of the single most important events in the history of physical therapy because it secured a reimbursable position for a nonphysician health professional within the traditional health care environment.

Under Medicare (Title XVIII of the Social Security Act), the cost of hospital care is provided for Social Security and Railroad Retirement beneficiaries aged 65 years and older. In addition, benefits are provided for persons entitled to a social security disability benefit (for 24 months), and certain persons (and their dependents) with end-stage renal disease. Those eligible for hospital benefits may enroll for medical benefits and pay a monthly premium and so may persons aged 65 years and older who are not eligible for hospital benefits. Medicare pays for all medically necessary inpatient hospital care for a specified number of days* per benefit period (a new benefit period begins after the patient has been out of the hospital for 60 days), during which the patient must pay a deductible for the year, a specified number of days of care in a nursing home as long as skilled nursing care is needed, visits by nurses and other health care professionals under the auspices of a home health agency, and certain aspects of hospice care.

Medicare is a very expensive system that may not be able to be supported in the future from the social security fund. "In 1988, nearly 52.7 billion was withdrawn from the hospital insurance trust fund for hospital and related benefits."[2(p691)] This high cost of a government-supported health care program will continue to be at the center of the debate in the United States regarding national health insurance.

The great majority of physical therapists continue to work in fee-for-service settings, including many hospitals, clinics, private practice, home health agencies, school systems, rehabilitation centers, specialized centers of care, sports physical therapy arenas, and industry. In addition to these traditional settings, physical therapists are also engaged in practice arrangements in complex organizational structures such as multihospital settings, corporate physical therapy, and managed health care environments.

The organizational structure is only one aspect of complexity in these settings. Increasingly, not only are the institutions organized as alternative health care systems, the internal organization is presented in a number of alternative structures, and the relationship of the physical therapy service to the institutions is presented in a variety of organizational alternatives.

· · · · · · · · · · ·
COMMUNITY HOSPITALS

Community hospitals are the hospitals that most people have become familiar with as they have encountered health care in their own community. These hospitals constitute the largest number of hospitals in the United States and account for the largest number of admissions. The majority of these hospitals are not-for-profit institutions, meaning that they do not have to pay tax on income or property and they do not distribute any profits to share holders at the end of the year. A small number of

---

*Medicare is a federal program administered by the Health Care Financing Administration (HCFA). It is the result of a law passed by Congress in 1965 that amended the Social Security Act and added Title XVIII (medicare). HCFA is the federal regulatory agency that administers the program on both a national and regional basis. That is, regulations are open to interpretation by the federal office, the regional office, and the third party that administers the program locally. As a law, Title XVIII is subject to congressional amendment as well as regulatory change. Therefore, the exact days of coverage as well as services covered are subject to change. For an accurate description of the benefits of the medicare program, the reader should secure a current copy of Title XVIII and amendments from HCFA, the local third-party payor, or a local health care provider.

community hospitals may be for-profit (proprietary) institutions, in which a single person or a group of people own the facility and share the profits. Specialized hospitals are developed in the same manner and include rehabilitation centers, Shriner's Burn Centers, and eye hospitals. Community hospitals are also often referred to as voluntary hospitals, because they have been developed by individuals within a community, not by a governmental agency, unlike military hospitals, state hospitals, or Veterans Administration hospitals.

Increasing competition, increasing cost, and decreasing resources placed many community health care systems in small or rural areas in jeopardy in the 1970s. This lead to major local or regional hospitals developing holding companies in which they could diversify and acquire for-profit operations and a variety of other hospitals or small community services. It is common now to see hospitals as systems rather than single institutions.

· · · · · · · · · · ·
MULTIHOSPITAL SYSTEMS

One of the primary goals of multihospital systems is to build a system that provides the continuum of care for its customers. That continuum of care may be age related (maternal and child health services to nursing home care) or procedure oriented (routine tests and procedures to the most sophisticated imaging and surgical procedures). Some hospitals have developed a regional cooperating system in which there are agreements of cooperation between facilities and each component agrees to focus services in certain ways that will support the system and allow the easy flow of patients between facilities. In most situations, however, the larger medical centers have actually diversified their operations and purchased the community facilities.

A hospital system may include the parent organization that is already a large referral hospital with a complex organizational structure (Fig 3–2), several smaller community hospitals, outpatient clinics in several communities, outpatient physical therapy practices (general and specialized), and several nursing homes. This level of complexity allows the hospital system to provide a full range of services to the client within the system without having to make referrals outside of the system. In order to make such a system work, it is carefully planned to maximize each type of facility. Local community hospitals may focus on specialized functions such as maternity care or sports medicine, which are relatively inexpensive, to delivery requiring low technology and less intensity of services; a larger community hospital may then take on another higher-level function in the system as the next step in care, providing more diagnostic and treatment facilities, while the parent facilities may provide the highest, most intense level of care. Multihospital systems are the wave of the future in hospital care. Independent community hospitals are too expensive for communities to support the level of care that they may want or need. As health care technology and specialization continue to expand, maintaining small health care facilities becomes more difficult for the individual practitioner and for the community.

As multihospital systems have grown, so have the large medical center and the physical therapy services needed to support large medical institutions. With the soaring health care costs of the 1970s and 1980s, hospitals were forced to look at the high cost of admitting patients to hospitals and consider other ways of providing care. Physicians were no longer allowed to admit a patient without authorization of the facility or the reimbursement agency. New services such as outpatient surgery, comprehensive outpatient rehabilitation facilities, and outpatient centers in chronic disease management (diabetes, arthritis, psoriasis, and kidney disease) have been developed to meet the needs of patients and health care providers in a more cost-effective mode.

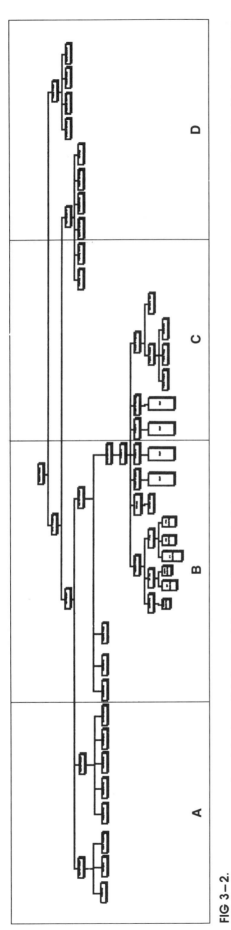

FIG 3–2.

A–D, large parent organizational structure within the hospital system. For exploded views, see next four pages (pp. 33–36). *OT* = occupational therapy; *CI* = clinical instructor; *COTA* = certified occupational therapy assistant; *PT* = physical therapist; *ATC* = clinical instructor; *PTA* = physical therapist assistant. *(Continued.)*

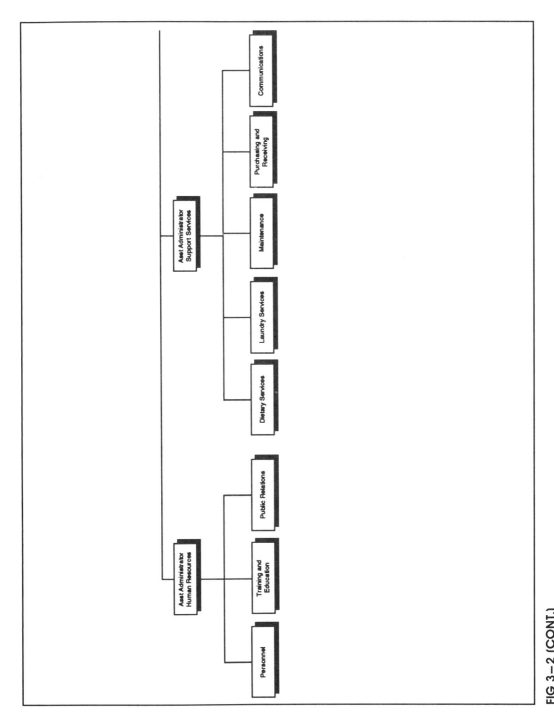

FIG 3–2 (CONT.)
Exploded view of box **A** (see p. 32) of large parent organizational structure within the hospital system. *(Continued.)*

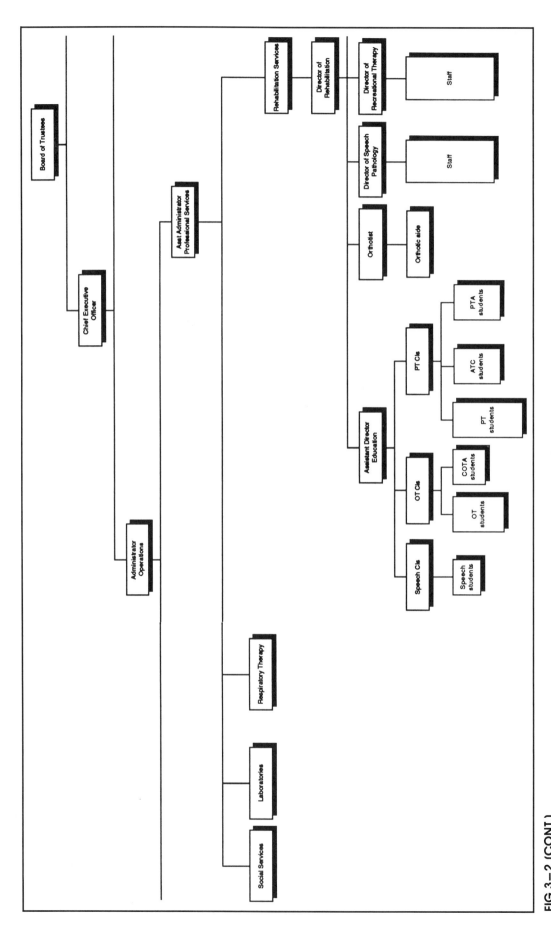

FIG 3–2 (CONT.)
Exploded view of box **B** (see p. 32) of large parent organizational structure within the hospital system. *(Continued.)*

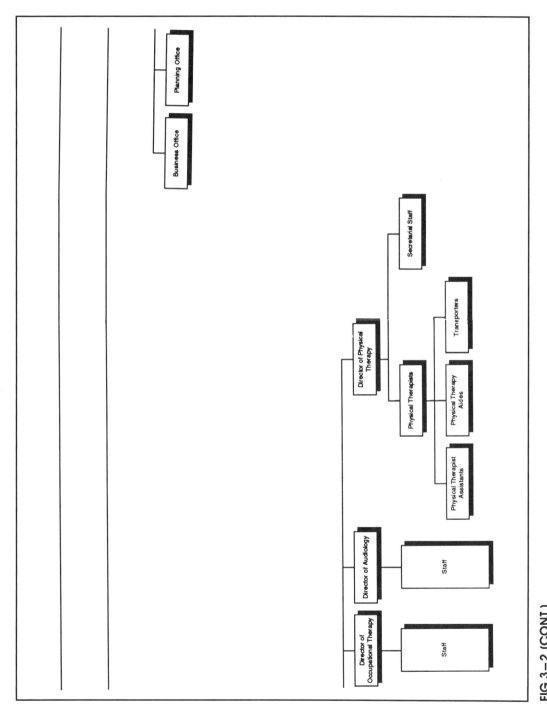

FIG 3–2 (CONT.)
Exploded view of box **C** (see p. 32) of large parent organizational structure within the hospital system.

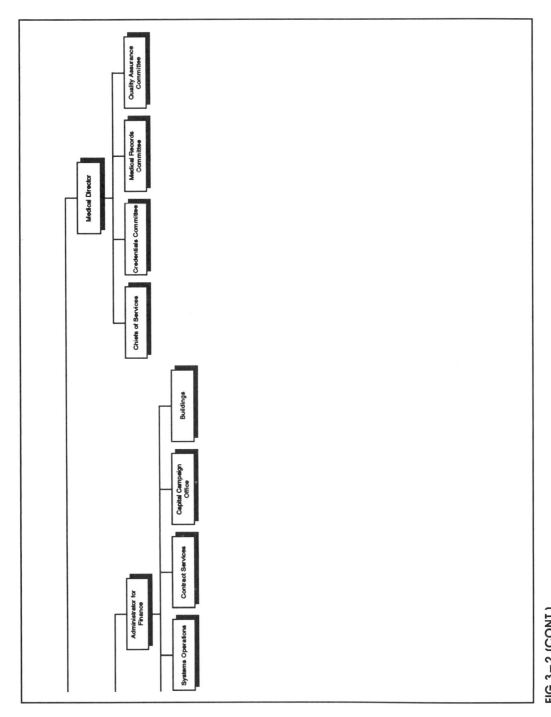

FIG 3–2 (CONT.)
Exploded view of box **D** (see p. 32) of large parent organizational structure within the hospital system.

OUTPATIENT SERVICES IN COMPLEX SYSTEMS

Managing the Outpatient Waiting List

One of the outcomes of the shift to outpatient care within the hospital and the shortage of physical therapists in hospitals is the growth of the outpatient waiting list. Many hospital-based physical therapy managers have developed strategies for dealing with waiting lists of 100 or more patients (Box 3–1). These strategies have included developing procedures for (1) prioritizing the outpatient referrals, (2) new start targets (how many patients can be started within an 8-hour day), (3) scheduling procedures for initial appointments, (4) reviewing urgent referrals, (5) appointment-keeping policies (including telephone contact with patients prior to the appointment to remind them of the appointment and policies regarding cancellation), and (6) peer review of patients who have been seen by the physical therapy service for more than 2 months.[3]

ORGANIZATIONAL RESTRUCTURING

Perhaps the most significant challenge for the institutionally based physical therapy manager is the need for aggressive intervention in developing new organizational structures, employment packages, and creative opportunities for the physical therapist. The most creative of these would be to design a structure that would allow the physical therapist to practice in a group practice arrangement similar to that of the physicians who provide medical services to the institution. Such an arrangement would provide maximal autonomy and the independence that physician staffs enjoy within an institution. The physical therapist could continue to serve the needs of the patient through a department structure just as surgeons meet the needs of the patients through a department of surgery, but would be given privileges instead of employment. Many physical therapists believe that as long as administrators think of physical therapists as employees, they cannot think of them as professionals.

Throughout the United States there are individual physical therapists as well as

---

BOX 3–1 WAITING LIST CRITERIA USED AT THE UNIVERSITY OF MICHIGAN OUTPATIENT SERVICE*

Emergent: Acute diagnosis requiring treatment within 24 hours
Urgent: Must be identified by the physician as urgent; must meet first three criteria of No. 1 subgroup
Number 1 priority
1. Patients whose safety would be jeopardized
2. Patients whose condition would worsen without physical therapy
3. Physical therapy is a prerequisite for return to work
4. If patient has been a number 2 priority for more than 6 weeks
5. Wheelchair and other similar prescriptions
Number 2 priority
All patients who do not fit into one of the above categories
Other considerations include policies regarding patient referrals from other institutions (health maintenance organizations) or programs (state-sponsored programs) that have special contracts for services with the physical therapy department.

*From Davidson G: Waiting List [audiotape presentation]. San Francisco, Calif, section on Administration, Combined Sections Meeting, American Physical Therapy Association, 1992.

managers of complex physical therapy practices who are developing a wide variety of contractual arrangements with hospitals. These arrangements place the physical therapist in a physical therapy practice environment for staff development, employment contracts, professional issues, and negotiations for resources, but within the institutional environment for the delivery of services.

Some physical therapy managers are trying to combine the principles of contractual practice while remaining an employee of the institution. The internal revenue service (IRS) is very clear about the criteria for independent contractors, and in most instances that means the individual cannot be both an employee and an independent contractor (Box 3–2). Before moving in this direction, the physical therapy manager must consult with an attorney familiar with IRS regulations related to employment contracts. "In October 1987, the IRS issued Internal Revenue Bulletin 1987–41 which specified twenty factors which the IRS will examine to determine whether an independent contractor or employee situation exists."[4(p37)]

The primary rules of thumb for the IRS are (1) the degree to which the independent contractor is integrated into the business operation, (2) the degree of risk of loss which the individual contractor takes in establishing and maintaining the business, and (3) the degree of direction and control the business has over the contractor.

Within the hospital department structure, creative structures are being experimented with throughout the country. For the most part these new structures are flattening the old hierarchical structure and providing opportunities for physical therapists to work with other departments in more creative ways. The product-line management system is one of the most creative approaches to challenging the strict confines of the hierarchical structure. That system is discussed in detail in the next chapter.

Many other flattened structures are being experimented with in health care organizations and within individual physical therapy departments. These include systems that flatten administrative structures external to the physical therapy department and systems that flatten the internal organizational structure of the physical therapy department. The internally flattened systems reduce the number of supervisory personnel and organize the staff into decision-making committees such as Space Utilization, Quality Assurance, Budget, Personnel, and Education. This is a design that looks at changing the management system *within* the physical therapy department to give the staff more control over internal decision making.

BOX 3–2 INTERNAL REVENUE INDEPENDENT CONTRACTOR CRITERIA*

1. Who provides instruction
2. Who provides training
3. How integrated is the worker into the business
4. Are the services rendered personally
5. Who hires, supervises, and pays assistants
6. Is there a continuing relationship
7. Who sets the hours of work
8. Is full-time work required
9. Is work done on employer's premises
10. Who sets the order or sequence of work
11. Are oral or written reports provided
12. Is payment by the hour, week, or month
13. Who pays for business and travel expenses
14. Who furnishes tools and materials
15. Has the worker made a significant investment
16. Does the worker realize profit or loss
17. Does the worker work for more than one firm at a time
18. Is the worker's service available to the general public
19. Who has the right to discharge
20. Who has the right to terminate

*From Contract Physical Therapy Services, American Physical Therapy Association, Alexandria, Va, 1990, p 37.

. . . .
MANAGED HEALTH CARE

The term *managed health care* refers to programs in which organizations seek to control (manage) the use of health care services by the patient. The organizational structure varies from the health maintenance organization (HMO) and preferred provider organization (PPO) to pretreatment reviews that are required by some third-party reimbursement agencies.

The fee-for-service structure of health care is based on the premise that the patient is free to choose a practitioner for health care and that there will be a one-on-one relationship between the patient and that practitioner. The patient pays for the service with private funds or through a variety of insurance programs administered by third-party reimbursement agencies.

Managed health care was inaugurated with the HMO. Regardless of the organizational structure, HMOs share the following five common characteristics.

"1. A defined population of enrolled members.

2. Payments by the members, determined in advance for a specific period of time and made periodically.

3. Medical services provided on a direct service basis rather than on an indemnity basis.

4. Services provided to patients by HMO physicians for essentially all medical needs with referrals to outside physicians being controlled by HMO physicians.

5. Voluntary enrollment by each family member."[5(p5)]

In the traditional HMO setting, the physician is the "gatekeeper" of the system. That is, the physician makes all decisions regarding care of the patient. The patient is not free to seek additional care or referrals to specialists without going through the patient's primary care physician within the HMO. The patient must also only use physicians and other health care providers who are affiliated with the HMO unless the specific services which the patient needs are not provided by the HMO. In a fee-for-service setting the patient pays for services after they are delivered, while in an HMO, the patient pays a set amount of money prospectively (before the services are rendered) similar to payments made to insurance companies.

In 1973 the Health Maintenance Organization Act was passed, which allowed HMOs that qualified to apply for financial incentives to deliver managed health care. This federal subsidy ended in the 1980s with the soaring cost of health care. By 1987 there were over 700 HMOs serving over 29 million people.

The goal of the practitioners within the HMO environment is to provide health care at the lowest cost. The impact on physical therapy in HMOs varies among the different structures, but for the most part, in those instances where physical therapy has proven to reduce costs, it is utilized. In the case of unproven interventions, physical therapists are encouraged to put the patient on home programs as soon as possible and to carefully document the outcome of the physical therapy intervention following the patient's progress after discharge. Although the HMO physician may be as interested in the quality of life as any other physician, the HMO physician is rewarded for not treating the patient, unlike the fee-for-service physician who is rewarded (paid) for treating the patient. Physical therapy managers within an HMO setting must master skills of triage and appropriate termination of care as well as the determination of the cost effectiveness of care.

In 1991, managed-care organizations demonstrated approximately a 12% decrease in health care costs. This decrease in costs is about the same as the health care expenditures experienced in fee-for-service settings. It is also estimated that approximately 75% of individuals who subscribe to HMO services are happy with the managed-care system.

Although HMOs are continuing to grow, there is increasing competition from a variety of other managed care organizations, particularly PPOs. A PPO is a group of health care providers (physicians, hospitals, clinics, physical therapists, and nurse specialists) who agree to provide care to a group of people for a negotiated fee for service that is less than the usual rate. The PPO arrangement allows the individual to continue to choose the health care provider while the organization controls costs. The PPO may be initiated by a third-party reimburser such as Blue Cross and Blue Shield, a hospital, a group of physicians, or a group of other health care providers such as physical therapists.

As large physical therapy corporations move into a community, many physical therapists have found that the PPO structure allows them to compete with the larger corporation and provide incentives for patients to seek physical therapy services from this group of providers. In some states, several physical therapy practices throughout the state have banned together in a state-wide PPO to provide cost-effective care.

SCHOOL SYSTEM PRACTICES

School systems have always been an attractive setting for physical therapists who specialize in pediatric care, because it is a setting in which the child can be observed and treated in a natural environment. The passage of PL 94-142, which ensured the equal educational opportunity for all handicapped children, lead to a significant influx of pediatric physical therapists into school systems. Under this law each public school system had to provide physical therapy, occupational therapy, and speech pathology services to handicapped children if those services were necessary to give the child an equal opportunity to take part in the public educational experience. For instance, if a handicapped child could not hold a pencil long enough to complete a test, then that child would be entitled to services to increase the grip, modify the pencil, or increase the child's endurance.

Physical therapists have become an integral part of the public school team of special educator, principal, parent, and special education coordinator to plan an appropriate educational plan for each handicapped child. Each year, the members of the educational and rehabilitation team working with the child meet with the parents to plan an Individual Educational Plan (IEP), in which goals are established for the academic year. This meeting is often highly emotionally charged. Parents are concerned about obtaining the maximum services for their child, and the school system is concerned about both the cost of services and the distribution of resources among all handicapped children.

In most instances physical therapists work closely with the classroom teacher, special education teacher, teacher aide, and parents to deliver services to handicapped children who are mainstreamed* in the public school system. The therapist evaluates the child and designs a program, which is then most commonly administered by the teacher or teacher aide. In some schools, physical therapist assistants

---

*The concept of mainstreaming means that handicapped children are placed within the public school system instead of a special school for handicapped children. Children may be placed in a special classroom for part of the day in which they are taught by special education teachers who can give the child special attention for special problems. The handicapped child is then placed in the regular classroom for part of the day to experience the social atmosphere of the classroom, to take part in education activities in which they are able, and to become a part of their peer group during home room activities, story time, recess, and lunch.

. . . .

BOX 3–3 FORCES LEADING TO HUMAN RESOURCE SHORTAGES IN PHYSICAL THERAPY

Markets
Public demands
Autonomy
Attractiveness
Shifts in health systems
Education programs
US population 18–23 declining
Regulations

are also working closely with the physical therapist to administer the physical therapy program.

The demand for physical therapists in the school systems is one of the forces leading to the human resource shortages in physical therapy (Box 3–3). Not only have the needs for physical therapists in schools created a new and expanding market, the existence of a law to protect handicapped children has made parents aware of the availability and need for physical therapists to deliver these services.

The most common arrangement for a physical therapist in the school system is as an independent contractor.

Oftentimes school systems are unable to find independent contractors and will seek services from hospitals, private practices, or faculty practices. The manager of the physical therapy services in the school system must apprise himself/herself of the laws governing services in school systems and be acutely aware of the difficult situation that the physical therapist will face when developing educational plans for individual clients. Although the physical therapist is an employee of the school system, that therapist must also be an advocate for the child and parent. Since parents are often forced to bring a suit against the school system to get adequate services, the therapist must be aware of the quasilegal situation that the IEP meeting represents and the vulnerability of the school system and the physical therapy practice in this situation. When the physical therapist is a member of a larger physical therapy practice, it is the responsibility of that therapist to keep the physical therapy manager informed regarding situations that may lead to legal action. It is fair to say that, as a school-based physical therapist, it is impossible to avoid being involved in legal action at some point.

CASE 3.1:

Urban Hospital in a Crisis

Cheryl Cooper, P.T., M.S.

It was time to prepare the operations budget for the next fiscal year, and the director of physical therapy at City Hospital was reflecting on a past year of difficulties and a year ahead of seemingly overwhelming challenges. This director, like so many others in the area, was finding her professional life full of hard decisions and ongoing frustration. Times had certainly changed, she thought. Where was physical therapy in urban, short-term care centers heading?

City Hospital had been open for patient care since the 1800s. After decades of fiscal mismanagement by the city and threats of closure, the hospital was bought by a large, nationally renowned hospital complex also located in the city.

The physical therapy department had maintained a low-profile image through most of the hospital's existence. Initially, the department primarily served the needs of the geriatric and long-term nursing home population that occupied one building on campus. As the acute hospital gained recognition for its physician group and the services offered, including the regional burn center, the number of referrals to the physical therapy department grew. With the purchase of the failing city facility came renewed confidence from the physician group and the community. Increased hospital admissions and visits to the outpatient clinics resulted in increasing numbers of referrals to the physical therapy department. Orthopedic staff joined the physician compliment referring from Rheumatology, Neurology, Medicine, and Burns. Referrals for outpatient physical therapy grew substantially.

The national and state trends in health care had also found their way into the physical therapy department.

1. The hospital's physician staff had affiliated itself with an HMO, with its governing group influencing referral and admission agreements with the hospital.

2. The state's medical assistance program was no longer paying for outpatient services delivered at a hospital. All outpatient services were to be delivered by community-based clinicians or private practitioners. Not only did this remove a volume of patients from the referral base, but it also created another market that would hire physical therapists.

3. Third-party payers in general were demanding more documentation to substantiate the bills being submitted. Even with the supporting documentation, the payers had markedly slowed the reimbursement to the hospital.

4. There was a significant move to direct most elective surgical procedures to outpatient areas.

5. The aging of the community population was resulting in an increasing number of chronically ill persons being admitted to the hospital.

6. The scarcity of nursing home beds meant that many patients needing "maintenance" care were occupying acute beds for longer periods.

7. A national and state economic recession, a state mandate to reduce health care costs, and a significant debt obligation for a rebuilding project had resulted in a devastating fiscal climate.

8. This hospital, like others, was following the general trend of business and private enterprise—it was flattening the organization and eliminating management positions. Managers and administrators were assuming more job responsibilities through the normal attrition of the organization.

9. The shortage of physical therapists, particularly those interested in acute care, had been felt in recent recruiting efforts to accommodate the significant increase in patient volumes.

10. In the economics of supply and demand, the therapists to be hired were commanding and getting high salaries from smaller facilities and private practices.

The director of physical therapy reflected on the situation in her department and made a list of the following significant issues needing attention.

1. The space in the department was totally inadequate for the activities performed there. At present, 42 staff members (6 aides, 2 secretaries, 3 managers, 2

speech pathologists, 11 occupational therapists, and 18 physical therapists) shared a space of 4,850 sq ft. While some treatment took place exclusively on the inpatient wards, a total of approximately 130 inpatients and outpatients from the 3 services combined were treated each day in the department. Patient safety had become a primary concern. Efficiency of the therapists was also affected by the poor physical setup.

2. The facility had failed to keep staff salaries growing at the pace of the local market for physical therapists—new graduates and experienced staff. The market provided many alternate opportunities for them. At present, the current starting salary would not attract candidates—even new graduates.

3. The rate of staff retention had been excellent to date. In spite of many operational challenges, staff experience overall averaged 7.5 years, with staff members staying in the facility an average of 6 years. With more years on staff, therapists were requiring more support for education, research, and professional development. Some therapists were seeking opportunities to "climb" the administrative ladder.

4. Productivity as a whole had declined, and the reasons needed to be examined. Some causes that came immediately to mind included the following: (1) Space did not allow therapists an opportunity to dovetail patient treatments effectively. (2) Documentation demands had increased. (3) The authorization procedures for HMO patients and recertification of medicare patients required extra paperwork and repeated phone calls to care sites and physicians. (4) A facility move to a centralized escort system meant relying on a group of workers with a high turnover rate and a variable level of commitment to the facility, their own department, and the rehabilitation section. (5) The staff heard little emphasis placed on productivity expectations from the department director. (6) Increased attention to reimbursement issues and questions from patients to therapists as to the prices for physical therapy treatment may have resulted in conservative billing of patients. (7) The highly motivated staff sought education, research, and developmental opportunities and activities that cut into patient treatment time.

The easy solutions to address many of these issues seemed simple—budget.

1. More salary monies were needed to keep up with the market salary and to allow hiring of more therapists to cover for staff development time.

2. A professional development program was needed to allow each staff member significant time for education—teaching and learning, research, and program development.

3. More supervisor/management positions would increase staff contact with management and involve therapists in the running of the department.

4. More education monies would support staff development activities.

5. More space and equipment were needed to accommodate more therapists and patients.

6. More technology to computerize documentation and recordkeeping was required for greater efficiency.

It was simple, all right. Money would solve the problems. Unfortunately, the director knew the hospital was limiting spending, not increasing it. She turned again to the blank budget forms and wondered how it was possible to balance the needs for the staff and the department with the limited resources of the organization.

Consider the obligations of the director of the service to both the institution and the staff. How could the department be restructured to meet the needs of the staff and the department? Given limited budget monies available, what creative steps could the director take to maintain her highly motivated staff and meet the needs of the referral sources? How does this case reflect the changing health care environment?

CASE 3.2:

School Case

Chris Pillow, P.T., M.A.

Kathy Smith, a physical therapist currently employed by Beta School District, services mainstreamed elementary and middle school children with physical disabilities and normal intelligence. She has 30 children on her case load and travels to approximately six schools throughout the week, with ½ a day reserved for paperwork and new evaluations. The six schools are within 10 miles of each other.

Ms. Smith feels that she is doing a good job since the children are making progress and the teachers praise her for her work and cheerful attitude. She has little interaction with the principals of the schools, except for passing remarks in the hall or school office. The Special Education Director, Ms. Jones, meets with her once a month, but Ms. Smith feels these meetings are not useful, since Ms. Jones is not sure why physical therapy is provided for the children, except because it is legally mandated by PL 94-142 and the State Special Education Law.

Jane, one of the children Ms. Smith currently services, is 11 years old with a medical diagnosis of spina bifida and an educational classification of physical or otherwise health impaired (POHI). She is mainstreamed full-time into the sixth grade and receives no additional academic support, although she is on the case load of the POHI teacher consultant. She is currently ambulatory at school with knee-ankle-foot orthoses (KAFOs) and forearm crutches, although she is slow and cannot always keep up with her friends when they walk quickly in the hall. She is independent with her crutches or wheelchair on all terrains and also in toilet needs. She uses her wheelchair for school field trips and outings with her family that require a lot of walking. She was discontinued from occupational therapy last year and receives direct physical therapy services once a week for 45 minutes. Her physical therapy goals include (1) improved endurance and speed of ambulation, (2) maintenance of strength, and (3) maintenance of range of motion.

According to PL 94-142, Jane is entitled to receive services, including physical therapy, to enhance her academic performance. Parents who are not satisfied with services offered to their children can ask for a state hearing at the school district's expense. Furthermore, all special education students must be completely re-evaluated and an individual educational plan conference held every 3 years. As part of the evaluation process, each team member must make recommendations for continued services. Jane is now in the process of being re-evaluated by all team members. At the staff meeting, the following is reported.

1. Jane's teacher reports that Jane is doing well academically, gets along well with her peers, and has her fair share of friends.

2. The physical education teacher states that Jane participates in gym to the best of her ability within the limitation of her disability.

3. The school psychologist has tested Jane and feels she is working up to her potential.

4. The occupational therapist reports that Jane continues to function well in her area and occupational therapy services are not recommended at this time.

5. The social worker states that Jane has met with her on several occasions. During their sessions Jane has said that she feels awkward being pulled out of her class for therapy services and that she is beginning to resent the use of her crutches because they do not always allow her to keep up with her friends. The social worker also states that Jane has expressed concern that her parents want her to continue physical therapy services since they feel she will lose much of her physical abilities. They feel this is especially important at this time since Jane will be transferring to the middle school next year.

6. Ms. Smith feels that Jane is functional in school and that she has reached her ambulation potential. She would like to discontinue direct physical therapy services and see Jane on a consultant basis once a month for the remainder of the current school year and once a semester when she goes to the middle school.

Following the meeting, Ms. Smith calls Jane's mother to discuss her plan for decreasing physical therapy services. Her mother is furious and tells Ms. Smith that her daughter is entitled to therapy services and that she will make sure that Jane continues to receive weekly physical therapy. Following this conversation, Ms. Smith is upset since she feels Jane's mother is questioning her professional judgment. In addition, she is beginning to have some doubts about her decision, since she knows that Jane will probably not be responsible enough to carry through with a home program that will help her maintain her present level of function. Ms. Smith also feels that she might continue to see Jane if she were working in a medical setting. As a result, she calls the special education director to elicit her opinion and is told that parents have a lot of power and the school district does not like attending hearings.

Consider the position of the physical therapist as both a patient advocate and a paid consultant to the school. Where does the physical therapist fit in the organizational structure of the school? Who is she responsible to? What obligations does the therapist have in this case? What are the obligations of the school and the parents? How are these obligations in conflict over this child? What would be the recommended course of action of the therapist?

References

1. Toffler A: *The Third Wave*. New York, NY, William Morrow and Co, 1980.
2. *Information Please Almanac.* Boston, Mass, Houghton Mifflin Co, 1992.
3. Davidson G: Waiting List [audiotape presentation]. San Francisco, Calif, Section on Administration, Combined Sections Meeting, American Physical Therapy Association, 1992. Produced by Infomedix, 12800 Garden Grove Blvd, Suite F, Garden Grove, CA 92643.
4. Staff: *Contract Physical Therapy Services.* Alexandria, Va, American Physical Therapy Association, 1991.
5. Cowan DH: *Preferred Provider Organizations.* Rockville, Md, Aspen Publications, 1984.

Suggested Readings

American Physical Therapy Association: *The Beginnings: Physical Therapy and the APTA.* Alexandria, Va, APTA, 1979.
Krumhansl B: *Opportunities in Physical Therapy.* Louisville, KY, Vocational Guidance Manuals, Inc, 1974.
Licht S: *Occupational Therapy Source Book.* Baltimore, Md, Williams and Wilkins Co, 1948.
Raffel MW, Raffel NK: *The U.S. Health System,* ed 3. Albany, NY, Delmar Pubs, 1990.
Staff: *1992 State Licensure Reference Guide.* Alexandria, Va, American Physical Therapy Association, 1992.

CHAPTER 4

Alternative Organizational Structures

. . . .

. . . .

INTRODUCTION

In the search for alternative organizational structures, health care managers will experiment with a variety of structures. One of the most creative methods of reorganizing the complex health care environment in the 1990s has been service line management. This is also referred to as product line management. There is a conceptual difference between products and services. From a physical therapy perspective, it is important to understand that health care services, not products, are being delivered. The important point of distinction is that services are provided coincidental to production and therefore have to be done correctly the first time.

Service line administration is the management of a family of products or services that differ from other lines according to the market served, competitors, resources utilization, and other characteristics. Each major service line structure lets the hospital maintain its functional organization while at the same time designating a person to have authority over and responsibility for a service line.[1] Service line is supposed to allow functional departments to exist, but in a different fashion. A service line manager can cross over into departments and work with individual managers and staff, but not disturb the professionalism and commaraderie or nature of professional service. Service line management causes a change because department members work more as a team with other disciplines in a manner different from the traditional patient team relationship.

BENEFITS OF SERVICE LINE MANAGEMENT

Some departments can be subsumed by others (i.e., social work by nursing), but over time, many of those departments are recreated when it becomes apparent that the functional unit of the department is still needed.

The benefits of service line administration include the following.

1. All aspects of the service are pulled together.

2. Guides new program development, profitability, analysis, implementation, and marketing under the guidance of one administrator.

3. A large production organization is broken into competitive units.

4. Services are divided into cohesive sets of programs targeted to specific markets that can be developed, planned, marketed, and accounted for in terms of profitability.

5. Departments can be evaluated as profit centers since they have identifiable cash flows comprised of revenues and expenses.

6. Growth is more easily accommodated. New departments can be added on a self-contained basis having a similar relationship to administration as existing departments.

7. Coordination between functions are facilitated for rapid response.

8. Client needs are the focus leading to greater customer service and satisfaction.

9. The hospital evaluates service lines according to a common set of internal and external factors.

10. Meets challenges for the future for resource allocation and profitability through competition.

11. Develops broadly trained administrators with new skills and new attitudes.

Service line administration results in increased market share, scrutinized operations, pruning where necessary, increased productivity, strengthening of the balance sheet, and increased cash flow.

The dominant messages of service line administration include the payers are driving the system, physician cooperation is required, and that good, timely decisions are the key to a successful response.

ENVIRONMENTAL FACTORS LEADING TO ALTERNATIVE ORGANIZATIONAL STRUCTURES

Several environmental factors have lead to alternative organizational structures. (1) The payer has become increasingly concerned about the cost of health care. In many states, relatively few citizens are supporting an elegant health care system, and they are increasingly concerned about the costs associated with that care. (2) There is an increasing competition for patients at all levels. The development of many community alternatives to hospital-based health care diverts many patients needing relatively few services away from hospital services. (3) Physicians are facing new pressures to earn money to cover the very high costs of care. (4) There is an increased concern for quality of care from the consumer, the provider, and the payers. (5) There is a limit on investments, given the down-shifting of the economy.[2]

GOALS OF THE ORGANIZATION

The goals for the organization which is considering service line management as an alternative structure are the following:

1. Must be customer (payer/patient) oriented.
2. Must gain increased physician involvement.
3. Must make decisions at the most appropriate organizational level.
4. Must meet the needs of those within the organization.
5. Must meet customer (patients, referral sources, insurance companies) needs.

ORGANIZATIONAL REQUISITES

In order to make service line management work in the organization, certain organizational requisites must be achieved. First, physicians must be incorporated into the operational management. That means improving resource allocation and utilization to encourage the physician to maintain services within the hospital environment. Clinical standards and the measurement of physician performance have to be established and then monitored and tied to the physician reimbursement system.[3]

A second organizational requisite is the support of decision making at the appropriate organizational level. That means looking at the layers of administration and restructuring to allow service line administrators to be creative and responsible for their operations.

The patient and payer also have to be oriented to service line management so that they understand the team, the billing mechanisms, and the organizational changes that they will encounter.

It is also critical to recognize the needs and potentials of people within the system and support individual and group problem solving and decision making as well as individual and professional development.

ORGANIZATIONAL STRUCTURE OF SERVICE LINE MANAGEMENT

Many hospitals will have a variety of service line configurations and a variety of numbers of service areas. One example of the configuration of this kind of a system is presented in Fig 4–1. From a physical therapy perspective, the physical therapists work with the service line members within specific service lines to the services provided within that line. From the perspective of professional development, education, and research, the physical therapist continues to work with the physical therapy department under the direction of the physical therapy manager.

The organizational chart for service line management can be considered as a typical organizational chart turned upside-down, with the patient on the top of the chart and the administration (base camp) on the bottom (Fig 4–2). There is great pressure to remove physical therapy managers within the physical therapy department in this system. If maintained in an altered supervisory position, the managers become the liaisons to the service line where they can negotiate on behalf of the physical therapy director. In a department that has more than one service (i.e., occu-

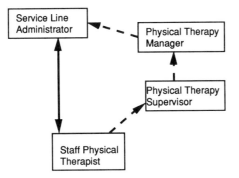

FIG 4–1.
Flow of information in service line administration.

pational therapy, physical therapy, speech), supervisors for each of these services can perform cross-functions and supervise a service line in which several different professionals may be utilized. Each department is then challenged to develop an organizational chart that directs the service delivery through the service line management system.

The flow of information occurs either directly from the service coordinator to the service line administrator or through the physical therapy manager to the service line administrator.

One of the greatest challenges to service line management is sorting out these lines of communication. If the physical therapy departmental structure and reporting relationships interfere with the efficient flow of information within the service lines, the benefits of service line management is lost. It must be clearly articulated that all

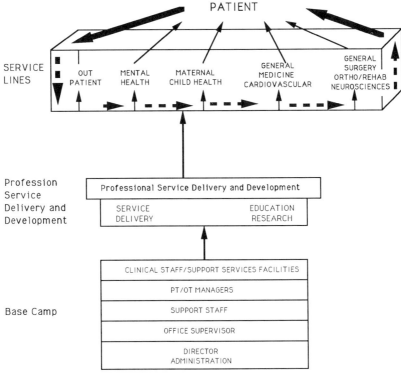

FIG 4–2.
Service line management configuration.

service-related communications must occur in the most direct line between the administrator of the service and the staff involved in the delivery of services.

Service line managers do not hire physical therapists or try to solve problems related to professional issues. This kind of activity still remains a part of the role of the physical therapy director/manager. The physical therapy manager/director must prepare the physical therapy service coordinator to become involved in operations decisions and become an effective team member.

· · · · · · · · · · ·

WORK OF THE SERVICE LINE ADMINISTRATOR AND COORDINATOR

The service line process changes relationships and attitudes. The service line administrator, by definition, is responsible for planning and delivery of assigned service line(s), defining service line costs, and determining service line profitability by type of service, payer, and physicians with other providers and coordinates the production of services with the hospital's functional administrator.[4]

Service line administrators are not in charge of functional departments. Functional directors/managers are still responsible for the operations of their departments, but service line administrators can cross functional department boundaries as they coordinate the operations components of their service.[5] In many instances, the service line administrator is dealing with services other than physical therapy, so the physical therapy manager should not feel threatened by the creation of a service line administrator. It is critical to be a part of the system instead of a barrier to the system. The physical therapy manager and staff must not assume there is a loss of authority and power. Power is dislodged, and it is the job of the physical therapy manager to find new ways to use the authority they have in this system.[6] It is important to remember that the service line administrator has a distinct job that involves many of the coordinating functions that are created by a system which cuts across functional departments. Although the job descriptions of these individuals may sound all-consuming (Box 4–1), they are not making the same professional decisions as the functional department manager (Box 4–1).

The service line administrator may have a difficult task if he or she is to be effective in this alternative organizational structure. Each of these administrators must accomplish the following.

1. Advocate for full-time workers for a particular set of services.

2. Be creative, flexible, and market oriented.

3. Set well-defined objectives of the service line.

4. Use the service line organizational structure for its intended purposes, not as a mechanism to "clean house."

5. Assess each service line and determine the appropriate approach.

6. Obtain commitment from the participants.

7. Establish goals that have a beneficial effect.

Effective service line administration must be based on well-documented analyses of service lines scrutinizing major issues such as resource utilization, market demand, and competition. To move to a service line management program it is critical to identify and understand the customers, to clarify the service strategy with the staff (understanding why the consumer will choose this institution), to educate the organization and gain commitment to the values inherent in this structure, to implement grassroots improvements, and to institutionalize the program.

There is a need for coordinated planning between the service line administrator

. . . .

BOX 4–1   JOB DESCRIPTION OF SERVICE LINE ADMINISTRATOR*

Qualifications

Education:—Baccalaureate degree with at least 3 years of comprehensive managerial experience in a health care setting

Advanced degree in an appropriate management or health science field is likely and will be helpful

Personal attributes:—Willingness to function in a setting with multiple reporting relationships

Ability to build a team of individuals from various disciplines in health care

Skills in organization, communication, leadership, and management

Understanding of managerial applications of automated data systems

Summary of Job Responsibilities

The administrator manages the service line. He/she leads the management team which plans, organizes, and operates the service line according to hospital goals, policies, and practices. Specific areas of responsibilities include, but are not limited to:

Developing strategies for continually improving the quality of services

Developing effective relationships with physicians, other health care providers, patients, and payers

Identifying and obtaining the people, equipment, data, and financial resources needed to deliver the service

Strengthening cooperation between the hospital and its physician staff around the delivery of services

Developing a business plan for the delivery of services

Preparing budgets that accurately reflect the goals of the service line

Monitoring and controlling costs to achieve efficient operations

Assuring that issues of professional practice are resolved in appropriate ways

Promoting collaboration and cooperation among service line staff

Encouraging cooperation with other service lines and support staff to achieve the hospital's goals

Serving on hospital-wide projects and committees

Promoting the interests of the hospital inside and outside the hospital

*Courtesy of the Medical Center Hospital of Vermont.

and the functional department managers. The service line administrator has a responsibility to develop budgets with functional department managers such as the physical therapy manager/director. In planning for the most efficient coverage of the service line, the service line administrator must develop productivity targets that are carefully coordinated with the physical therapy staffing pattern. If there is a conflict between the service line targets and the staffing needs, then those issues have to be negotiated between the service line administrator and the physical therapy manager/director.

This system is set up to encourage negotiation and problem solving at the service level. Service coordinators are designated within the functional department to provide services within the service line (Box 4–2) and supervise the delivery of (physical therapy) services. For instance, a rehabilitation service line may need seven to ten physical therapists working within the service line. The service coordinator coordinates the delivery of physical therapy services within this service line. The service coordinators in physical therapy also develop programs while the physical therapy director/manager negotiates the budget to deliver the services.[7] The service coordinator does none of the paperwork traditionally delegated to supervisory jobs. This person is totally responsible for providing services, attending meetings, and co-

· ·

BOX 4–2 CHARACTERISTICS OF THE SERVICE COORDINATOR*

Maturity
Have a settling affect on younger clinicians
Enhance problem solving; serve as a resource
Have seasoned time management skills
Can manage uncomfortable or stressful situations

Clinical Skills
Experience to draw upon for evaluation and problem solving
Versatile in treatment approaches and techniques
Innovative and risk taker

Communications
Contacts with service line colleagues are meaningful and timely
Documentation is a model
Understands the environment and is system adaptable
Participates effectively, collaborates with ease

Assignments
Develops specific interests and skills to an elegant generalist or a specialist
Can contribute to the quality of care through clinical studies or research
Shares knowledge and experience effectively

Evaluation
Willingly participates in continuous quality assurance
Can recognize and apply cost-containment opportunities
Willingness to be evaluated
Can accept and adapt to change and acquire and apply new skills

*Adapted from Feitelberg SB: *Product Service Line Management: Its Impact on Physical Therapy*, audiotape. 1991 Combined Sections Meeting, American Physical Therapy Association, Orlando, Fla.

ordinating the staff in the provision of services. Traditionally, there are the same
number of coordinators as the number of service lines unless there are lines that do
not use any physical therapy. If service lines are very large (orthopedics), it may be
necessary to have more than one coordinator for that line.

· · · · · · · · · · ·
CONTROLLING AND SHARING FUNCTIONS TO REACH COLLABORATIVE OUTCOMES

It is possible for functional departments to maintain control of and develop programs outside of service lines. For example, an outpatient back program may remain
under the direction of the physical therapy manager if the back program is successfully (effectively and efficiently) managed from physical therapy and provides customer satisfaction.

Nursing has established one model in which all of the education and research
activities of the nursing department are placed into a common center within the hospital. The establishment of such a center is funded by external activities and agencies. Some physical therapy departments are moving in the same direction, using
continuing education funds as the start-up funds for the establishment of similar centers.

The service line model allows a degree of flexibility for senior therapists within
a service line who are responsible for advanced patient care and recognizes them as

stable and mature members of the staff. Advanced clinicians devote a portion of their time to clinical research and must be funded within the base camp concept through formula funding or through outside funding sources.[7]

Service line organizational structures in rehabilitation-related services are experiencing mixed success in complex health care organizations. Some of these programs appear to fail because the service line administrator is not sensitive to professional issues, and is not a skilled negotiator among professionals, and therefore compromises the program. The most successful of these programs are in organizations in which a physical therapist or a like professional is the service line administrator or in which the service line administrator and director/manager of the physical therapy department have developed a strong working relationship. In these situations, the professional issues of physical therapy are dealt with by the physical therapists, not by the service line administrator.

It also appears that some of these systems are failing because the service line administrators and service coordinators do not have the human resource skills to effectively manage the requisite for elegant teamwork. Service line management is highly dependent on human resources, and the administrator and coordinators of these service lines must be very skilled at facilitating and managing communications to develop and maintain an effective team.

Some service line structures fail because there is a lack of committment on the part of the major referral source, which is most often the medical staff. A critical participant in the service line is the physician, whose traditional attitudes and behaviors (Box 4–3) present certain barriers to be overcome to facilitate service line management.[8]

It is incumbent upon the hospital administration to improve the relationship of the referral source with the hospital and other health professionals in order to accomplish the goals of the service line. The referral source (physician) will be most likely to embrace the service line structure if the quality of the medical care is improved by the structure, the service line is well equipped and adequately staffed, the service line enhances the hospital's image in the community, there is ease in referring patients into the system, there is an atmosphere of collegiality, and there is an opportunity to provide input to the policies and governance of the service line.[9]

Service line administration presents many challenges to directors and managers of physical therapy as well as other services.[10] The physical therapy manager must provide information in different ways and expect that the information will be subjected to more scrutiny and sharing among a wider variety of professionals. The physical therapy aspect of the service must be carefully articulated within the service,

· ·

BOX 4–3 SERVICE LINES AND THE REFERRAL SOURCE ATTITUDES AND BEHAVIORS

1. Want to maintain autonomy
2. Want a voice in the governance of the service line
3. Interested in the quality and service offered
4. Want to enhance their reputation and that of institution
5. Concerned with competition from colleagues, groups
6. Want to provide exclusive services and have contracts
7. Look for convenience and a sense of belonging
8. Impatient with the misuse of time.
9. Have high expectations of support services at all levels
10. Often lack administrative and marketing knowledge
11. Resent bureaucracy that slows service delivery

and the appropriate priority for physical therapy must be set by the service line administrator and the team through a negotiated process. There is a need to define costs in relation to the benefits of the service effectively delivered within a system that measures the quality of outcomes. These tasks are typical management responsibilities, and although the information may have to be collected and targeted in some new ways, the task of collecting and analyzing the information is not new to physical therapy managers.

Perhaps the most difficult task of the physical therapy manager is coping with the changing use of power and authority, collaborating and negotiating, and integrating professional/ethical issues into the service line approach.[8] The physical therapy manager must focus on facilitating and coaching members of the department and leading the staff in adjusting to new reporting relationships.

The physical therapy manager often uses protocols as a way of merging quality with costs.[11] The protocol (ie, total hip protocol) reflects the management of a disease process or a symptom complex, including expected time periods during which the patient will achieve certain milestones (Box 4–4). The service line manager attaches resource needs and costs to each of the milestones, and from that information the expected cost of the delivery of services for specific diagnostic categories is computed. Critical path techniques are an expanded method for examining a protocol.

Protocols are updated periodically to include data that are missing and eliminate nonapplicable data, to incorporate new knowledge, to eliminate or correct previous knowledge that is no longer valid, and to retain relevance and focus. The management of the hip replacement, for example, is then a team protocol that is constantly updated and gives the starting point for a consistent data base, insures thoroughness, facilitates the audit of care and performance, encourages continued learning through problem solving, contributes to identifying allocations of resources, and provides a baseline for constructing the costs of a service.

Most physical therapy departments have protocols but few truly merge those protocols with other services. Service line management encourages physical therapy to creatively negotiate the manner in which aspects of the physical therapy–specific protocols will be incorporated into the team protocols. This gives a baseline for developing costs and quality assessment.

The Joint Commission on the Accreditation of Healthcare Organizations is now focusing on continuous quality improvement. Service line management must provide outcome data and incorporate the patient and family into the system. The therapist cannot always determine if the service was effective at the point that the patient is discharged. The service line members must creatively determine how to collect quality data over time following discharge involving the patient, family, community, and employer and use the data analysis for program review.

Service lines are here because there is a movement away from reimbursement as we now know it. The system has to be replaced. We have moved to prospective payment and fixed-price systems. The physical therapy manager is now dealing with managed care. The administrator is finding that he or she must have information regarding the cost of treating the individual patient in the system.

- -

BOX 4–4 TOTAL HIP PROTOCOL (EXCERPT OF ONE ACTIVITY)

Ambulation:		
Patient upright with maximal assistance	Patient upright with moderate assistance	Patient upright with minimal assistance
Day 1 _____	Day 2 _____	Day 3 _____

Cost analysis is needed to adopt, maintain, and discontinue services. As difficult as it is, there must be discontinuation of services. There has to be a process to compare treatments and evaluate alternative protocols to seek standardization and quality and define quality as minimal quality.[7] Nothing less than this is adequate. Standard treatment protocols have to look at all direct and indirect costs.

To measure a service from admissions to discharge requires an organizational scheme that makes this possible. Service line can maintain certain values and practices that are proven, but it does require a significant change in traditional health care delivery relationships.[9]

The new relationships concern professional and team power and practices. Individuals must learn to give power to others, work with a variety of professionals in new ways, and reach commitment, trust, and success. To succeed, they have to socialize the staff and students, which requires an understanding of the economics of health care. They must have managerial responsibilities as autonomous practitioners from the time that they graduate, change professional behavior especially in working with teams, aquire critical measurement capabilities, and be able to make choices about providing and not providing care, and to always keep the patient as the center of service management.[12]

References

1. MacStravic R: Product-line administration in hospitals. *Health Care Manage Rev* 1986; 11:35–43.
2. Ciole R: *The New Medicine.* Rockville, Md, Aspen Publications, 1990.
3. Zelman W, McLaughlin C: Product-line in a complex marketplace: Matching organizational strategy to buyer behavior. *Health Care Manage Rev* 1990; 15:9–14.
4. Fottler M, Repasky L: Attitudes of hospital executives toward product-line management: A pilot survey. *Health Care Manage Rev* 1988; 13:15–22.
5. Goodrich R: St. Luke's hospital reaps benefits by using product management. *Mod Health Care,* Feb 15, 1985, pp 157–158.
6. Kotter J: Power, dependence, and effective management. *Harvard Business Rev* 1977; 55:125–136.
7. Feitelberg SB: *Product/Service Line Management: Its Impact on Physical Therapy,* audiotape. 1991 combined sections meeting, American Physical Therapy Meeting, Orlando Fla.
8. Valentine S: *Physician Bonding.* Rockville, Md, Aspen Publications, 1990.
9. Goldsmith J: A radical prescription for hospitals. *Harvard Business Rev,* May-June 1989, pp 104–111.
10. Nordstrom R, Allen B: Cultural change vs. behavioral change. *Health Care Manage Rev* 1987; 12:43–49.
11. Schermerhorn J: *Management for Productivity,* New York, John Wiley, 1983.
12. Cleverly W: Product costing for health care firms. *Health Care Manage Rev* 1987; 12:39–48.

Bibliography

Egli H: A product line approach to rehabilitation. *Physical Therapy Forum* 1990; 9:1–6.
Kotler P: *Marketing Management.* Engelwood, NJ, Prentice Hall, 1980.
Nackel J, Fenaroli P, Kis G: Product-line performance reporting: A key to cost management. *Health Care Financial Manage* 1987; 41:54–62.
Orloff T: Hospital cost accounting: Who's doing what and why? *Health Care Manage Rev* 1990; 15:73–78.
Romito D: A critical path for CVA patients. *Rehabil Nursing* 1990; 15:153–156.
Shelly J, Stefan D: Product-line management. *The Pyramid* 1989; 18(special issue):1–7.
Zelman W, Parham D: Strategic, operational, and marketing concerns of product-line management in health care. *Health Care Manage Rev* 1900; 15:29–35.

CASE 4.1:

Oceanview Community Hospital

Donald Jackson, P.T., M.S.

Oceanview Community Hospital (OCH) is a relatively small 225-bed hospital located in a predominantly residential Los Angeles suburb with many large industries on its periphery. The Board of Directors of the hospital is composed of prominent executives and physicians of the community. Until 3 years ago, the executive director of OCH was the wife of the executive director of one of the nearby major industries.

The hospital, although it had a reputation for providing quality care for its patients, was falling further and further into debt. The Board of Directors, realizing this, made a move to bring in a young executive director with a broad background in hospital administration and management. The new executive director then surrounded himself with three young hospital administrators who were also extremely well qualified with excellent backgrounds in modern management techniques (Fig 4–3).

The associate executive director in charge of patient care services, John Doe, recognized that the department heads of some of the patient care services were weak in management and administration. As time progressed, however, he noted that the director of physical therapy, in particular, had a great deal of difficulty in planning budgets, allotting time for administrative responsibilities, and managing departmental personnel.

The director of respiratory therapy, on the other hand, because of previous management experience in a major department store chain, was able to develop budgets realistically and seemed to be able to manage his personnel effectively. When the director of the physical therapy department resigned a few months later, the associate executive director determined it was time to make a managerial change. He elected to appoint the director of respiratory therapy to a new position that he called director of therapy services. The respiratory therapy supervisor was promoted to manager of respiratory therapy, and the vacated position in physical therapy was termed manager of physical therapy. As applicants interviewed for the physical

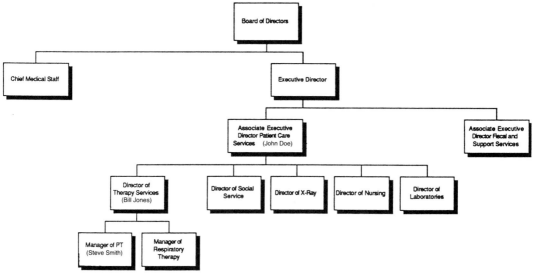

FIG 4–3.
Organization chart of Oceanview Community Hospital. *PT* = physical therapy.

therapy position, it was made clear that they would be working under the director of therapy services, Bill Jones.

Bill, after three or four interviews with prospective applicants, selected Steve Smith, a young therapist with only 3 years of experience, but who had demonstrated a great deal of leadership in his previous position and was already well known among physical therapists in the Los Angeles area. Steve came highly recommended, and he demonstrated an air of confidence that appealed to Bill immediately.

When Steve took the job, he knew he was to be the only physical therapist on the staff for at least 6 months. The department had been running 6 days a week with the previous therapist working Monday through Friday. On Saturday the department was run by one of two physical therapist assistants.* Steve informed Bill that it was not legal for a physical therapy department to be open without a physical therapist on the premises, and, in addition, Steve explained that in the event of an accident, the hospital would be liable if there was not a physical therapist in the building. Bill explained that the current budget did not allow for the addition of any help, and that if Steve could straighten out the budget, he could promise him an additional therapist in 6 months. Steve, not wanting the department to be open without a physical therapist on the premises, elected to work 6 days a week for the first 6 months.

Steve was very well liked by his staff, and they were eager to work for him. He made many changes in departmental operating procedures, including regular staff and inservice meetings that were set up for the purpose of keeping the staff abreast of changes and for delivering continuing education programs for members of the department. He also became actively involved in other aspects of patient care within the hospital, and within the first 4 months he had spoken with each of the physician groups in the hospital. Referrals from physicians for physical therapy care began escalating to an all-time high, and by the end of the second month the physical therapy department had met the budget for the first time in 2 years.

The department continued to meet its budget for the next 4 months, and by the end of the 6 months, the department was close to operating in the black for the fiscal year. At this time, Steve approached Bill in his office.

Steve: Bill, in looking over our budget reports you can see that in 5 of the last 6 months the physical therapy department has been able to meet its budget and we're nearing our budget for the fiscal year.

Bill: I can't compliment you enough on the work you've been able to do for this department. I was just talking to John the other day, and he is extremely pleased with the way things are going. Of course I gave you all the credit for the success. He said he was very pleased with the direction of the physical and respiratory therapy departments since I took over as director of therapy services.

Steve: As you know I've been working 6 days a week for the last 6 months because, as I pointed out to you earlier, this department cannot be open legally without a physical therapist on the premises. Since we've been able to meet the budget for 5 of the last 6 months, I would like to start advertising for a staff physical therapist.

Bill: As you pointed out, we're just now starting to creep into the black in terms of our annual budget. If we hire another therapist now it will blow the budget. If I bring it up to John he's going to reject the idea immediately. I don't see any way we can hire another therapist at this point in time.

Steve: The reason we are hitting black is because I've been working 6 days a week in order to pull the ends together in terms of both patient care and management of the department.

---

*In the State of California, physical therapist assistants are not required to be graduates from an accredited program. Many still receive their background through on-the-job training programs. The law in California governing the practice of physical therapy also states that physical therapist assistants will work under the direct (on-site) supervision of the physical therapist.

Bill: I realize the job you've been doing, Steve, and I know it's been a hard 6 months for you. I would recommend that you have your physical therapist assistants alternate weekends and you take the weekends off.

Steve: You know I won't do that.

Bill: That's the way the department ran for 3 years previously. There's no reason we can't do it again now. John just would not accept the idea of hiring another therapist at this time.

Steve left the meeting angry, realizing that Bill was not about to approach John about hiring another therapist. At the same time Steve felt he could not continue to work 6 days a week or keep pushing himself as hard as he had over the past 6 months. During his 6 months at Oceanview, he had made many friends among the medical staff and with three members of the Board of Directors. He knew that if he approached them properly they would be more than happy to support his cause. But at the same time he felt that this was not the ethical solution to the situation. He also knew that John would not be open to discussing the matter with him at the present time. Steve felt that if he did go to the medical staff or to any of the members of the Board of Directors for support there might be repercussions from Bill for going over his head. Steve elected to approach Bill again to try to gain his support.

Steve: As you can see by these reports our daily census for physical therapy treatments has increased significantly over the past 6-month period. Currently I am personally seeing 12 patients a day by scheduling one patient every half hour. During the remaining 2 hours I attend to the other activities that are necessary to run the department. The assistants are doing a good job with the patients they're treating, however, we're beginning to treat patients who require the skills of a professional physical therapist. I'm finding it more difficult to devote time to all these patients. In addition, I will not leave the department open without a physical therapist on the premises. That means that until I can get some more help I will continue to work 6 days a week. As you know I find this a very discomforting situation. I feel it's a situation that we need to investigate in order to find the most equitable solution.

Bill: I've already given you the solution, Steve. Either continue to work 6 days a week, or let one of the assistants run the department on Saturday. That's the only alternative.

A few minutes after his discussion with Bill, Steve ran into John in the hall.

Steve: John, I need to talk to you right away. There's a situation developing that should be brought to your attention.

John: If it has to do with the physical therapy department, I'll hear about it through Bill. Besides, I'm leaving town in 10 minutes for an important meeting. If, after talking to Bill, I feel the situation requires your consultation, I'll arrange to meet with you in my office.

Later that day Steve discussed his problem with one of his influential friends on the medical staff. His friend expressed a desire to bring the situation to the attention of the chief of the medical staff. Steve could see a potential powder keg developing. Steve knew he could get his way through the medical staff, but he also knew that if he approached the situation in this manner he would never be able to develop a trusting relationship with John or other members of the administration. Steve continued to search for a solution to his problem.

Consider the issues of restructuring the department in this case. When individuals who are not professionals (physical therapists) are responsible for the administration of the department, how should professional issues such as unsupervised physical therapist assistants be handled? When the organizational structure was flattened, should there have been mechanisms put in place for the manager of physical therapy to talk directly to the hospital administrator? What are the problems of communication posed by this case? How could these problems be managed successfully?

CHAPTER 5

Law and Regulations in Physical Therapy

I. Illegal practice and malpractice
   A. Statutory laws
      1. Professional licensing laws
      2. Nondiscrimination laws
   B. Common law
      1. Malpractice
      2. Business practices

II. Accrediting agencies
   A. Joint commission on the accreditation of healthcare organizations
   B. Commission on the accreditation of rehabilitation facilities
      1. Work hardening standards development and debate
      2. Accreditation criteria

III. Regulatory agencies
   A. Health care financing administration
      1. Level 1 review
      2. Level 2 review
      3. Level 3 review
   B. State department of public health
   C. Occupational safety and health administration
   D. Worker's compensation
   E. Internal revenue service: independent contractor status

IV. Professional standards
   A. Guides to personnel utilization
   B. Code of ethics and guides of conduct
   C. Standards of practice
   D. Specialization

V. Institutional standards
   A. Practice privileges
   B. Immunizations

VI. Case
   A. Hiring practices: case 5.1

VII. Legal and regulatory definitions

VIII. Appendices
   A. Appendix 5.1: schema for medicare reimbursement
   B. Appendix 5.2: guide for professional conduct
   C. Appendix 5.3: guide for conduct of the affiliate member
   D. Appendix 5.4: standards of practice for physical therapy

· · · · · · · · · · ·

One of the most challenging and important roles of the physical therapy manager is the knowledge and observation of laws and regulations regarding the practice of physical therapy related to the specific institution in which the service is located.

· · · · · · · · · · ·

ILLEGAL PRACTICE AND MALPRACTICE

Some of the laws that govern physical therapy come from statutes (statutory law) which are passed by legislatures. Other laws come from common law principles that have evolved from legal decisions.

Statutory Laws

Statutory laws that have an impact on physical therapy include licensure laws, worker's compensation law, medicare/medicaid, nondiscrimination laws (Rehabilitation Act of 1973, civil rights laws, Americans With Disabilities Act [ADA]), copyright law, anti-trust laws (Sherman Act and related state anti-trust laws), Federal Trade Commission Act), tax codes, licensure laws applying to businesses (permits, zoning laws), criminal laws (controlled substance laws, mail fraud, assault, battery), and corporate business laws. Tort reform rests in this area and proposes the enactment of legislation that will dictate how malpractice claims will be administered in the future. The proposed tort reform laws are extensions of the Federal Tort Claims Act and the Uniform Commercial Code.

The statutory law discussion in this chapter will be limited to professional licensing laws and nondiscrimination laws. Although the other areas of statutory law are of importance, the physical therapy manager is encouraged to seek the advice of a lawyer specializing in the specific kind of law in which advice is needed.

Professional licensing laws

Ironically, Texas was the last state to require state licensure for physical therapists, although it was "in 1873, the first state to establish a state board of medical examiners."[1(p26)] The original medical licensure laws were enacted to protect the public against exploitation by quacks and commercial opportunists as well as professional incompetence. These early laws laid the groundwork for licensure laws in physical therapy that present minimal standards of practice as indicated by graduation from an accredited program in physical therapy, successful completion of a national licensing examination, and the ethical and legal minimums related to the continuing practice of physical therapy. Licensure is a mechanism used to determine a minimal standard of educational preparation and to establish the rights, responsibilities, and limitations of the professional's practice. Historically, physical therapists were originally credentialed nationally through the Physical Therapy Registry by meeting minimal educational standards and passing a national examination. The movement to achieve licensure laws in all states in physical therapy began in the 1920s and ended in the 1960s. Over the years the laws have been modified to reduce the limitations placed on the practice of physical therapy—the elimination of a need for a referral, the definition of the scope of practice from a modality-driven practice to a practice defined by evaluation and physical treatment, and the inclusion of provisions of supervision of the physical therapist assistant.

Licensure of physical therapists occurs through state practice acts that either stand alone or are included within the medical practice act within the state. All states require that the applicant be a graduate of an accredited educational program in physical therapy and that the applicant demonstrate successful completion of the national licensing examination for physical therapists. In those states where physical therapist assistants are licensed or registered, the process is the same.

Once solely the responsibility of the profession through the American Physical Therapy Association (APTA), the development of the physical therapy licensure examination and related activities are now being assumed by the newly formed Federation of State Boards of Physical Therapy.* This federation is modeled after the Federation of State Medical Boards and is responsible for the development, administration, revision, and confidentiality of the national licensing examination used by all states. Each state obtains the licensure examination from the federation on a fixed schedule determined by the federation. The federation, in turn, contracts with a testing agency to develop and score the test. In addition, it is forming a national network of state boards and is considering computer networking with all boards and developing a national data base in order to track physical therapy practice within the United States. This data base will also include disciplinary actions taken against physical therapists so that those actions can be accurately reported from state to state as physical therapists relocate. All states belong to the Federation of State Boards of Physical Therapy.

The obtaining of a physical therapy license is the first professional responsibility of the physical therapist. The license to practice physical therapy provides both privileges of practice as well as the limitations of that practice. *Physical therapy managers must assume the full responsibility of informing applicants of their responsibilities to acquire a license (or temporary license) prior to beginning employment.* Too many managers in physical therapy either do not ask for proof of licensure or actually indicate to the new employee that it is acceptable to begin employment without due notification of licensure (full or temporary) within the jurisdiction. Physical therapy managers must realize that such practices are not only unethical, but unlawful. As physical therapy moves toward a more autonomous practice, it is anticipated that the profession will require full licensure before the individual is allowed to practice. *Temporary licensure is a remnant of dependent practice. As long as physical therapists (new graduates and physical therapists seeking endorsement) feel that they can engage in practice under supervision without being licensed, they are not willing to take full responsibility as a professional.*

As a way of demonstrating a high regard for licensure and in order to invite patient questions about the standards of practice, the physical therapy manager should consider creative ways of prominently displaying the licenses and certifications of staff physical therapists and physical therapist assistants. Displaying these documents along with diplomas, codes of ethics, and the patient's bill of rights in physical therapy may increase questions from patients, but at the same time will educate them as to the standards of the profession.

One of the aspects of physical therapy laws that is changing rapidly is the re-

---

*For more information about the Federation of State Boards of Physical Therapy, contact the Division of Professional Relations at the American Physical Therapy Association, 1111 N Fairfax St, Alexandria, VA 22314; telephone: 1-800-999-APTA.

quirement for a physician referral in order to practice physical therapy. Maryland was the first state to pass direct access legislation in 1979, allowing the physical therapist to both evaluate and treat the patient without physician referral. Currently, it is legally permissible to evaluate a patient without physician referral in over 40 states and to evaluate and treat a patient in nearly 30 states. In 11 states in which treatment without referral is allowed, there are specific restrictions or qualifications imposed on the physical therapist. For instance, one state specifies two levels of physical therapist, with special practice requirements of a level II therapist in order to treat patients without referrals.

The number of states passing direct access legislation is changing rapidly. Although the state law may allow practice without referral (direct access), third parties may not agree to pay without a physician referral. In all states that have passed this legislation, there is a concerted effort to compel the insurance commissioner or individual third parties to pay for physical therapy services without physician referral. It is the responsibility of the physical therapy manager to understand the state laws that govern physical therapy practice in the jurisdictions in which the practice(s) is located and the ruling of the insurance commissioner and/or insurance companies and managed-care facilities regarding the relationship of reimbursement to physician referral.

As of 1992, physical therapist assistants are regulated through state law and administrative rules in 40 states. In states where the physical therapist assistant is licensed or regulated, the physical therapy manager must be particularly aware of the restrictions of practice imposed on the physical therapist assistant, such as the nature of the supervision necessary and the degree to which the physical therapist assistant may take part in evaluation and program planning. Although Arizona was the first state to regulate the physical therapist assistant in 1952, APTA policies did not describe the physical therapist assistant until 1967. The physical therapist assistant officially became a part of the association in 1973 when the affiliate member category of the association was created. As the name implies, the physical therapist assistant was intended to be regulated as a health care worker responsible to the physical therapist. Unfortunately, supervision requirements in state laws range all the way from on-site supervision by a physical therapist to supervision by a physician with no physical therapist involvement.

Complaints can be made against physical therapists who are practicing outside of the professional licensing laws for physical therapy within the state. For instance, some states restrict the practice of physical therapy to practice by referral from a physician. If a physical therapist accepts and treats a patient without a physician referral in such a state, the physical therapist is practicing illegally in that state and is subject to penalties imposed by the licensing board. These penalties vary from reprimands and fines to suspension and revocation of license. The licensing board is empowered by the state with rights and responsibilities to act as a judicial body in determining the facts of wrongdoing and imposing penalties in the name of the state. Members of these boards are appointed through a governor's appointment process. Boards are administrative arms of the state and are governed by both state laws governing professional practice as well as administrative rules that further define the laws. Usually these boards are housed in state departments of health with close ties to the attorney general's office. The board may be assigned an assistant attorney general to offer counsel in the investigation of claims, conduct of public and private hearings, determine the facts of law, and determine the appropriate level of penalty to be imposed by the board (in essence, by the state).

The physical therapy community is represented in several ways on these boards. In some instances, a physical therapist sits on the Medical Board, with all of the rights and responsibilities of any other board member. There may also be a physical therapy advisory committee to the board, an advisory committee to a regulatory agency or department (Department of State), or an independent physical therapy licensing board. Twenty-four states currently have independent physical therapy boards that have all of the rights and responsibilities described above.

One of the reasons physical therapy has advanced as far as it has in relation to similar professional groups is because of its early involvement in licensure. Whenever questions arose over the past 70 years regarding rights and responsibilities of the profession, the fact that physical therapists were licensed professionals was a key determinant of expanding those rights and responsibilities.

A number of state and federal laws govern the practice of business in the United States. Statutory laws govern the nature of partnerships, articles of incorporation, sales of goods, establishment and maintenance of credit, payment of taxes, and zoning laws that define the nature of the business allowances (size of business, parking requirements, size of structures, flow of traffic) in a community. Like all laws, the laws that govern these areas have "at least eight major functions: (1) to keep the peace, (2) to influence and enforce standards of conduct, (3) to maintain the status quo in certain aspects of society, (4) to facilitate orderly change, (5) to allow for maximum self-assertion by the individual, (6) to facilitate planning and the realization of reasonable expectations, (7) to promote social justice, and (8) to provide a mechanism for compromise solutions between polar principles and positions."[2(p2)]

Nondiscrimination laws

Several US laws prevent a facility from discrimination against employees with regard to race, color, religion, gender, or national origin if it receives a particular level of federal support, affects commerce, or is considered to be a public institution. Title VII of the 1964 Civil Rights Act prohibits a private employer who employs 15 or more persons, all educational institutions, state and local government, public and private employment agencies, and labor unions with 15 or more members from discriminating against job applicants and employees because of race, color, sex, religion, or national origin. Regulations regarding the Civil Rights Act are developed and enforced by the Justice Department and Equal Employment Opportunity Commission, which was greatly strengthened and expanded under the Equal Employment Act of 1972.

The Equal Pay Act of 1963 required all employers subject to the Fair Labor Standards Act to provide equal pay for men and women performing similar work.

Executive order no. 11246 was issued in 1965, requiring affirmative action programs by all federal contractors and subcontractors and requires that firms with contracts over $50,000 and 50 or more employees develop and implement written programs for affirmative action. These requirements include identifying areas of minority and female underutilization.

The Age Discrimination and Employment Act of 1967 prohibits employers of 25 or more persons from discriminating against persons from 40 to 70 years of age in any area of employment.

Title IX, the Education Amendments Act of 1972, prohibits discrimination on the basis of sex against employees or students of any educational institution receiving federal financial aid. This act lead to the disintegration of many men's and women's colleges and opened admissions to both sexes.

The 1973 Rehabilitation Act imposed regulations through the Department of Labor, which required all federal contractors (with contracts over $2,500) to have an affirmative action plan that included handicapped workers. Part of the act is also regulated by the Department of Health and Human Services (HHS) and the Rehabilitation Services Administration under the Department of Education, which states that the act applies to institutions receiving medicare, medicaid and other federal support.[3(pp191–192)]

The Education for All Handicapped Children Act of 1974 (Public Law 94-142) entitles all school-aged children to a free and appropriate education in the least restrictive environment regardless of the severity of the disability.

From an employee perspective, if an institution has 25 or more employees, compliance with the Americans With Disabilities Act was mandatory by July 1992. This legislation goes much further than the 1973 Rehabilitation Act. For the employer this means that pre-employment physicals are no longer allowable for the purpose of denying employment. The employer may use the physical after employment as a placement physical. That is, based on the physical, the employer will decide the degree to which the employee must be preconditioned for the job or the degree to which the work site must be modified.*

It is critical that the physical therapy manager understand the nature of the institution and the degree to which the institution subscribes to the nurturing of a multicultural organization. The intent of current laws and regulations is that the institution go beyond creating an affirmative action plan that stops discrimination. The intent of the law is that organizations use the plan to correct past discriminatory actions (Box 5–1).

Discrimination laws and regulations also relate to individual access to services in the community and therefore relate to the acceptance and treatment of clients. Some private facilities that are specialized in their function are not bound by laws or regulations to accept clients that need services outside their specialty. For instance, children's hospitals are exclusively devoted to the care of children and are therefore not obligated to accept adult patients. A private facility also can deny access to patients who cannot afford to pay if the facility does not accept assignment for medicare or medicaid patients; is not a public, state, or county facility; or if the institution does not have any agreements with the community regarding indigent care. Public facilities are required to accept patients regardless of their ability to pay and may have agreements with surrounding communities or their Board of Trustees to accept a particular number of indigent patients from their area. Although policies regarding the acceptance of indigent patients may cause a significant degree of internal and external debate related to the institution's obligations to care for the ill and the patient's rights to access health care, it is the responsibility of the manager to understand the facility's regulations and standards related to these issues and to abide by those regulations. Employees should understand that if they do not agree with restrictions related to the acceptance of clients at that institution and they are unable to change those policies, they should not continue to work at that institution.

Common Law

Common law areas that have an impact on physical therapy include tort law (negligence, professional liability), contract law (employment contract, service contract), liable and slander, and real property law (buildings, land). Common law cannot be amended as statutory law can be amended.

Malpractice

Physical therapists are personally responsible for both negligence and other principles of liability that result in malpractice. Negligence usually occurs as a result of failure to carry out professional duties or breach of conduct, in which a direct cause

---

*This new legislation will become another market for physical therapists as consultants to assess the physical condition of the employee and to assess the ergonomics of the work site. Since it applies to all businesses in the United States, the market potential for physical therapists is large, although unmeasured at this point. As the profession experiences increasing shortages of physical therapists, the Americans With Disabilities Act legislation will have even more impact on that shortage than any previous legislation.

BOX 5-1 ELIMINATING DISCRIMINATORY PRACTICES*

1. Avoid stereotyping women, minorities, and the handicapped
2. Identify the facility as an equal opportunity employer
3. Documents should recognize a diverse patient population and be produced in the languages most common to the community
4. Avoid word-of- mouth recruitment, which is discriminatory
5. Employment advertising, applications for employment, and all employee forms should state that the facility considers all applicants regardless of race, color, religion, creed, national origin, gender, disability, age, marital or veteran status, or sexual orientation; advertising should be placed in vehicles that will reach the minority population
6. All reference to points of discrimination should be avoided during employment interviews; managers may ask about the applicant's legal status in the United States, command of English as a primary language, record of convictions of felonies, educational status, and employment history (including firings)
7. Prepare employees equally when mentoring for leadership or management positions
8. Review all policies within the facility and eliminate any restrictions or barriers for women, minorities, and the handicapped
9. Make both a personal and formal commitment to diversity
10. Become involved in all aspects of the community; provide services and recruit in the ethnic communities
11. Involve the ethnic communities in new projects, volunteer opportunities, tours of physical therapy, and sponsorship of promising students
12. Confront biases when they become apparent
13. Invite feedback from women, minority, and handicapped patients regarding the individual, organizational, and structural barriers that they encounter in the department
14. Acquire information related to the major minority groups in the community and sensitize the staff to the culture of those groups.
15. Recognize cultural difference among the staff; encourage staff to share cultural perspectives with each other

*Adapted from Feitelberg SB: *Meeting the Challenge of Cultural Diversity in Health Care,* monograph. Chicago Area Director's Forum, Burlington, Vt, p 12.

of injury can be ascribed to the professional that results in harm to the individual. In tort law, if there is no harm, there is no valid claim of negligence.

When physical therapists are employees in an employer-employee relationship, they will always be responsible for personally negligent actions, but claims of injury will often fall under the doctrine of *respondeat superior* (let the superior respond), which means that the employer is responsible for the actions of the employee if injury is incurred under usual work conditions. Most physical therapists still work for employers, even if the employer is another physical therapist, so this doctrine provides significant protection for most therapists. The common reference to this doctrine is that the injured party goes after the deep pockets. It is true that institutions and businesses generally carry a greater amount of liability insurance than the individual professional, and the individual will be more likely to recover greater awards by suing the employer. However, the point of law is that since the employer benefits from the work of the employee, the employer also accepts the liabilities of the employee.

There are situations that are covered by the doctrine of *res ipsa loquitur* (the thing speaks for itself), in which negligence has occurred at the hand of the physical therapist without any contribution by the patient but was not an act of personal negligence. "The doctrine of *res ipsa loquitur* comes to the aid of the injured person who can show: (1) that the event that caused the injury was one that would not normally happen in the absence of negligence and (2) that the defendant had exclusive control over the instrumentalities which caused the harm. This doctrine then shifts the burden of explanation to the allegedly negligent party who in order to escape liability must show that the duty of due care was met."[2(p11)] The most common example of such a situation occurs when there is injury from a piece of equipment that may break and hit the patient. The piece of equipment may have been recently purchased and therefore would not be expected to break, the physical therapist may use reasonable care in positioning the patient and the equipment, and all paperwork related to the safety of the equipment may be in order. The burden will be on the physical therapist to justify the degree to which the equipment was tested in simulated situations to assure its stability. The accident would not have happened if the physical therapist had not positioned the equipment and the patient had not been in the care of the physical therapist, so the court would be inclined to consider the patient entitled to some compensation for the injury.

Malpractice is actually a term used to describe the constellation of wrongs or injuries that might accrue through the professional-patient relationship. Malpractice claims are made when, in the course of performing responsibilities in carrying out the duties of the physical therapist to do no harm (nonmaleficence), the physical therapist fails to perform that duty, causing harm. Although there are many other ethical principles that can be violated in caring for patients such as acting without consent, breaking of confidentiality, and lack of respect for privacy, most claims against physical therapists involve doing harm to the patient. The most severe of these harms, such as sexual or physical abuse of patients, may also become actions whose legal outcome will be decided in civil courts, in which the physical therapist is vulnerable to significant fines and loss of freedom.

Typically, physical therapy claims most often involve harm to patients from a failure to adequately monitor the condition of the patient and include burns, infections, opening of wounds, torn soft tissues, and injuries resulting from falls. Secondary reasons for claims against physical therapists are the failure to treat the patient properly and failure to maintain equipment. Also, a much smaller number of claims against physical therapists result from failures to refer or follow physician's orders and sexual misconduct. "Almost 70% of the professional liability claims examined arose from an activity in a physical therapy clinic and/or office. Other settings in which claims arose include hospitals, nursing homes, private residences, health clubs, and schools."[4(p4)] In all of these instances, the degree to which the therapist was negligent in the performance of the duty to the patient will be closely examined as will the patient's responsibilities. In some instances, when patients fail to follow orders or directions, both parties may be deemed negligent in the action and the resultant injury.*

There are procedures that the physical therapy manager can reinforce to reduce malpractice claims (Box 5–2).[5]

Most physical therapists who work in health care institutions do not feel the need to purchase malpractice insurance. They feel confident that if a malpractice situation develops, it will be the result of the normal practice of physical therapy under the employer-employee arrangement and therefore be covered by the employer. It

---

*Exceptional resources are available to the manager and practitioner through the American Physical Therapy Association (APTA) regarding risk management and malpractice issues. A comprehensive guide entitled *Risk Management: An APTA Malpractice Resource Guide* was produced in 1990 and can be purchased from the APTA, 1111 N Fairfax St, Alexandria, VA 22314. In addition, the Judicial Committee of the APTA and the Division of Health Policy and Practice have produced a number of documents, including a bibliography on liability, malpractice, and risk management that may be obtained by contacting information services or the Division of Health Policy and Practice at 1-800-999-APTA.

· ·

BOX 5–2   PRACTICE PROCEDURES FOR PHYSICAL THERAPISTS TO REDUCE MALPRACTICE CLAIMS*

1. Accept only those patients within your area of expertise
2. Screen patients for the potential of litigation
3. Establish a support system so that the patient always has someone to contact in the event it is after office hours or you aren't available
4. Develop a protocol for handling each patient, including a consent form for treatment

5. Exercise sound judgment in decisions involving patient treatment
6. Terminate patients in a responsible fashion
7. Avoid improper conduct
8. Clarify all situations that may appear to be improper, illegal, or unethical
9. Resolve problems quickly

*Adapted from Connolly J: *Risk Management Resource Guide.* Alexandria, Va, American Physical Therapy Association, 1990, pp 2.4–2.5.

would be ideal for all physical therapists to carry malpractice insurance. Although many physical therapists may be an agent of the hospital or other health care institution, the physical therapist is still personally liable in a malpractice suit.

There are times in which the actions of the physical therapist may be interpreted to be outside the coverage of the institution; the physical therapist will then be responsible for payment of claims related to those activities. For instance, a physical therapist was practicing in an acute care facility within a state where physician referral was not required. The therapist was performing bedside treatment to a patient who had had a stroke. The patient in the next bed said that she was uncomfortable and asked the physical therapist to help her to move her leg. The therapist adjusted the patient's leg, placing it on a pillow as requested by the patient. The patient had had a femoral artery graft 3 days previously. The graft became occluded that night, and the patient was rushed to surgery for a replacement graft. The patient claimed that the physical therapist placed her leg too high and caused a kink in the graft, leading to the occlusion. The institution decided that the physical therapist was functioning outside of the common protocols of the facility and attempted to absolve itself of responsibility for the actions of the physical therapist.

As of 1990, all persons paying malpractice claims must submit the information to the National Practitioner Data Bank. This data bank is provided under the Health Care Quality Improvement Act of 1986 within the federal Health Resources and Services Administration. All hospitals must check the data bank against all practitioners who have clinical privileges or are on the medical staff of the hospital. Other health facilities are encouraged to use the data bank when hiring new health care professionals. (A data bank help line can be accessed at 1-800-767-6732.)[6(p1/36)] Managers should note that if a check of the data base is activated, the person whose name is being checked is notified of the inquiry. This is a measure that protects the individual against inappropriate or capricious investigation.

Business practices

In business situations, common law principles govern the nature of contractual arrangements, as well as the owning and managing of property. Physical therapy managers must be aware of all statutory laws and common law principles that govern the operation of the business as well as the conduct of the professionals who work within the business. The physical therapy manager should seek guidance from lawyers specializing in business law when developing contracts, buying property, and establishing leases.

Regulations emanate from accrediting bodies, laws (including professional licensing laws and regulations), regional and state regulatory agencies such as medicare and medicaid, professional codes of ethics and guides of professional conduct, and internally or corporately generated standards of operation.

. . . .
ACCREDITING AGENCIES

Joint Commission on the Accreditation of Healthcare Organizations

The Joint Commission on the Accreditation of Healthcare Organizations (JCAHO) is a "private, not-for-profit organization [which] sets standards and accredits 84 percent of the nation's general hospitals, as well as long term care facilities, psychiatric hospitals, substance abuse programs, outpatient surgery centers, urgent care clinics, group practices, community health centers, and hospices. In 1988 it added a home care accreditation program. The Joint Commission is governed by a 22-member Board of Commissioners composed of one public member and representatives from the American College of Physicians, the American College of Surgeons, the American Dental Association, the American Hospital Association and the American Medical Association."[1(p171)] As can be seen by the constituency of this group, this is a physician and hospital administration–dominated group. The JCAHO "developed from the Hospital Standardization Program established by the American College of Surgeons in 1918. Over the years, the American College of Surgeons became unable to financially support itself and decided to broaden its base. A new organization, the JCAHO, was founded to encourage the voluntary attainment of uniformly high standards of institutional medical care."[7(p595)] Joint Commission review teams are usually composed of physicians, hospital administrators, and nurses. Physical therapy is represented by the APTA on some of the Professional Technical Advisory Committees of JCAHO, such as the Long Term Care Professional Technical Advisory Committee and the Rehabilitation Professional Technical Advisory Committee. The newly established TriAlliance made up of the presidents of the APTA, the American Occupational Therapy Association, and the American Speech, Language, and Hearing Association provide ongoing input to JCAHO regarding standards of rehabilitation services in health care organizations. Hospitals and other agencies seek accreditation on a voluntary basis. However, federal programs such as medicare and state programs such as medicaid require the facility to be accredited by an unbiased recognized agency, so it is to the advantage of the facility to seek accreditation. Also, "the Joint Commission has agreements with about 40 states in which accreditation may fulfill all or part of the state licensing requirements."[1(p172)] (For more information on JCAHO, including standards and criteria, the reader may wish to contact the Joint Commission on Accreditation of Healthcare Organizations at 1 Renaissance Blvd, Oak Brook Terrace, IL 60181.)

Commission on the Accreditation of Rehabilitation Facilities

The Commission on Accreditation of Rehabilitation Facilities (CARF) was established in 1966 "under the operational auspices of the Joint Commission on the Accreditation of Hospitals (previous name of JCAHO) and remained under their auspices until December, 1971, when it became a fully independent voluntary accreditation agency."[8(p107)] CARF is a not-for-profit organization that provides voluntary accreditation for rehabilitation facilities and recently began accrediting Work Hardening Programs.

CARF is made up of a commission that consists of sponsoring members and associate members. The APTA is a sponsoring member of the commission along with other organizations such as the American Academy of Neurology, American Academy of Orthotists and Prosthetists, American Academy of Physical Medicine and Rehabilitation, American Hospital Association, American Occupational Therapy Association, American Speech-Language-and-Hearing Association, Association of Rehabilitation Nurses, and a number of other similar groups. The associate members include organizations such as the American Academy of Pain Medicine, American Congress of Rehabilitation Medicine, American Society of Hand Therapists, American Spinal Injury Association, and several other organizations.

The Board of Trustees of the commission is composed of one person appointed by each sponsoring organization and an equal number of at-large trustees.

CARF is responsible for developing standards and accrediting a wide variety of programs, including the following:

1. Comprehensive inpatient rehabilitation.
2. Spinal cord injury programs.
3. Chronic pain management programs.
4. Brain injury programs.
5. Outpatient medical rehabilitation.
6. Work hardening programs.
7. Infant and early childhood developmental programs.
8. Vocational evaluation.
9. Work adjustment.
10. Occupational skill training.
11. Job placement.
12. Work services.
13. Supported employment.
14. Industry-based programs.
15. Personal and social adjustment services.
16. Community living programs.
17. Respite programs.
18. Alcoholism and other drug-dependency rehabilitation programs.
19. Community mental health organizations.
20. Psychosocial rehabilitation programs.

Work hardening standards development and debate

The Board of Trustees of CARF names a number of board committees to establish standards in its various arenas. The newest committee of the Board is the National Advisory Committee for Work Hardening Standards. This committee is responsible for developing standards, sending them out for field review, collating the results, and making decisions regarding the feedback and then drafting final standards for consideration by the Board of Trustees. The APTA also has a representative on this advisory committee and engages in regular discussions with the CARF executive staff regarding the development of standards, conflicts with standard development and existing programs, and a myriad of other issues.

The current CARF standards manual describes work hardening programs as follows:

"Work Hardening programs, which are interdisciplinary in nature, use conditioning tasks that are graded to progressively improve the biomechanical, neuromuscular, cardiovascular/metabolic, and psychosocial functioning of the person served in conjunction with real or simulated work activities. Work hardening provides a transition between acute care and return to work while addressing the issues of productivity, safety, physical tolerances, and worker behaviors. Work hardening is a highly structured, goal-oriented, individualized treatment program designed to maximize the person's ability to return to work."[9(p71)]

By interdisciplinary, CARF defines an interdisciplinary team, which should include an occupational therapist, a physical therapist, a psychologist, and a vocational specialist. In addition, CARF suggests that several other services should be provided or formal arrangements made for physician services and rehabilitation nursing.

Prior to the involvement of CARF in work hardening programs, physical therapists often delivered work hardening in a single discipline environment. The physical therapy community is now engaged in a definition of the single discipline (physical therapy) approach as work conditioning, which can be delivered in the *individual discipline environment*. The APTA, through a committee that is concerned with issues related to industrial physical therapy, is in the process of conducting a field review on work conditioning guidelines that parallels the efforts of CARF in defining work hardening. The physical therapy community believes that over 90% of patients who seek physical therapy following an industrial accident will return to work following work conditioning, and only 10% of the patients will go on to require the multidisciplinary work hardening approach.

Accreditation criteria

The following criteria must be met in order to be eligible for, obtain, and/or retain accreditation by the commission (Box 5-3).

Like many accrediting bodies, CARF functions under both criteria and standards. The standards are derived from professional consensus through a process of field review and serve as guidelines for the on-site visitors in determining whether a facility is able to carry out its mission and serve its intended clientele. The degree to

- -
BOX 5-3 CARF ACCREDITATION CRITERIA*

1. The organization demonstrates that the persons served are the focus of control for all decisions affecting them; the organization also demonstrates that persons served are involved in individual program planning, decision making, and implementation that affect the services they will receive
2. The organization is involved in a process of maximizing the functioning of the persons served, either within the organization or through linkages with other agencies
3. The organization provides services that are designed to enhance the independence, self-sufficiency, and productivity of the persons served
4. The organization, through a team approach, is involved in a process of providing goal-oriented, comprehensive, and coordinated services, either within the organization or through linkages with other agencies
5. The organization provides services that are individually tailored, integrated, and coordinated. The mechanism by which this will be achieved is in writing

6. The organization adopts policies and implements mechanisms necessary to preserve the basic human rights and dignity of those served within the scope of its programs
7. The organization provides persons served the opportunity to move into other programs and levels inside or outside the organization when appropriate
8. The organization demonstrates responsible financial management in order to operate viable programs
9. The organization has all legally required licenses and/or certificates
10. Any applicable certification by the Wage and Hour Division of the US Department of Labor is maintained
11. The organization meets the Special Policy on Accessibility
12. The organization meets the Special Policy on Input From Those Served
13. The organization meets the Special Policy on Safety
14. The organization meets the Special Policy on Program Evaluation

*From the Commission on Accreditation of Rehabilitation Facilities (CARF): *1991 Standards Manual for Organizations Serving People With Disabilities.* Tucson, Ariz, CARF, 85711, p 3.

· ·
BOX 5–4   CARF ACCREDITATION GUIDELINES*

Accreditation Outcomes

In addition to meeting each of the accreditation criteria, an organization should demonstrate, through a site survey, that it meets the standards established by the commission. While an organization may not be in full compliance with every applicable standard, the accreditation decision is based upon the balance of an organization's strengths with those areas needing improvement. The following guidelines are used by the commission staff, surveyors, and trustees in determining the accreditation outcome.

3-Year Accreditation

The organization meets each of the accreditation criteria and shows substantial fulfillment of the standards. Its programs and practices are designed and implemented to benefit the people with disabilities whom it serves. Its program, personnel, and documentation clearly indicate that present conditions represent an established pattern of total operation and that these conditions are likely to be maintained and/or improved in the foreseeable future.

1-Year Accreditation

The organization meets each of the accreditation criteria. Although there are deficiencies in relation to the standards, there is evidence of capability and commitment to correcting the deficiencies and progress in their correction. On balance, the program is benefiting its clientele, and there is apparent protection for their health, welfare, and safety.

Nonaccreditation

The organization has major deficiencies in several areas of standards, and there are serious questions as to the rehabilitation benefits, health, welfare, or safety of its clientele; the organization has failed to bring itself over time into substantial conformance with the standards; the organization has failed to meet each of the accreditation criteria.

An organization may be considered to be functioning between the 3-year and 1-year levels previously described because of certain problem areas. In this instance, accreditation for 1 year shall be awarded.

***From the Commission on Accreditation of Rehabilitation Facilities:** 1991 Standards Manual for Organizations Serving People With Disabilities. Tucson, Ariz, CARF, 1991, p 7.*

which an institution meets both the criteria and standards determines the tenure of the accreditation granted by the agency (Box 5–4).

· · · · · · · · · · ·
REGULATORY AGENCIES

Presently, major reimbursement for health care costs is provided under the Social Security Act and its accompanying amendments (Title XVI, XVIII, and XIX).

The regulations that govern the amendments are developed and administered through federal regulatory agencies (Fig 5–1), which then contract with state-based agencies to administer the program for the federal government. For instance, supplemental security income is administered through the state vocational rehabilitation agencies, medicare is administered through fiscal intermediaries and carriers, and medicaid is administered through the state department of health in some states.

Health Care Financing Administration

The Health Care Financing Administration (HCFA), an agency under the Department of HHS oversees the medicare program under Title XVIII of the Social Security Act.

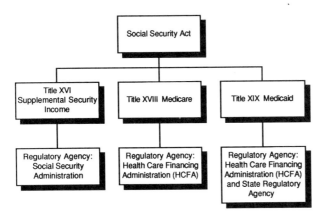

FIG 5–1.
Major health care reimbursement legislation and regulatory agencies.

HCFA contracts to administer the medicare program through fiscal intermediaries and carriers (generically known as payers) such as Blue Cross and Blue Shield or through commercial insurance companies such as Travelers Insurance Company (Appendix 5.1). For the purposes of medicare, intermediaries are organizations that will process bills of providers who are considered to be facilities, whereas carriers are organizations that will process bills of providers who are considered to be individuals or group practices. When one agency serves as both an intermediary and a carrier, it does so under two separate contracts with the government to provide these services. In addition to the regulations that are a direct result of HCFA actions, the payer may provide further regulations, coding systems, and interpretations on a regional or state basis. It is the responsibility of the physical therapy manager to understand the regulations of the payer as well as HCFA in the jurisdictions in which the facility operates.

Each fiscal payer develops its own processes of review of claims. For the most part, these reviews are conducted in a variety of levels.

Level 1 review

This is the review of claims by the computer or clerical staff. The computer or clerk looks for the status of the insured person, completeness of the claim, and whether the claim is logical. That is, given a specific Current Procedural Terminology (CPT) code, do the procedures fit the diagnosis? Services that are well documented and fall within the guidelines of the agency will be paid. Claims that are incomplete or unclear in relation to the agency guidelines will be denied or referred to a level 2 review.

Level 2 review

This is a personal review by a claims reviewer who is usually a nurse or other professional employed by the agency. The reviewer "looks at the claim's medical documentation to judge whether individual circumstances support payment."[10] If the claims reviewer cannot decipher the claim or match it to the agency requirements with a high degree of confidence, the claim will be referred to a level 3 review.

Level 3 review

This review is supervised by the medical director of the agency. It may be conducted by a specialty firm contracted to perform level 3 reviews or it may be conducted by a physical therapist who is contracted (either individually or through the state chapter of the APTA) by the agency to review claims for their appropriateness in relation to both the agency standards and the standards of practice within the profession.

If a claim is denied at the level 3 review, a provider may, under certain factual circumstances, take the matter to the courts. By certain factual circumstances, it is meant that the provider has documents that demonstrate a real or implied contractual relationship between the provider and the payer. The issue under consideration, then, is a breach of that contract by nonpayment of what the provider identifies as a valid claim.

For the most part, physical therapists or physical therapy practices do not have real contracts with payers, although facilities such as hospitals may have contracts. The physical therapist applies for provider status and is therefore permitted to submit claims on behalf of the insured. It is the patient (the insured) who has a real contract with the payer and is therefore the party most likely to appeal an unpaid claim through the court system.

HCFA has recently developed a set of medicare edits to be used for a level 2 medical review for outpatient physical therapy reimbursement. A level 2 review occurs when a bill is denied if the claim falls outside the expected level of care for a specific diagnosis. The edits set limits regarding the number and frequency of reimbursable physical therapy treatments within the medicare program (Table 5–1), although technically HCFA admonishes third-party reimbursers not to deny a bill solely on the basis that it exceeds the edits. These edits were developed intuitively without adequate data available to determine if the number of treatments would result in the appropriate effect for the specific category of patient. The edits have been negotiated with the APTA but still remain unsubstantiated. There is a great need for the physical therapy manager to recognize the importance of clinical data related to outcomes and to collect these data on all major diagnostic categories of patients treated in the facility by physical therapists.

TABLE 5–1.   Partial Listing of Medicare Edits*

Edit ID No.	Diagnosis	ICD-9-CM†	No. of Visits	Duration (mo)
1	Cancer	162.0–163.9	7	1
		165.0–165.9	24	2
2	Parkinson's disease	332.0–332.1	13	1
3	Meningitis	320.0–323.9	16	2
	Huntington's chorea	333.4–333.7	16	2
	Multiple sclerosis	340	16	2
4	Cerebrovascular accident, acute	436.0	32	3
	Concussion	850.4	32	3
5	Transient ischemic attack	435.0	7	1
6	Paralytic syndromes	344.0–344.9	39	4
	Spinal cord injury	952.0–952.9	39	4
7	Late effects, polio	138	19	2
	Peripheral nerve injury	953.0–957.9	19	2
8	Diabetes	250.7	13	1
	Lymphedema	457.0–457.9	13	1
9	Diabetes with ulcer	250.8	29	2
	Hansen's disease	030.0–030.9	29	2
	Cellulitis	681.0–682.9	29	2

*From *Medicare Intermediary Manual: Part 3—Claims Process*, HCFA publication 13—3. Washington, DC, Health and Human Services, 1988, revision 1398. There are 26 categories of medicare edits and hundreds of diseases and symptoms covered in these categories. This representation covers only nine of the categories and does not depict all of the diseases or symptoms covered. Newer revisions depict duration in days rather than months.
†ICD-9-CM is the International Classification of Diseases-9-Clinical Manifestations codification system. Unlike the older ICD system, the ICD-9 system classifies symptoms such as weakness, swelling, and contractures as well as traditional disease entities. This classification system is traditionally used in billing by physical therapists and other disciplines and is also used to collect and report clinical outcome data in individual departments as well as publications.

Although there is no central mechanism for collecting, storing, or analyzing such data on a national level, this information will provide critical substantiation as physical therapy seeks reasonable recognition by a growing number of reimbursement agencies.

HCFA has also established medicare limits for physical therapists in independent physical therapy environments. In addition to a 30-day recertification process in which the physician must review the patient's progress and recertify the need for physical therapy, a $750 limit is placed on the medicare patient receiving care from an independent practitioner. At 1992 costs, patients often incur several hundred dollars of physical therapy services during the evaluation process and cannot complete the course of treatment with that private practitioner. Under the current guidelines, the patient could leave that physical therapist when the dollar limit is reached and seek care at an institutionally based physical therapy program without an imposed dollar limitation. This limit reduces the medicare patient's ability to select a practitioner of choice and hampers the private practice–based physical therapist from engaging in a practice that would be highly dependent on medicare-age patients (i.e., arthritis).

A discussion of medicare would be incomplete without mention of medicare abuse and fraud. Many health care providers, including physical therapists, have been indicted for both Medicare fraud and abuse and have been heavily fined, imprisoned, and/or lost their professional licenses to practice. Abuses of medicare, as a federally regulated program, carry very heavy penalties. Common abuses in physical therapy include treating groups of patients simultaneously and billing each patient for individual care, billing a nursing home or home health agency for treatment time when the therapist is not on site, and billing patients for procedures that were never performed. Medicare fraud includes purposely writing progress notes that, instead of reflecting the progress of the patient, reflect progress necessary to continue reimbursement; inaccurate billing; and escalated billing in order to collect usual and customary fees.

It is the responsibility of the physical therapy manager to walk a fine line between collecting all fees due the institution for services rendered, teaching therapists to write appropriately phrased notes for reimbursement agencies, and to monitor and reinforce honesty in the recording of patient progress and services rendered. Young therapists often see the reimbursement agency as the enemy, as an agency that limits the patient's rights to appropriate care. It is a challenge to teach the therapist the obligations to the patient, the institution, and the reimbursement agency when delivering physical therapy services.

State Department of Public Health

Departments of public health are state agencies that are closely related to the Centers for Disease Control (CDC) and are responsible for immunizations, tracking and controlling epidemics, and providing public health services to all needy citizens within the state. These services include large maternal and child health clinics, administering federal programs such as Women, Infants, and Children (WIC); crippled children's clinics (a remnant of the polio epidemics); and other wellness clinics as well as the coordinated care of indigent families.

Medicaid is usually administered in the state by the State Department of Public Health. Medicaid regulations and reimbursement levels are highly variable from one state to another and are very dependent on other costs incurred by the Public Health Department of the individual state and the legislative levels of funding of this department.

"Medicaid, authorized by Title XIX of the Social Security Act, is a federal-state financed program which pays for health services for the categorically needy and the medically needy. The categorically needy are those receiving public assistance from the Aid to Families with Dependent Children (AFDC) program and those who receive Supplementary Security Income (SSI) because they are aged, blind, or disabled. The medically needy are those who have enough money to live on, but not enough to pay for medical care."[1(p257)]

In many states medicaid-supported programs and individuals are severely underfunded, and funds often run out long before the end of the fiscal year. In addition to traditional medical, nursing, and rehabilitation services covered by this agency, durable medical equipment (DME) is also funded. The variable level of funding within the fiscal year presents a burden to both the client and the health care and DME provider when the continuation of care to chronically ill patients must either be terminated or become the fiscal responsibility of the provider to continue care. Although it is possible to imagine the termination of some aspects of physical therapy when funding is no longer available, it is less plausible to discontinue oxygen, stoma supplies, transcutaneous electrical nerve stimulation (TENS) units, wheelchairs, and portable commodes.

Occupational Safety and Health Administration

In 1970 the Occupational Safety and Health Act was passed to ensure the safety of the workplace for every employee. The Occupational Safety and Health Administration (OSHA) was created in the Department of Labor from this act to develop standards and regulations that are legally enforceable. These standards relate to the safety of structures, including regulations such as building codes, heating and plumbing standards, and structural safety.[11] In addition, OSHA has developed regulations related to hazardous substances and safe machinery operation (Box 5–5).

Given the epidemic of acquired immune deficiency syndrome (AIDS) in the United States, OSHA has expanded its regulations to include more rigorous standards for handling blood products and for detecting and controlling bloodborne

• •
BOX 5–5   COMMON AREAS OF OSHA STANDARDS AND REGULATIONS*

Air monitoring
Asbestos
Back safety
Chemical safety
Confined spaces
Drugs in the workplace
Emergency response and cardiopulmonary resuscitation
Employee assistance
Environmental protection
Ergonomics
Eye/vision
Fire
Hazardous materials
Health promotion
Hearing conservation
Indoor air quality
Protective equipment
Respiratory protection

*Adapted from 1991 subject index. *J Occup Health Safety* 1991; 60:28–29. *OSHA* = Occupational Safety and Health Administration.

. . . .
BOX 5–6   OSHA CATEGORIES OF RISK FOR BLOODBORNE PATHOGEN EXPOSURE*

Category I	Employees may be routinely exposed to bloodborne pathogens
Category II	Employees are not usually exposed, but may be exposed under certain conditions
Category III	Employees are never exposed

*Adapted from Rekus JF: Bloodborne pathogens. *J Occup Health Safety* 1991; 60:32. OSHA = Occupational Safety and Health Administration.

pathogens (malaria, syphilis, brucellosis, hepatitis B, human immunodeficiency virus). OSHA has divided personnel into three categories of risk for bloodborne pathogen exposure (Box 5–6).

Worker's Compensation

All large employers (more than ten employees) or high-risk employers must take part in worker's compensation by paying a percentage of salary to the worker's compensation board of the state. This percentage payment is based on the risk rating of the job or institution. Any injury that arises from or in the course of employment can be claimed through worker's compensation. Physical therapists, physical therapists assistants, and physical therapy aides are at risk for a variety of musculoskeletal injuries, particularly low-back strain. Although there is no national data available, the 1991 House of Delegates of the APTA passed a motion requiring the Board of Directors of the APTA to identify and investigate the most common health risks of physical therapists.

The risks that are being investigated are not only the risk of musculoskeletal injury, but also the risks associated with the use of equipment such as diathermy and ultrasound and a myriad of electrical equipment. Physical therapists may also be exposed to a variety of chemicals in the manufacture of splints and casts. A long-standing concern of female physical therapists has been the risk associated with wave transmission by diathermy and ultrasound and the effects of these wave transmissions on the therapist during pregnancy.

As computers become more of an integral part of the practice of physical therapy, there will be the same level of risk to physical therapists of discharge from the computer as is experienced by other professions that have a high level of computer use.

It is the responsibility of the physical therapy manager to (1) assess the environmental risks to the physical therapy staff, (2) inform the employee of risks, (3) minimize the risks as much as possible, (4) keep accurate records of exposure, and (5) encourage regular medical assessment of staff members related to environmental exposure. In some instances the manager may sense pressure from the institution not to pursue medical follow-up or maintain records of exposure, since such records clearly link the institution to potential claims of harm. The physical therapy manager must weigh the obligations to the institution against obligations to the employee and the profession when confronted with such a dilemma.

Internal Revenue Service: Independent Contractor Status

When the physical therapist functions as an independent contractor, all Internal Revenue Service (IRS) requirements for independent contractors must be met. Most importantly, the physical therapist must demonstrate no employer-employee relationship, including being bound by protocols and procedures of the institution that would limit the independence of the individual.

The IRS has challenged the independent contractor status of physical therapists in home health agencies due to the strict regulations to be followed in meeting medicare requirements, which significantly reduces, from the IRS perspective, the independent nature of the practice of physical therapists in these settings. This challenge has been successfully met several times in court, and physical therapists continue to maintain independent contractor status in home health agencies.

In addition, physical therapists, like physicians, who are independent contractors actually have a contract with the patient rather than the health care facility. However, if, in the course of caring for the patient, the physical therapist relies on the institution to perform certain functions for the patient, the health care facility also takes on a measure of responsibility and liability for the patient's care. When an injury results from that care, the injured party may make claims against both the independent contractor and the health care facility.

PROFESSIONAL STANDARDS

Professional standards that are developed by associations are only binding on members of the association. In the case of the APTA, approximately 70% of physical therapists and 20% of physical therapist assistants in the United States belong to the association. The association, however, does have a significant impact on the practice of physical therapy, and its standards are often adopted by individuals and organizations.

Guides to Personnel Utilization

Some states carefully detail the practice of the physical therapist assistant in legislation and in so doing determine the legal authority and limitations of practice in which the physical therapist assistant may engage.

Appropriate utilization of the physical therapist assistant is further defined by the House of the Delegates (06-88-14-25) of the APTA (Box 5–7).[13]

The physical therapy aide is not covered by licensing laws other than the fact that in those states where physical therapist assistants are licensed, the physical therapy aide may not be called a physical therapist assistant. In some facilities, however, they are referred to as physical *therapy* assistants.

The physical therapy manager must be aware of these legal restrictions and requirements and institute policies and procedures that guarantee the adherence to both the laws and administrative rules governing the legal practice of physical therapy, including the practice of the physical therapist and the physical therapist assistant. In addition, it is important that the physical therapy manager seek interpretations of laws and regulations whenever the practice of physical therapy is pushing the limits of those laws and regulations.

Codes of Ethics and Guides of Conduct

Codes of ethics of professions specify the moral role of the professional and help the individual professional to understand how to act as a professional. According to the literature related to the development of professions, the existence of a code of ethics is one of the hallmarks of a true profession. The House of Delegates of the APTA established a code of ethics for its members shortly after the association was

. . . .

BOX 5-7   UTILIZATION OF THE PHYSICAL THERAPIST ASSISTANT

Definition

The physical therapist assistant is a health care worker who assists the physical therapist in the provision of physical therapy. The physical therapist assistant is a graduate of a physical therapist assistant associate degree program accredited by an agency recognized by the Secretary of the United States Department of Education or the Council on Postsecondary Accreditation.

Utilization

The physical therapist assistant is required to work under the direction and supervision of the physical therapist. The physical therapist assistant may perform physical therapy procedures and related tasks that have been selected and delegated by the supervising physical therapist. Where permitted by law, the physical therapist assistant may also carry out routine operational functions, including supervision of the physical therapy aide or equivalent, and documentation of treatment progress. The ability of the physical therapist assistant to perform the selected and delegated tasks shall be assessed on an ongoing basis by the supervising physical therapist. The physical therapist assistant may, with prior approval by the supervising physical therapist, adjust a specific treatment procedure in accordance with changes in patient status.

When the physical therapist and the physical therapist assistant are not within the same physical setting, the performance of the delegated functions by the physical therapist assistant must be consistent with safe and legal physical therapy practice and shall be predicated on the following factors: complexity and acuity of the patient's needs; proximity and accessibility to the physical therapist; supervision available in the event of emergencies or critical events; and type of setting in which the service is provided.

The physical therapist assistant shall not perform the following physical therapy activities: interpretation of referrals; physical therapy initial evaluation and re-evaluation; identification, determination, or modification of plans of care (including goals and treatment programs); final discharge assessment/evaluation or establishment of the discharge plan; or therapeutic techniques beyond the skill and knowledge of the physical therapist assistant.*

*From *Definition and Utilization of the Physical Therapist Assistant, HOD 06-88-14-25.* Alexandria, Va, American Physical Therapy Association, 1988.

founded in 1921. This code guides the behavior of its members and sets standards of conduct for the whole profession. The code of ethics has changed considerably over the years, and like many other professional codes of ethics, its development has been driven by incidents and by the changing practice environment. At one point it was unethical to work independent of a physician according to the code of ethics, and physical therapists who were becoming more autonomous were, in the early 1970s, in danger of being in violation of the code. If they continued to pursue independent practice, these individuals were likely to be expelled from the association.

The code of ethics now has eight ethical principles by which the physical therapist must practice (Box 5–8). This code of ethics is only binding on members of the professional association, but is also embraced by many institutions and state administrative bodies.

The code of ethics is further defined by the "Guide for Professional Conduct of the American Physical Therapy Association." The guide assists in the interpretation of the code of ethics through further description of ethical behaviors within each principle (see Appendix 5.2 at the end of this chapter).

The practice of the physical therapist assistant is guided by the standards of ethical conduct for the physical therapist assistant (Box 5–9). Just as the code of ethics of the physical therapist is explicated by the guide for professional conduct, the stan-

. . . .
BOX 5–8   CODE OF ETHICS*

Preamble

This code of ethics sets forth ethical principles for the physical therapy profession. Members of this profession are responsible for maintaining and promoting ethical practice. This code of ethics, adopted by the American Physical Therapy Association, shall be binding on physical therapists who are members of the association.

Principle 1

Physical therapists respect the rights and dignity of all individuals.

Principle 2

Physical therapists comply with the laws and regulations governing the practice of physical therapy.

Principle 3

Physical therapists accept responsibility for the exercise of sound judgment.

Principle 4

Physical therapists maintain and promote high standards for physical therapy practice, education, and research.

Principle 5

Physical therapists seek remuneration for their services that is deserved and reasonable.

Principle 6

Physical therapists provide accurate information to the consumer about the profession and about those services they provide.

Principle 7

Physical therapists accept the responsibility to protect the public and the profession from unethical, incompetent, or illegal acts.

Principle 8

Physical therapists participate in efforts to address the health needs of the public.

Adopted by the House of Delegates
June 1981
Amended June 1987
June 1991

*From the American Physical Therapy Association, 1111 N Fairfax St, Alexandria, VA 22314.

dards of ethical conduct for the physical therapist assistant are interpreted by the guide for conduct of the affiliate member (see Appendix 5.3 at the end of this chapter).

Standards of Practice

Many facilities use the APTA standards of practice in defining the practice and administration of physical therapy. These standards can be found in Appendix 5.4 at the end of this chapter. If an institution does not use these specific standards, it is important to develop standards of practice in order to relate the physical therapy service to the mission statement of the facility and other standards of care

· ·
BOX 5–9   STANDARDS OF ETHICAL CONDUCT FOR THE PHYSICAL THERAPIST ASSISTANT*

Preamble
Physical therapist assistants are responsible for maintaining and promoting high standards of conduct. These standards of ethical conduct for the physical therapist assistant shall be binding on physical therapist assistants who are affiliate members of the association.

Standard 1
Physical therapist assistants provide services under the supervision of a physical therapist.

Standard 2
Physical therapist assistants respect the rights and dignity of all individuals.

Standard 3
Physical therapist assistants maintain and promote high standards in the provision of services, giving the welfare of the patients their highest regard.

Standard 4
Physical therapist assistants provide services within the limits of the law.

Standard 5
Physical therapist assistants make those judgments that are commensurate with their qualifications as physical therapist assistants.

Standard 6
Physical therapist assistants accept the responsibility to protect the public and the profession from unethical, incompetent, or illegal acts.

Adopted by House of Delegates
June 1982
Amended June 1991

*From the American Physical Therapy Association, 1111 N Fairfax St, Alexandria, VA 22314.

within the facility. Such standards should form the foundation for the evaluation of the service.

Both the practice of physical therapists and physical therapist assistants are defined in practice acts within the state and in a variety of documents. However, the role of the physical therapy aide is often left to interpretation by the facility.

Specialization

The American Board of Physical Therapy Specialties (ABPTS) identifies and defines physical therapy specialty areas and formally recognizes physical therapists who have attained advanced clinical knowledge and skills in those areas. The ABPTS sets rigorous standards for recognition that include not only content expertise but evidence of research and educational activities within the content area. Specialists are required to pass a national specialty examination to maintain specialty status. Although any physical therapist may discuss the focus of their practice as their specialty, only ABPTS-certified physical therapists may use the initials CS after the letter, specifying their specialty. For instance, a cardiopulmonary certified specialist may sign documents as John Smith, P.T., M.S., C.C.S. The full list of certified specialties now recognized by ABPTS is as follows: cardiopulmonary certified specialist, or CCS; electrophysiologic certified specialist, or ECS; neurologic certified specialist, or NCS; orthopaedic certified specialist, or OCS; pediatric certified specialist, or PCS; and sports certified specialist, or SCS; and geriatric certified specialist, or GCS.

INSTITUTIONAL STANDARDS

Practice Privileges

This issue has been dealt with in Chapter Two, but deserves some repetition here. Regulation of practice privileges has traditionally focused on physicians as a mechanism for the institution to engage in credentials review and to monitor and discipline the practice of medicine within the institution. As an autonomous professional, the physician found this to be an acceptable level of regulation as a mechanism for gaining access to the use of the institution to care for his patients. Physical therapy is in the position of evolving into an autonomous profession, and as such still may have physical therapist employees within an institution in which other physical therapists are seeking practice privileges. At the present time, practice privileges for physical therapists are most often successfully sought in rural communities where there are no institutionally based therapists and little competition, and in situations where physician groups who have a business or consulting relationship with particular physical therapy practices seek physical therapist privileges through the physician credentialling bodies. This later situation causes great concern on the part of the institutionally based therapist since it poses many potential and real problems. It sets up a group of consulting physical therapists who have no relationship to existing services, it establishes an elitist layer of physical therapists in the system in that these therapists are treated as consultants by the institution and the physician groups with all the prestige and rights that comes from moving from an employee status to a consultant status with none of the responsibilities of the institutionally based therapists, and it seriously divides the patient population into those whom the consultants choose to treat and the rest of the patient population, which may be the more ill, less well insured, more challenging portion of the population.

Immunizations

Individual institutions will also have regulations that the physical therapy manager must be aware of and enforce. For instance, many hospitals require inoculation against hepatitis B prior to employment. If it is not explicitly stated, the manager should determine if this also applies to students, volunteers, or part-time employees on- and off-site and institute mechanisms to assure that each person in the department is properly immunized.

Of national concern and debate is the testing of employees for human immunodeficiency virus (HIV) either as a pre- employment requirement or as a matter of course for all employees. With the passage of the Americans With Disabilities Act legislation, pre-employment screening to determine employment status will be prohibited. However, administrators will still be able to test employees to assess risk. Managers must again be aware of the institutional regulations and institute mechanisms to assure compliance. This is an area where the manager may also be intimately involved in the debate of ethical concerns. The debate centers on the individual's right to privacy and the institution's (and its clients') right to know. Once a regulation has been determined, the institutional regulation overrides the individual's rights if the individual wants to work in the particular institution.

•••••• CASE 5.1 ••••••

Hiring Practices

Jane Walter, P.T., Ed.D.

In January 1991, Jane Doe, P.T., who was serving a 4-year term on the Physical Therapy Board, attended the opening of a local physical therapy practice. As she made her way to the hydrotherapy area, Sue Smith, a physical therapist assistant, greeted her warmly and proceeded to tell her about the hydrotherapy area. Sue stated that she had moved to the area 6 months ago and had been working in City Physical Therapy for John Adams for 3 months (since the new practice opened). Although Jane did not say anything at the time, she could not recall Sue's name or her application for a physical therapist assistant license. Jane had been instrumental in writing and promoting the licensure law for physical therapist assistants. There was a provision for temporary licensure given a physical therapist as a sponsor and supervisor during the temporary licensure period. The normal waiting time for full licensure for either physical therapists or physical therapist assistants was 4 months in the state, so many people planning to move to the state decided to forego the temporary licensure and applied directly for a full license.

Jane called the licensure office the next day to inquire about Sue's license. She was told that there was no temporary or full license issued to Sue, and, as a matter of fact, there was no application on file.

Jane called John. She rather awkwardly thanked him for the invitation to the open house the night before and then related to him how she had come to inquire about Sue. Jane informed John that Sue would have to revert to practicing as a physical therapist aide, that she must immediately apply for a license, that both Sue and John may be asked to appear before the board, and that Sue was in danger of either not being given a license or being placed on probation.

John was insensed. He felt that Jane had overstepped her bounds. He had invited her to the open house as a colleague, not as a member of the board. He felt that as a colleague she should inform Sue of the importance of getting her license as soon as possible, but that threatening denial of licensure or probation was petty and uncalled for.

Jane went on to tell John that unfortunately, the board would probably also take some action related to his role in this situation and could even place him on probation or suspend his license for hiring a subordinate without a license.

Jane wrote up her observations and an account of her conversations with Sue and John and sent them to the board office to be distributed to the board members, asking that this issue be placed on the agenda for the next meeting. Several days later, Jane received a copy of a letter sent to the board.

Consider the legal rights and responsibilities of the staff therapist and the supervisory therapist. Does John Adams have an obligation to assure the proper credentialling of his personnel? Are there issues of confidentiality here? Does the therapist have a right to work if the board cannot provide her with a timely response to her request for a temporary license? Is John Adams justified in his outrage?

••••••••••• LEGAL AND REGULATORY DEFINITIONS[2(p2)]

Acceptance: The actual or implied receipt and retention of something that is offered.

Administrative agencies: Agencies of the federal government that deal with specialized subject matter areas and that possess quasijudicial powers in their areas of subject matter expertise.

CITY PT
Our City, HH
John Adams, P.T.
Jan 17, 1991

Board of Physical Therapy
One State Street
Our City, HH

Dear Board Members,

I received a telephone call from Jane Doe, P.T., this morning, telling me that the physical therapist assistant whom I hired 3 months ago (Mrs. Sue Smith) is not licensed in the state and that she had to stop practicing as a physical therapist assistant immediately and proceed to secure her license. While I agree that Mrs. Smith, P.T.A., should apply for her license as soon as possible, I am confident that neither she nor I have intentionally broken any laws or placed any of my patients in jeopardy.

I have practiced in this state for 15 years and have just opened my third office. I have 15 staff members and clerical staff who work for me, and I have never had any kind of complaint filed against me. As in other situations, all of Mrs. Smith's patients are evaluated by a physical therapist, and there is a physical therapist on site at least 60% of the time. Mrs. Smith has 8 years' experience as a physical therapist assistant and has exceptional references.

I see no reason for Mrs. Smith to stop practicing while her application is being processed. Mrs. Smith will appear at your office on Monday with a temporary license application in hand. If you would be able to issue her temporary license that day, then we will be in compliance with your regulations.

If you have any questions about this situation, please do not hesitate to contact me.

Sincerely,

John Adams, P.T.
Owner
City PT

Antitrust laws: Statutes designed to protect commerce from illegal restraints and monopolies.

Bilateral contract: Each of the contracting parties makes a promise.

Bill of lading: The written evidence of a contract for the carriage and delivery of goods.

Blue Cross/Blue Shield: Not-for-profit tax-exempt insurer whose authority comes from special state legislative statutes and insurance regulations under the state Insurance Commission.

Breach of contract: Wrongful act or omission of another in derogation of his or her contractual obligations.

Carrier: From an insurance perspective, an organization that will process bills of providers who are considered to be individual or group practice providers.

Competitive torts: Torts relating to unfair methods of business.

Contract: A promissory agreement between two or more persons that creates, modifies, or destroys a legal relation.

Copyright: The legally protected right to literary property that is extended by statute to the author or originator of certain literary or artistic productions.

Corporation: An artificial person or legal entity created by authority of the laws of a state or country.

Deed: Written document signed by the owner of real property, transferring ownership of that real property to another person.

Deep pockets: A slang expression meaning the party in a suit or potential suit with the greatest financial resources.

Easement: A right held by one person to use the land of another in some specified way.

Eminent domain: Power of the government to take private property for public use.

ERISA: Employer Retirement Income Security Act. A federal financing act under the US Department of Labor that governs self-insurance programs.

Executory: A contract is said to be executory until all of the parties have fully performed their responsibilities under the contract; at that point it becomes an executed contract.

Express contract: Terms, conditions, and promises specifically set forth in words.

FTC Act: Federal Trade Commission Act. An act of Congress establishing the FTC and entrusting it with certain powers and responsibilities. The FTC has included the enforcement of anticompetitive practices by health professionals among its duties and has been involved in several hospital privilege disputes.

Implied contract: Essential elements are not set forth in words but must be determined from the circumstances, general language, or conduct of the parties.

Intermediary: From the insurance perspective, an organization that will process bills of providers who are considered to be health care facilities.

Land contract: Contract for the sale of land whereby the buyer enters into possession and is entitled to the usual requisites of ownership but that allows the seller to retake ownership and possession if the buyer defaults on his or her obligations under the contract of sale.

Law: The ethical minimum of society to be obeyed by all citizens and subject to sanctions and legal consequences.

Lease: An agreement that produces the landlord-tenant relationship.

Lien: An encumbrance placed on property to secure payment or the performance of an obligation.

Limited partnership: Partnership that contains one or more limited partners in addition to its general partners.

Mechanic's lien: Lien on real property to secure payment of a monetary obligation arising out of the performance of labor or supplying of materials used in erecting or repairing a building or similar structure on the real property.

Mortgage: A conditional conveyance of property to serve as security for the payment or performance of some obligation.

Negligence: Failure to do some act that the ordinary reasonable man would do or would not do; the result of which is to cause injury to some person or property.

Negotiation: Process by which the owner of a negotiable instrument passes full ownership and rights to another person under such circumstances that the latter becomes a holder.

Partnership: Voluntary contract between two or more persons to combine some or all of their labor, skill, money, and property to carry on a business and to split profits and losses.

Patent: A grant made by the government to an inventor, giving the inventor the exclusive right to make, use, and sell his or her invention for a specified number of years.

Property: The generally exclusive right to possess, enjoy, and dispose of a thing or bundle of legal rights.

Quitclaim deed: A deed of conveyance that purports to convey only those rights and interests the conveyancer actually has and which contains no promise or assurance that the person has any rights or interests to convey.

***Res ipsa loquitur*:** The thing speaks for itself. The rebuttable presumption that the defendant was negligent since he or she was in control of the instrument causing the injury, and the accident was one that would not normally occur in the absence of negligence.

***Respondeat superior*:**   Let the superior respond. When in an employer-employee relationship, the employer is liable for the actions of the employee.

Title: Ownership right to property.

Torts: A violation of a civil duty imposed by law and owed to members of society.

Unenforceable contract: Meets the basic requirements for a valid contract, but the courts are forbidden by statute or rule of law to enforce.

Unilateral contract: Only one of the parties makes a promise.

Valid contract: Meets all of the legal requirements for a contract and is enforced by the courts.

Void contract: No legal force or effect and therefore not really a contract.

Voidable contract: Binds one of the parties to the transaction but gives the other party the option of either withdrawing from the contract or of insisting on compliance with the contract.

Zoning: The use of the police power to divide a governmental unit into various districts that are subject to regulations as to the size, type, and use of building within that district.

References

1. Raffel MW, Raffel NK: *The U.S. Health System,* ed 3. Albany, NY, Delmar Pubs, 1990.
2. Barnes AJ: *Business Law.* Homewood, Ill, Learning Systems Co, 1981.
3. Hickok RJ: *Physical Therapy Administration and Management.* Baltimore, Md, Williams and Wilkins, 1982.
4. Horting M. *Understanding Professional Liability, Today's Student PT.*Alexandria, Va, American Physical Therapy Association, 1989, p 4.
5. Connolly J: *Malpractice, Risk Management Resource Guide.* Alexandria, Va, American Physical Therapy Association, 1990.
6. Staff: Malpractice cases, adverse actions must be reported to new data bank, *PT Bull* 1990; 5:3.
7. Wong SG: Historical perspective of optometrists' and other health professionals' involvement in hospitals. *J Am Optom Assoc* 1988; 59:594–597.
8. Cull JG, Hardy RE: *Administrative Techniques for Rehabilitation Facility Operations.* Springfield, Ill, Charles C Thomas, 1974.
9. Commission on Accreditation of Rehabilitation Facilities: *1991 Standards Manual for Organizations Serving People with Disabilities.* Commission on Accreditation of Rehabilitation Facilities, 101 N Wilmot Rd, Suite 500, Tucson, AZ 85711.
10. Rasmussen B: *Claims Review and PTs, Insurer Briefing on Physical Therapy Issues.* Alexandria, Va, American Physical Therapy Association, 1991.
11. 1991 subject index. *J Occup Health Safety* 1991; 60:28–29.
12. Rekus JF: Bloodborne pathogens. *J Occup Health Safety* 1991; 60:32.
13. *Definition and Utilization of the Physical Therapist Assistant, HOD 06-88-14-25.* Alexandria, Va, American Physical Therapy Association, 1988.

········
APPENDIX 5.1
·········

Schema for Medicare Reimbursement

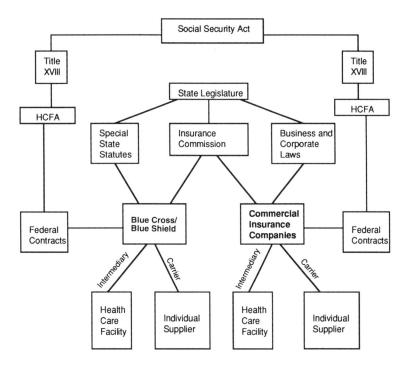

········
APPENDIX 5.2
·········

*Guide for Professional Conduct**

··········
PURPOSE

This guide for professional conduct (guide) is intended to serve physical therapists who are members of the American Physical Therapy Association (association) in interpreting the code of ethics (code) and matters of professional conduct. The guide provides guidelines by which physical therapists may determine the propriety of their conduct. The code and the guide apply to all physical therapists who are association members. These guidelines are subject to changes as the dynamics of the profession change and as new patterns of health care delivery are developed and

---

*Printed by permission of the American Physical Therapy Association.

accepted by the professional community and the public. This guide is subject to monitoring and timely revision by the Judicial Committee of the association.

• • • • • • • • • •
INTERPRETING ETHICAL PRINCIPLES

The interpretations expressed in this guide are not to be considered all inclusive of situations that could evolve under a specific principle of the code but reflect the opinions, decisions, and advice of the Judicial Committee. While the statements of ethical principles apply universally, specific circumstances determine their appropriate application. Input related to current interpretations, or situations requiring interpretation, is encouraged from association members.

Principle 1

Physical therapists respect the rights and dignity of all individuals.

1.1 Attitudes of Physical Therapists
A. Physical therapists shall recognize that each individual is different from all other individuals and shall respect and be responsive to those differences.
B. Physical therapists are to be guided at all times by concern for the physical, psychological, and socioeconomic welfare of those individuals entrusted to their care.
C. Physical therapists shall be responsive to and mutually supportive of colleagues and associates.

1.2 Confidential Information
A. Information relating to the physical therapist-patient relationship is confidential and may not be communicated to a third party not involved in that patient's care without the prior written consent of the patient, subject to applicable law.
B. Information derived from component-sponsored peer review shall be held confidential by the reviewer unless written permission to release the information is obtained from the physical therapist who was reviewed.
C. Information derived from the working relationships of physical therapists shall be held confidential by all parties.
D. Information may be disclosed to appropriate authorities when it is necessary to protect the welfare of an individual or the community. Such disclosure shall be in accordance with applicable law.

Principle 2

Physical therapists comply with the laws and regulations governing the practice of physical therapy.

2.1 Professional Practice

Physical therapists shall provide consultation, evaluation, treatment, and preventive care in accordance with the laws and regulations of the jurisdiction(s) in which they practice.

Principle 3

Physical therapists accept responsibility for the exercise of sound judgment.

3.1 Acceptance of Responsibility

A. Upon accepting an individual for provision of physical therapy services, physical therapists shall assume the responsibility for evaluating that individual; planning, implementing, and supervising the therapeutic program; re-evaluating and changing that program; and maintaining adequate records of the case, including progress reports.

B. When the individual's needs are beyond the scope of the physical therapist's expertise, the individual shall be so informed and assisted in identifying a qualified person to provide the necessary services.

C. When physical therapists judge that benefit can no longer be obtained from their services, they shall so inform the individual receiving the services. It is unethical to initiate or continue services that, in the therapist's judgment, either cannot result in beneficial outcome or are contraindicated.

D. Physical therapists shall maintain the ability to make independent judgments, which must not be limited or compromised by professional affiliation, including employment relationships.

3.2 Delegation of Responsibility

A. Physical therapists shall not delegate to a less-qualified person any activity that requires the unique skill, knowledge, and judgment of the physical therapist.

B. The primary responsibility for physical therapy care rendered by supportive personnel rests with the supervising physical therapist. Adequate supervision requires, at a minimum, that a supervising physical therapist perform the following activities:

1. Designate or establish channels of written and oral communication.
2. Interpret available information concerning the individual under care.
3. Provide initial evaluation.
4. Develop a plan of care, including short- and long-term goals.
5. Select and delegate appropriate tasks for the plan of care.
6. Assess competence of supportive personnel to perform assigned tasks.
7. Direct and supervise supportive personnel in delegated tasks.
8. Identify and document precautions, special problems, contraindications, goals, anticipated progress, and plans for re-evaluation.
9. Re-evaluate, adjust plan of care when necessary, perform final evaluation, and establish follow-up plan.

3.3 Provision of Services

A. Physical therapists shall recognize the individual's freedom of choice in selection of physical therapy services. Professional affiliations, including employment relationships, may not limit access to services.

B. Physical therapists' professional practices and their adherence to ethical principles of the association shall take preference over business practices. Provisions of services for personal financial gain rather than for the need of the individual receiving the services are unethical.

C. Overutilization caused by continuing physical therapy services beyond the point of possible benefit or by providing services more frequently than necessary for maximum therapeutic effect is unethical.

D. If physical therapy services are misused, the physical therapist(s) involved must accept responsibility for the misuse.

3.4 Referral Relationships

A. In a referral situation where the referring source specifies the treatment program, extension of physical therapy services beyond the proposed treatment program shall be undertaken in consultation with the referring source.

B. Physical therapists may suggest to the referring source the possibility of referring the person under care to a qualified individual whose services may be beneficial.

C. When there is no referral, physical therapists shall refer persons under their care to other qualified individuals if symptoms or conditions are present that require services beyond the scope of their expertise or for which physical therapy is contraindicated.

3.5 Practice Arrangements

A. Participation in a business, partnership, corporation, or other entity does not exempt the physical therapist, whether employer, partner, or stockholder, either individually or collectively, from the obligation of promoting and maintaining the ethical principles of the association.

B. Physical therapists shall advise their employer(s) of any employer practice that causes a physical therapist to be in conflict with the ethical principles of the association. Physical therapist employees shall attempt to rectify aspects of their employment which are in conflict with the ethical principles of the association.

Principle 4

Physical therapists maintain and promote high standards for physical therapy practice, education, and research.

4.1 Continued Education

A. Physical therapists shall participate in educational activities that enhance their basic knowledge and provide new knowledge.

B. Whenever physical therapists provide continuing education, they shall ensure that course content, objectives, and responsibilities of the instructional faculty are accurately reflected in the promotion of the course.

4.2 Review and Self-Assessment

A. Physical therapists shall provide for utilization review of their services.

B. Physical therapists shall demonstrate their commitment to quality assurance by peer review and self- assessment.

4.3 Research

A. Physical therapists shall support research activities that contribute knowledge for improved patient care.

B. Physical therapists engaged in research shall ensure:
1. The consent of subjects;

    2. Confidentiality of the data on individual subjects and the personal identities of the subjects;

    3. Well- being of all subjects in compliance with facility regulations and laws of the jurisdiction in which the research is conducted;

    4. The absence of fraud and plagiarism;

    5. Full disclosure of support received;

    6. Appropriate acknowledgment of individuals making a contribution to the research.

C. Physical therapists shall report to appropriate authorities any acts in the conduct or presentation of research that appear unethical or illegal.

4.4 Education

A. Physical therapists shall support quality education in academic and clinical settings.

B. Physical therapists functioning in the educational role are responsible to the students, the academic institutions, and the clinical settings for promoting ethical conduct in educational activities. Whenever possible, the educator shall ensure:

    1. The rights of students in the academic and clinical setting;

    2. Appropriate confidentiality of personal information;

    3. Professional conduct toward the student during the academic and clinical educational processes;

    4. Assignment to clinical settings prepared to give the student a learning experience.

C. Clinical educators are responsible for reporting to the academic program student conduct which appears to be unethical or illegal.

Principle 5

Physical therapists seek remuneration for their services that is deserved and reasonable.

5.1 Fiscally Sound Remuneration

A. Physical therapists shall never place their own financial interest above the welfare of individuals under their care.

B. Fees for physical therapy services should be reasonable for the service performed, considering the setting in which it is provided, practice costs in the geographic area, judgment of other organizations, and other relevant factors.

C. Physical therapists should attempt to ensure that providers, agencies, or other employers adopt physical therapy fee schedules that are reasonable and that encourage access to necessary services.

5.2 Business Practices/Fee Arrangements

A. Physical therapists shall not:

    1. Directly or indirectly request, receive, or participate in the dividing, transferring, assigning, rebating of an unearned fee.

    2. Profit by means of a credit or other valuable consideration, such as an unearned commission, discount, or gratuity in connection with furnishing of physical therapy services.

B. Unless laws impose restrictions to the contrary, physical therapists who provide physical therapy services in a business entity may pool fees and moneys received. Physical therapists may divide or apportion these fees and moneys in accordance with the business agreement.

C. Physical therapists may enter into agreements with organizations to provide physical therapy services if such agreements do not violate the ethical principles of the association.

5.3 Endorsement of Equipment or Services

A. Physical therapists shall not use influence upon individuals under their care or their families for utilization of equipment or services based upon the direct or indirect financial interest of the physical therapist in such equipment or services. Realizing that these individuals will normally rely on the physical therapists' advice, their best interest must always be maintained as well as their right of free choice relating to the use of any equipment or service. While it cannot be considered unethical for physical therapists to own or have a financial interest in equipment companies, or services, they must act in accordance with law and make full disclosure of their interest whenever such companies or services become the source of equipment or services for individuals under their care.

B. Physical therapists may be remunerated for endorsement or advertisement of equipment or services to the lay public, physical therapists, or other health professionals provided they disclose any financial interest in the production, sale, or distribution of said equipment or services.

C. In endorsing or advertising equipment or services, physical therapists shall use sound professional judgment and shall not give the appearance of association endorsement.

Principle 6

Physical therapists provide accurate information to the consumer about the profession and about those services they provide.

6.1 Information about the Profession

Physical therapists shall endeavor to educate the public to an awareness of the physical therapy profession through such means as publication of articles and participation in seminars, lectures, and civic programs.

6.2 Information about Services

A. Information given to the public shall emphasize that individual problems cannot be treated without individualized evaluation and plans/programs of care.

B. Physical therapists may provide information about themselves to the public to facilitate the pubic selection of a physical therapist.

C. Physical therapists shall not use, or participate in the use of, any form of communication containing a false, plagiarized, fraudulent, misleading, deceptive, unfair, or sensational statement or claim.

D. Physical therapists shall not compensate or give anything of value to a representative of the press, radio, television, or other communication medium in anticipation of, or in return for, professional publicity in a news item.

E. A paid advertisement shall be identified as such unless it is apparent from the context that it is a paid advertisement.

Principle 7

Physical therapists accept the responsibility to protect the public and the profession from unethical, incompetent, or illegal acts.

7.1 Consumer Protection

A. Physical therapists shall report any conduct that appears to be unethical, incompetent, or illegal.

B. Physical therapists may not participate in any arrangements in which patients are exploited due to the referring sources enhancing their personal incomes as a result of referring for, prescribing, or recommending physical therapy.

7.2 Disclosure

If the physical therapist is involved in an arrangement with a referring source in which the referring source derives income from the physical therapy service, the physical therapist has an affirmative obligation to disclose to the patient that the referring practitioner derives income from the provision of the physical therapy service.

Principle 8

Physical therapists participate in efforts to address the health needs of the public.

Issued by Judicial Committee
American Physical Therapy Association
October 1981
Amended January 1983
January 1984
January 1985
January 1987
January 1989
July 1990
January 1991
July 1991

· · · · · · · · ·
APPENDIX 5.3
· · · · · · · · ·

*Guide for Conduct of the Affiliate Member**

· · · · · · · · · · ·
PURPOSE

This guide is intended to serve physical therapist assistants who are affiliate members of the American Physical Therapy Association (APTA) in the interpretation of the

---

*Reprinted with permission of the American Physical Therapy Association.

Standards of Ethical Conduct for the Physical Therapist Assistant, providing guidelines by which they may determine the propriety of their conduct. These guidelines are subject to change as new patterns of health care delivery are developed and accepted by the professional community and the public. This guide is subject to monitoring and timely revision by the Judicial Committee of the association.

· · · · · · · · · · ·
INTERPRETING STANDARDS

The interpretations expressed in this guide are not to be considered all inclusive of situations that could evolve under a specific standard of the Standards of Ethical Conduct for the Physical Therapist Assistant but reflect the opinions, decisions, and advice of the Judicial Committee. While the statements of ethical standards apply universally, specific circumstances determine their appropriate application. Input related to current interpretations, or situations requiring interpretation, is encouraged from APTA members.

Standard 1

Physical therapist assistants provide services under the supervision of a physical therapist.

1.1 Supervisory Relationships

Physical therapist assistants shall work under the supervision and direction of a physical therapist who is properly credentialed in the jurisdiction in which the physical therapist assistant practices.

1.2 Performance of Service

A. Physical therapist assistants may not initiate or alter a treatment program without prior evaluation by and approval of the supervising physical therapist.

B. Physical therapist assistants may, with prior approval by the supervising physical therapist, adjust a specific treatment procedure in accordance with changes in patient status.

C. Physical therapist assistants may not interpret data beyond the scope of their physical therapist assistant education.

D. Physical therapist assistants may respond to inquiries regarding patient status to appropriate parties within the protocol established by a supervising physical therapist.

E. Physical therapist assistants shall refer inquiries regarding patient prognosis to a supervising physical therapist.

Standard 2

Physical therapist assistants respect the rights and dignity of all individuals.

2.1 Attitudes of Physical Therapist Assistants

A. Physical therapist assistants shall recognize that each individual is different from all other individuals and respect and be responsive to those differences.

B. Physical therapist assistants shall be guided at all times by concern for the dignity and welfare of those patients entrusted to their care.

    C. Physical therapist assistants shall be responsive to and supportive of colleagues and associates.

2.2 Request for Release of Information

Physical therapist assistants shall refer all requests for release of confidential information to the supervising physical therapist.

2.3 Protection of Privacy

Physical therapist assistants must treat as confidential all information relating to the personal conditions and affairs of the persons whom they serve.

Standard 3

Physical therapist assistants maintain and promote high standards in the provision of services giving the welfare of patients their highest regard.

3.1 Information About Services

Physical therapist assistants may provide consumers with information regarding provision of services within the protocol established by a supervising physical therapist.

    Physical therapist assistants may not use, or participate in the use of, any form of communication containing a false, fraudulent, misleading, deceptive, unfair, or sensational statement or claim.

3.2 Organizational Employment

Physical therapist assistants shall advise their employer(s) of any employer practice that causes them to be in conflict with the Standards of Ethical Conduct for the Physical Therapist Assistant.

3.3 Endorsement of Equipment

Physical therapist assistants may not endorse equipment or exercise influence on patients or families to purchase or lease equipment except as directed by a physical therapist acting in accord with the stipulation in paragraph 5.3.A. of the Guide for Professional Conduct.

3.4 Financial Considerations

Physical therapist assistants shall never place their own financial interest above the welfare of their patients.

3.5 Exploitation of Patients

Physical therapist assistants shall not participate in any arrangements in which patients are exploited. Such arrangements include situations where referring sources enhance their personal incomes as a result of referring for, delegating, prescribing, or recommending physical therapy services.

Standard 4

Physical therapist assistants provide services within the limits of the law.

4.1 Supervisory Relationships

Physical therapist assistants shall comply with all aspects of law. Regardless of the content of any law, physical therapist assistants shall provide services only under the supervision and direction of a physical therapist who is properly credentialed in the jurisdiction in which the physical therapist assistant practices.

4.2 Representation

Physical therapist assistants shall not hold themselves out as physical therapists.

Standard 5

Physical therapist assistants make those judgments that are commensurate with their qualifications as physical therapist assistants.

5.1 Patient Treatment

Physical therapist assistants shall report all untoward patient responses to a supervising physical therapist.

5.2 Patient Safety

Physical therapist assistants may refuse to carry out treatment procedures that they believe to be not in the best interest of the patient.

5.3 Qualifications

Physical therapist assistants may not carry out any procedure that they are not qualified to provide.

5.4 Discontinuance of Treatment Program

Physical therapist assistants shall discontinue immediately any treatment procedures that in their judgment appear to be harmful to the patient.

5.5 Continued Education

Physical therapist assistants shall continue participation in various types of educational activities that enhance their skills and knowledge and provide new skills and knowledge.

Standard 6

Physical therapist assistants accept the responsibility to protect the public and the profession from unethical, incompetent, or illegal acts.

6.1 Consumer Protection

Physical therapist assistants shall report any conduct that appears to be unethical or illegal.

Issued by Judicial Committee
American Physical Therapy Association
October 1981
Amended January 1983
January 1984
July 1988
January 1989
July 1991

APPENDIX 5.4

Standards of Practice for
Physical Therapy*

PREAMBLE

The physical therapy profession is committed to provide an optimum level of care and to strive for excellence in practice. The House of Delegates of the American Physical Therapy Association (APTA), as the responsible body representing this profession, attests to this commitment by adopting, publishing, disseminating, and applying the following Standards of Practice. These Standards of Practice are the profession's statement of conditions and performances that are essential for quality physical therapy. They provide a foundation for assessment of physical therapy practice.

ADMINISTRATION OF PHYSICAL THERAPY SERVICE

I. Purposes and goals.
   A written statement of purposes and goals exists for the physical therapy service which reflects the needs of the individuals served, the physical therapy personnel, the facility, and the community.
   Define scope and limitation of service.
   Contain current description of purpose.
   List objectives and goals of services provided.
   Are appropriate for the population (community) served.
   Provide a mechanism for annual review.
II. Organizational plan.
   A written organizational plan exists for the physical therapy service.
   Describes the interrelationships within the overall organization.
   Provides for direction of service by a physical therapist.
   Defines supervisory functions within the program/service.
   Reflects current personnel functions.
III. Policies and procedures.
   Written policies and procedures, which reflect the operation of the service, exist and are consistent with the purposes and goals of the physical therapy service.
   Address pertinent information about the following:
   Clinical education.
   Clinical research.
   Criteria for access, initiation, and termination of care.
   Equipment maintenance.
   Infection control.

---

*Reprinted with permission of the American Physical Therapy Association.

Job description.
Medical emergencies.
Patient care policies and protocols.
Patient rights.
Personnel-related policies.
Quality assurance.
Recordkeeping.
Safety.
Staff orientation.
Supervisory relationships.
Meet requirements of external agencies and state laws.
Meet requirements of overall organization.
Are reviewed on a regular basis.

IV. Administration.

A physical therapist is responsible for the direction of the physical therapy service.

Assures that the service is consistent with established purposes and goals.

Assures that the service is provided in accordance with established policies and procedures.

Assures compliance with local, state, and federal requirements.

Complies with current APTA Standards of Practice and Guide for Professional Conduct.

Reviews and updates policies and procedures as appropriate.

Provides appropriate education, training, and review of physical therapy support personnel.

V. Staffing.

The physical therapy personnel are qualified and sufficient in number to achieve the purposes and goals of the physical therapy service.

Meets legal requirements regarding licensure and/or certification of appropriate personnel.

Provides expertise appropriate to the case mix.

Provides adequate staff-to-patient ratio.

Provides adequate support staff to professional staff.

VI. Physical setting.

1. The physical setting is designed to provide a safe and effective environment that facilitates the achievement of the purposes and goals of the physical therapy service.

Meets all applicable legal requirements for health and safety.

Meets space needs appropriate for the number and type of patients served.

2. Equipment is safe and sufficient to achieve the purposes and goals of the physical therapy service.

Meets all applicable legal requirements for health and safety.

Meets equipment needs appropriate for the number and type of patients served.

Provides for routine safety inspection of equipment by a qualified individual.

VII. Fiscal affairs.

Fiscal planning and management of the physical therapy service is based upon sound accounting principles.

Include preparation and use of a budget.

Conform to legal requirements.

Are accurately recorded and reported.

Provide for optimum use of resources.

Include a plan for audit control.

Establish the basis for a fee schedule consistent with cost of service and within customary norms of fair and reasonable.

VIII. Quality assurance.

A written plan exists for the assessment of, and action to assure, the quality and appropriateness of the physical therapy service.

Provides for a current written plan for assessment of the service.

Provides evidence of ongoing review, evaluation of the service.

Resolves identified problems.

Is consistent with requirements of external agencies.

IX. Staff development.

A written plan exists that provides for appropriate ongoing development of staff.

Is reflected by evidence of ongoing service education or attendance at continuing education activities.

PROVISION OF CARE

X. Informed consent.

XI. Initial evaluation.

The physical therapist performs and records an initial evaluation and interprets results to determine appropriate care for the individual.

Is initiated prior to treatment.

Is performed by the physical therapist in a timely manner.

Is documented, dated, and signed by the physical therapist who performed the evaluation.

Identifies physical therapy needs of the client.

Includes pertinent information of the following:

History

Diagnosis

Problem

Complication and precautions

Physical status

Functional status

Critical behavior/mentation

Social/environmental needs

Provides sufficient data to establish immediate goals.

The physical therapist shall render care within the scope of the physical therapist's education and experience. Appropriate referral to other practitioners shall be made when necessary.

The physical therapist utilizes objective measures to establish a baseline at the time of the initial evaluation.

XII. Plan of care.
1. The physical therapist establishes and records a plan of care of the individual, based on the results of the evaluation.
   Includes realistic goals and expected outcome.
   Is based on identified needs.
   Includes effective treatment method, frequency, and duration.
   Recommends appropriate coordination of care with other professionals/services.
   Is documented, dated, and signed by the physical therapist who established the plan of care.
2. The physical therapist involves the individual/significant other in the plan, implementation, and revision of the treatment program.
3. The physical therapist plans for discharge of the individual taking into consideration goal achievement, and provides for appropriate follow-up or referral.

XIII. Treatment.
1. The physical therapist provides or delegates and supervises the physical therapy treatment consistent with the results of the evaluation and plan of care.
   Is under the ongoing personal care or supervision of the physical therapist.
   Reflects that delegated responsibilities are commensurate with the qualifications of the physical therapy personnel.
   Is altered in accordance with changes in individual status.
   Is provided at a level consistent with current physical therapy practice.
2. The physical therapist records, on an ongoing basis, treatment rendered, progress, and change in status relative to the plan of care.

XIV. Re-evaluation.
The physical therapist re-evaluates the individual and modifies the plan of care as indicated.
   Is performed by the physical therapist in a timely manner.
   Reflects that the individual's progress is reassessed relative to initial evaluation and plan of care.
   Is documented, dated, and signed by the physical therapist who performed the evaluation.

. . . .
EDUCATION

XV. Professional development.
The physical therapist is responsible for his/her individual professional development and continued competence in physical therapy.

XVI. Student.
The physical therapist participates in the education of physical therapy students and other student health professionals.

RESEARCH

XVII. The physical therapist utilizes research findings in practice, promotes and encourages or participates in research activities.

COMMUNITY RESPONSIBILITY

XVIII. The physical therapist participates in community activities to promote community health.

LEGAL/ETHICAL

XIX. Legal.
The physical therapist fulfills all the legal requirements of the jurisdictions regulating the practice of physical therapy.

XX. Ethical.
The physical therapist practices according to the code of ethics of the APTA.

CHAPTER 6

Information Management in Physical Therapy

I. **History of computing**

II. **Computing and the economic development of the United States**

III. **Information management in physical therapy**
   A. Hardware
   B. Software

IV. **Ethics of computing**

V. **Computer applications in physical therapy practice**

VI. **Decision making regarding computer systems**

VII. **Definitions**

HISTORY OF COMPUTING

Several innovations in the 1800s in information machines such as the typewriter, the adding machine, and the slot machine (Box 6–1) laid the groundwork for information processing.[1(p147)] They were advances in technology that reduced human error and stored information efficiently and would lead to the development of the computer—the machine that changed the world.

Although managers often mean computer technology when they speak about managing information, information management is a science that extends beyond computer hardware, requiring a "management system and human engineering to determine the manner in which information will be collected, stored, and retrieved. Furthermore, it requires a systematic planning process to assure that each component of the organization and each phase of the organization's development will fit into the system. Richard Nolan of the Harvard Business School has defined six stages of growth of information management within an organization.[2(p127)] These six stages are: initiation, contagion, control, integration, data administration, and maturity.[3(p87)] Every organization grows at varying rates and may have components at different stages of growth in information management as it strives to develop a system which supports the primary mission of the organization."[2(p128)]

The first computer generation ended in 1959 as the integrated circuit was developed and "vacuum tubes, punched cards and machine codes [gave] way to second-generation transistors, magnetic tape, and procedural languages in computer design and operation."[1(p15), 4(pp89–131)] The computer chip,[5(p21)] and the development of the

. . . .

BOX 6–1 COMPUTER TIMELINE

500 BC	Abacus originates in Egypt
1430	Quadrant developed in Europe
1614	John Napier develops idea of logarithms
1622	William Oughtred develops the slide rule
1642	Blaise Pascal builds first mechanical calculating machine
1780	Benjamin Franklin discovers electricity

First-Generation Computers

1801	French silk weaver Joseph-Marie Jacquard invents a punched-card operated loom
1822	Charles Babbage designs the Difference Engine to calculate logarithmic tables (machine never built)
1831	Michael Faraday builds first electrical generator
1833	Charles Babbage designs first general-purpose computer—the analytical engine
1854	George Boole creates Boolean algebra
1855	George and Edvard Scheutz build first practical computer based on Babbage's design
1886	William Burroughs develops first mechanical adding machine
1890	Herman Hollerith's electromechanical punched card tabulator used to compile US census
1895	Charles Fey invents first slot machine (forerunner to arcade games)
1903	Nikola Tesla patents electrical logic circuits
1924	Thomas Watson Sr. becomes CEO of IBM
1928	Vladimir Zworykin invents cathode-ray tube
1936	Konrad Zuse designs Z1 computer with keyboard input, mechanical switches, and a row of light bulbs to flash answers
1938	Hewlett Packard founded
1939	George Stibitz builds complex number calculator at Bell Labs (first digital computer)
1945	John von Neumann sets precepts for a stored-program computer
1947	Transistor invented at Bell Labs
1951	Univac I delivered to US Bureau of Census—first US commercially produced computer
	Wang Labs founded
1952	Univac predicts Eisenhower's victory
1955	First commercially available computer (Univac)
1956	"Artificial intelligence" coined at Dartmouth (John McCarthy)

Continued.

computer language BASIC (Beginner's All-Purpose Symbolic Instruction Code) in 1964 revolutionized the computer industry. Computers were more manageable in size, language, and cost. The first commercial minicomputer was produced in 1964 by Digital Equipment Corporation.[6(p15)] The third generation of computers was "underway, with integrated circuits, floppy disks, and nonprocedural languages becoming prominent in computer construction and usage"[1(p15)] by 1967. The introduction of the Apple II personal computer (Apple Computer, Inc) in 1977 and the Radio Shack TRS-80 microcomputer (Tandy Corporation) a year later, followed by the introduction of the IBM PC in 1980 ushered in the personal computer.[1(p15)] In 1984, Apple again revolutionized the computer industry with the introduction of the MacIntosh, a user-friendly computer that allowed the user to issue commands using a mouse and pull-down menu schema that bypassed the need to learn keyboard commands, the more traditional method for initiating computer functions. It is this fifth generation of computer—the microcomputer—which has the potential to revolutionize society.[5(p24), 7(p1)] Given that organizations have historically responded to

. . . .
BOX 6–1 COMPUTER TIMELINE (CONT.).

Second-Generation Computers

1959   Integrated circuit developed by Jack Kilby at Texas Instruments and Robert Noyce of Fairchild Semiconductor
1961   Patient monitoring system at National Institutes of Health Clinics
1964   First criminal prosecution for computer crime (5 years for stealing $5 million of software)

Third-Generation Computers

1964   First commercial minicomputer (Digital)
1965   BASIC developed by John Kemeny and Tom Kurtz
1968   Dendral—first medical diagnostic computer program
        Automated Laboratory Systems Committee makes decisions regarding laboratory computing

Fourth-Generation Computers

1971   Floppy disk introduced by IBM
1974   Banks begin to experiment with automated teller machines
1975   First personal computer (PC) developed by Ed Roberts and Bill Yates of Massachusetts Institute of Technology
1977   Apple II—Steve Wozniak and Steve Jobs (founders of Apple) TRS-80 introduced by Radio Shack
1979   Wordstar released

Fifth-Generation Computers

1981   IBM PC debuts with Microsoft's MS-DOS
1982   *Time* magazine names the computer its Man of the Year
        Jimmy Carter first president to use word processor to write memoirs
1983   First touch-screen computer
1984   Macintosh introduced (mouse, pull-down menus)
        Introduction of supercomputer
1990   Introduction of notebooks and powerbooks (notebook-sized portable computers)

societal changes and needs, such a revolution in society has had a significant effect on organizations as well.

"In *The Gutenberg Galaxy,* Marshall McLuhan reduced the Western intellectual tradition to a single hypothesis: that the invention of movable type in the 15th century has been the main force in shaping Western culture."[5(p2)] "Microcomputers represent a critical force that is bringing to an end typographic culture and creating in its place a post-typographic culture and consciousness."[5(p4)]

The industrial revolution extended the individual's power over the environment. The invention of vehicles such as trains and steamboats allowed people to move beyond the limitations imposed on them by their human size and strength, as did the use of new and complex machines in the manufacturing of goods. In similar ways, the computer revolution of the past few decades has extended human power, emancipating the power of the brain.[5(pp16,17)]

Futures authors such as Toffler[8] and Naisbitt[9(p181)] have speculated on the trends and growth of computer technology and its effects on society. Each has foreseen the potential of remote access to information through complex societal networking—which on one hand provides the benefit of freeing the individual from traveling to work, businesses, schools, entertainment, and other sites of human interaction, and on the other hand, firmly establishes the potential for isolation from human interaction, reason, and inspiration.

Toffler develops this theme further and speculates on the emergence of the "electronic cottage,"[8] in which the individual can access all services and information and in essence never has to leave his home—which has become a central communications center.[8(pp181–193)] Naisbitt continues this hypothesis and introduces the dialectic of high tech vs. high touch and the probability that human beings are likely to always maintain and increase human contact in certain realms of their lives as others become more dehumanized and decentralized.[9] This concept of high tech vs. high touch is very important in a profession such as physical therapy, which has always been highly involved with touching patients. The development of computerized exercise equipment in the field is enticing the therapist away from subjective assessments and treatments by offering more objective measurements of progress. Physical therapists must become involved in the decision making regarding the development of computerized clinical systems so that there is a balance between the objectivity of high technology and the subjectivity of touching, since both of these concepts have a place in the healing process.

· · · · · · · · · · ·
COMPUTING AND THE ECONOMIC DEVELOPMENT OF THE UNITED STATES

Toffler describes three major time periods ("waves") in American culture (Fig 6–1).[8] During the first wave (up to about 1900), culture was agrarian based and family centered. The industrial revolution ushered in the second wave (1900 to about 1980), characterized by a massive move from rural to urban areas and away from the family and toward the media and experts as primary sources of information.[10(p37)] During this time, the individual centered himself around the workplace, whereas in the previous wave the home and community served as focal points. Toffler discusses this wave as a truly revolutionary one because it was so dramatically different from the first wave and because it caused significant shifts in the economy and structure of the culture. The third wave (1980 to some future date) is characterized by a movement toward greater personal autonomy and the growth of information management and the provision of services to support the individual.[8] There will be a trend toward a greater percentage of leisure hours and the need therefore to accomplish the same amount of work in less time. He describes the "features of the Third Wave civilization [as more] consonant with those of First Wave civilization . . . they imply the possibility of change with less, not more, disruption, pain, and future shock. . . . And so, not merely in the fields of energy or technology, agriculture or economics,

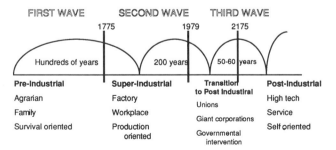

FIG 6–1.
Three waves of economic and social development of the United States. (Adapted from Toffler A: *The Third Wave.* New York, NY, William Morrow and Co, Inc, 1980.)

but in the very brain and behavior of the individual, the Third Wave brings the potential for revolutionary change."[8]

High technology is not just changing technologically driven professions such as engineering and mathematics. It is transforming our lives and has great potential to escalate that transformation. Through massive national and international networks of services, it has the potential of increasing the individualistic nature of our culture or, by allowing the individual greater freedom to work at a site distant from the traditional work site, to encourage the individual to remain closer to the family and to make career decisions that are least disruptive to the family.

· · · · · · · · · · ·

INFORMATION MANAGEMENT IN PHYSICAL THERAPY

Within physical therapy, computer systems are used to manage waiting lists, schedule patients, maintain records, billing, conduct clinical research, monitor patient progress on computerized exercise and testing equipment, and to perform a myriad of managerial functions such as maintaining staff records, monitoring productivity, analyzing department functions, and developing and maintaining the budget and a wide variety of communication functions. According to a study of over 500 physical therapy practices in Missouri, Illinois, and Indiana, the primary use of computers in physical therapy is in the management of the practice (Table 6–1).[11]

As health care managers have begun to computerize department operations, the most common error observed is the acquisition of the computer hardware (computer, hard drive, keyboard, mouse) as the first step making sure that the hardware is compatible with hardware in other departments within the system. Once the hardware is in place the manager proceeds to find software that will most closely fit the needs of the department and then decide which functions will be computerized and who will use the computer. This is exactly the opposite approach to take when faced with the problem of computerizing any function. The manager should first decide which functions *must* be computerized and which personnel are responsible for those functions, then find software that will accomplish that function, and then make hardware decisions based on the hardware needed to run the software. Compatibility with other departments is important if the function that must be computerized cuts across departments and there is a need for personnel to enter data using the

TABLE 6–1. Primary Use of Computers by Physical Therapy Managers: Results of the Gogia and Braatz Study[11]

Computer Application	% of Respondents
Entering charges on the hospital system	72
Recording patient charges	65
Receive M.D. orders from ward	59
Patient billing	38
Patient records	33
Cybex data reduction and interpretation	21
Word processing	19
Practice analysis and management reports	16
Telecommunications	14
Quality assurance activities	11
Accounts receivable	01
Accounts payable	01
Budgeting	01
Insurance claim processing	01
Electronic mail service	01

same software. If it is possible to purchase compatible software, it will reduce the training time and expenses associated with teaching personnel to use new software and hardware.

In physical therapy, one of the most common functions that managers want to computerize is patient and therapist scheduling. The first comercially produced software is just becoming available for this function. The California Chapter of the American Physical Therapy Association has launched a project to develop scheduling software, and many managers have developed their own internal programs to meet their unique needs.

Because so little physical therapy software is available, it is very difficult for physical therapist managers to find software that meets the needs of the department. Physical therapy is in the *stage of initiation* in development as a profession that uses information management from a practice and education perspective and in the *mature stage of development* from a research perspective. In research, physical therapists are able to use well tested and highly developed software because the research functions used are the same as those within many other fields such as math, physics, engineering, statistics, and sociology. Computer technology was developed for the researcher and is highly sophisticated to handle almost any research function within a quantitative domain. Qualitative research functions are now being addressed by software that is being developed primarily for anthropology and sociology and allow the investigator to store, retrieve, and analyze field notes and interviews.

Hardware

Computer hardware varies from mainframe computers, which are the largest type of computer, usually capable of serving many users simultaneously, with a processing speed about 100 times faster than that of a microcomputer to personal computers (PCs) and portable computers. Whereas the original mainframe computers occupied a whole building when they were first introduced, small companies and individual departments can now house mainframe computers in an average office space. In most institutions individual departments do not house mainframe computers. They are housed centrally where they can be more easily maintained and accessed by a number of users. These computers may be used for billing, scheduling clinic visits, maintaining medical records, and maintaining the institution's inventory. Individual departments then access the mainframe using passwords that give access to particular data.

The most common denominator in computing today is the PC. In many instances the PC is more powerful than the original mainframe computers and is able to store large data bases. When data are unique to a specific unit within a health care institution, it is usually maintained on a PC within that unit. Managers are responsible for acquision and maintainence of the hardware, software, and data. Computer specialists are hired as consultants to develop software, maintain hardware, troubleshoot, and assist the manager in buying and maintenance decisions.

Computer hardware is the physical appartus of computing. In a PC it commonly includes the central processing unit and hard disk, the monitor, the disk slots, the keyboard, and the mouse. There are a number of peripherals that can be connected to this basic hardware such as modems, compact disk players, and external disk drives.

A very large variety of PC hardware is available, but perhaps the most common hardware purchased are IBM and IBM-compatible systems and Apple systems.

The primary decisions that must be made when selecting hardware include the capacity of the memory and the size of the monitor. Memory is the storage facility of a computer and is applied only to internal storage as opposed to external storage, such as disks or tapes. The capacity of the memory will depend on the functions that the individual computer is to perform. In most instances 2 to 4 megabytes (MB) of memory is adequate for word processing, graphics, and small data bases. The most common disk storage size is now a 40-MB hard drive, although 80-MB hard drives are commonly used when the computer user needs a large storage capacity for data bases or desktop publishing.

Monitor sizes vary as much as television screen sizes vary. Monitors can be produced by the company making the basic hardware or from other companies that make compatible equipment. The traditional monitor is adequate for most functions. A larger screen is desirable if the department plans to use desktop publishing. Desktop publishing is the use of hardware and software to produce market-quality publications such as newsletters, flyers, and patient education materials. Producing quality desktop publications is easier if an entire page of text can be viewed on the screen. Therefore, a monitor for this operation should be purchased as recommended for the particular publication software. In some instances, these monitors may be as large as the publication being produced. The rule of thumb is that as the size of the monitor increases, the resolution should also increase so that the operator can predict the final product from the image on the screen. Therefore, when purchasing larger monitors for the computer, buy the highest resolution possible.

Computer hardware operating systems are becoming more and more compatible with each other, which increases their ability to interpret information from one system to another. It is very likely that in the next 20 years we will see absolute compatibility.

Software

A wide variety of software is available to the physical therapy manager. Although company names and special features may vary, there are specific categories of software to be considered when analyzing the needs of the department (Box 6–2). Many software programs perform only one function such as word processing. Decisions regarding which of these programs to purchase are driven by the features of the program, the cost, and the licensing agreements available.

Features of a word processing program, for example, include advanced capabilities such as footnoting, sorting by letters and numbers, creating columns, and wrapping text around graphics. It is the responsibility of the manager to understand the

---

BOX 6–2 CATEGORIES OF COMMERCIAL SOFTWARE

Word processing
Spread sheets
Graphics
Business applications
Virus protectors
Screen protectors
Data bases
Statistical packages
Computer-assisted design (CAD)
Computer-assisted manufacture (CAM)
Computer-aided instruction (CAI)
Games
Desktop publishing
Personal information managers
Calendars and schedules

needs of the staff and professionals in the department and purchase the appropriate software in the appropriate quantities. For example, perhaps the secretary is the only person who needs the most sophisticated word processing program, but all of the professionals have to be able to bring their work to that person for formatting and final copy. The manager would purchase the most sophisticated word processing program for the secretary, making sure that the word processing packages purchased for the professionals were compatible with the secretary's hardware and software.

More expensive software programs are commonly integrated with other programs such as a graphics or spread sheet program. Many business software packages are integrated and allow the user to work easily from word processing, to spread sheet, to graphics programs using one data entry point. In such a package, the individual may enter a set of data and then ask to have it displayed in a spread sheet or graphic format or printed out as a report. Similar integrated packages are being developed in physical therapy practice, where data are entered related to a patient's progress; they are then available as a data point in a department data base, as a progress note, and as a graphic displaying the patient's progress. IBM's introduction of Windows has also made it possible for the computer user to easily integrate several software programs and therefore customize their needs without purchasing integrated software. As Windows continues to be perfected, the need for integrated software will decrease.

· · · · · · · · · · ·
ETHICS OF COMPUTING

Our society is one in which children are introduced to computers at a very young age as a game to be mastered, a puzzle to be solved, or a code to be broken. This game mentality extends to computer use as the child grows to an adult, with little or no introduction to concepts of the individual's social responsibility related to computing. Breaking the code or finding the back door to computer software becomes a game, and few individuals relate to these activities as computer crime. Breaking into a piece of software, personal files, or bank statements is no different than physically breaking into a locked office or filing cabinet. Illegally copying software is the same as illegally copying a book from cover to cover. The ease with which software can be copied and the nature of the software as a vehicle for doing work on the computer confuses the legal and moral issues for many individuals. Many pieces of software allow the individual to word process or file or analyze data, and the individual often feels that he/she has a right to use these tools. Software tools should be thought of as very good pens, slide rules, calculators, or typewriters. Just as the individual would not think of stealing these tools, neither should the individual consider stealing software.

Licensing agreements raise many moral and legal issues. If a department manager wants to make word processing available to all of the staff, then specific licensing rules must be adhered to in order to legally use the software. For instance, if the manager purchases one word processing program, that program may only be legally loaded onto one computer. If that computer is part of a network, then the software must be loaded on the computer in such a fashion that only one user could access the program at a time. However, if the manager needs 14 staff members to access the software from a common network, the facility may be able to purchase a site license. Word processing software often costs between $300 and $500. A site license for the software to be used by 15 people may cost the institution $3,000, leading to a savings of $1,500 to $2,000.

The manager may be tempted to allow the software to be copied and used by all staff members. This is both morally wrong and illegal. It is no different than plagiarism. It is computer crime. Society is beginning to differentiate between the ethical and legal issues related to computers. Many issues have already been clearly defined by the courts as computer crimes.* Examples of computer crimes include copying software and breaking into files. Yet in many health care institutions, professionals and staff are encouraged to copy software in order to save money, since group purchasing decisions were made based on hardware costs without adequate budgeting for software. Health care institutions must identify the legal issues related to computer use and provide opportunities to deal with the moral dilemmas that high technology brings to the institution. Students emerging from the university must also be prepared to meet their moral and legal obligations to society, and one arena in which these students will be challenged is the interface of high technology and society.

It is the responsibility of the manager to understand that the true cost of computing is not in the capital outlay for the hardware. The continuing costs of purchasing the right software, upgrading software, adding peripherals, paper costs, cartridges for the laser printers, training of personnel, cost of consultants, and equipment repair are costs that will exceed the original capital expenditures. The most frustrating situation for a staff is to have the hardware without adequate budget support to maximize the use of the system. When making the decision to computerize, the manager must carefully consider true start-up costs and annual costs to operate the system. When considering engaging in a new function for the department such as building a data base or implementing desktop publishing, the manager should plan on hiring consultants to help to set up the basic software, train the primary and secondary users, and serve as an ongoing consultant to the primary users. Such training costs can easily account for thousands of dollars of expenditures, but the results will be rewarding.

In general, the more that physical therapy functions are the same as or similar to functions performed in other disciplines, the more likely there will be computer software to perform those functions. For instance, many word processing programs can be used for generating notes and reports. Software companies are now beginning to develop software specifically for physical therapy. A new bar code scanning program called SOAP NOTES allows the therapist to scan specific categories and procedures that are transformed into a prose SOAP note by the computer. Forms-based documentation such as manual muscle testing forms or back assessment forms can be turned into prose notes using another software program called Ghost Writer.

· · · · · · · · · · ·
COMPUTER APPLICATIONS IN PHYSICAL THERAPY PRACTICE

Increasingly, computer-operated testing and exercise equipment is finding its way into physical therapy practice. The introduction of the electronic goniometer, three-dimensional motion analysis, and the ground-breaking work resulting in computer-generated ambulation in paraplegics will revolutionize physical therapy practice and clinical research. As the field continues to advance in this area, this equipment poses three potential problems for the manager. First, physical therapists who are not computer literate will not use this equipment to its potential or continue to explore the boundaries of its applicability. The profession has reached the point where computer literacy must be one of the foundations of the professional's skills. How-

---

*References 12 (p. 14), 13 (pp. 63–64), 14 (p. 141), 15 (p. 12), 16 (p. 2), 17 (pp. 53-55), 18 (p. 66), 19 (p. 17), and 20 (p. 9).

ever, of over 100 physical therapy educational programs in the United States, fewer than 20 teach computer applications in physical therapy. Therefore, it is incumbent on the manager to provide a means for therapists who are not computer literate to learn how to operate basic computer systems and to make sure that the rest of the professional staff is continuing to set positive examples of the value of computer literacy to good patient care. Second, it introduces another source of ongoing costs for repair, maintenance, and support. And finally, it raises questions related to high tech vs. high touch. The manager must engage the staff in regular discussions about the importance of human touch and the subjective vs. objective needs of the discipline and the patient.

There has been significant technological progress in computing in general as well as in the use of high technology in physical therapy. "Technological progress requires more analytical decision making. Today numerous turnkey systems are designed for specific management uses, including many intended specifically for the health care field, such as scheduling systems, inventory systems, physician office recordkeeping and billing systems, claims preparation and processing systems, not to mention interfaces that exist between microcomputer systems and larger institutional systems in hospitals and other health care facilites."[21(p11)]

DECISION MAKING REGARDING COMPUTER SYSTEMS

Not too long ago, the best advice a manager could get about a computer system was to "try one out." This is no longer an option. If the physical therapy manager is unfamiliar with computer systems, the best approach is to hire a computer consultant to help make the best decision regarding the system that meets the needs of the particular department or practice. The role of the manager will be to conduct a very careful needs analysis of the department from an information management perspective. The following questions would be helpful in beginning that needs assessment.

Research

- Is there a need to document clinical outcomes?
    For the individual patient?
    For the entire unit?
    Is there a plan in place?
    Would a clinical data base be helpful?
    How will patient progress be measured after the patient is discharged?
    Would it be helpful to have computer mailing lists and the opportunity
       to merge addresses with individual letters?
- Is the professional staff engaged in clinical research?
    Is there a need for statistical packages?
    Is there a need for a data base management program?
- Is the quality assurance program in place?
    Should it be computerized?

Education

- Is the department engaged in producing educational materials? For professionals? For patients? Volume?
- Does the department produce a newsletter? Volume?
- Does the department produce flyers? Volume?
- Is there a need to document student physical therapist outcomes over time? Would a data base be helpful?

Communications

- What is the volume of correspondence?
- What is the volume of reports? What kind of reports?
- Would it be helpful to have reports on the computer?
- What is the nature of the mailings that go out of the department during a 1-week period?
- Does the department use a FAX machine? For what?
- Would it be helpful to communicate directly by computer in addition to FAX? With whom? Other departments? Other facilities? Third-party reimbursers? Referral sources?
- How are progress notes processed? What is the volume?

Business Functions

- How is professional and patient scheduling performed? Volume? Does it involve more than one site?
- What is the volume of patients per day?
- How is billing done? Would it be helpful to enter billing data directly into the institution's billing data base?
- Budgeting, planning, and revisions of budget? What role does the physical therapy manager play? Is a spread sheet used? How are reports generated? What is the nature of the reports?
- How accessible is current information?
- How are cost and utilization of resources tracked?
- How are time and productivity tracked?

Practice

- What computerized equipment is used in the department?
- How are progress notes written?
- How are data maintained and reported?
- What demographic data are maintained on patients?
- How are patients scheduled?
- How is productivity recorded and reported?
- What data are maintained on patients regarding history of illness and claims history?
- How is information maintained and updated on referring sources? Referral facilities? Discharge facilities?

The computer consultant will then analyze the computer resources already available in the facility, the possibility of networking with these systems, the compatibility of various programs, and the relative costs of working in a network environment.

When analyzing the needs of the department, the manager must not overlook low technology as a part of the system. One of the common complaints of computerizing a system is that the increased efficiency does not decrease the volume of work. Individuals still work as hard, they just work faster. A major consideration of the manager is to plan an operation that is efficient and well paced. Pacing will help to alleviate burnout. For instance, the manager may want to institute a plan to speed up billing or the authorization process by computer networking with the billing office and the third-party reimburser. However, if the department already has a 100-person waiting list, the manager may not want to develop a more efficient method of receiving referrals without finding a way to increase productivity. The manager must play a key role in developing a needs assessment for the department, analyzing the plan from the computer consultant, and deciding which aspects of the computer plan to put in place. If networking is to be a part of this plan, then the manager must consult with other managers, since computer networking is often a part of institutional planning, requiring compatible telephone systems and meeting wiring codes. If the plan the physical therapy manager considers goes beyond networking and appears to have significant implications for other departments (outcome assessment), persons in higher administration should be consulted so that these plans can be considered in light of the overall objectives of the institution.

· · · · · · · · · · ·
DEFINITIONS

Algorithm: A step-by-step procedure for solving a problem; programming languages are essentially means of expressing algorithms.

Analog computer: A computer in which continuous physical variables such as the movement of gears or the magnitude of voltage represent data.

Artificial intelligence (AI): The branch of computer science that attempts to create programs capable of emulating such human characteristics as learning and reasoning.

ASCII: The acronym for American Standard Code for Information Interchange, a widely used system for encoding letters, numerals, punctuation marks, and signs as binary numbers.

Backup: A copy of a program or data file made as insurance in case the original gets lost or damaged.

BASIC: Beginner's all-purpose symbolic instruction code—variation of FORTRAN computer language developed in 1965 by John Kemeny and Tom Kurtz at Dartmouth College. Encouraged widespread use of computing through a simple programming language.

Baud: A term used in describing data transmission rates, usually 1 bit per second.

Binary code: A system for representing things by combinations of two symbols, such as 1 and 0, TRUE and FALSE, or the presence or absence of voltage.

Binary: Having two components or possible states.

Bit: The smallest unit of information in a binary computer, represented by a single 0 or 1. The word "bit" is a contraction of "binary digit."

Bomb: A program "bombs" when it fails spectacularly. Programmers "bomb" a computer system when they deliberately write a program that will disrupt the system.

Boolean algebra: A method of expressing the logical relationships between entities such as propositions or on-off computer circuits; invented by the 19th century English mathematician, George Boole.

Bug: Error in a program that keeps it from working properly.

Bus: A set of wires for carrying signals around a computer.

Byte: A sequence of bits, usually eight, treated as a unit for computation or storage.

CAD/CAM: Two separate topics, but usually spoken as one word. CAD (Computer-Aided Design) today consists mostly of fancy drafting aids used to lay out printed circuit boards and integrated circuit chips. CAM (Computer-Aided Manufacture) is the use of computers to manage and control a factory's operations.

CD-I (compact disk-interactive): A CD-ROM format capable of storing audio, animated, textual, and graphics data; intended for use with a special player attached to a television set.

CD-ROM (compact disk read-only memory): A type of compact disk used to store text or graphics in digital form.

Chip: An integrated circuit on a fleck of silicon, made up of thousands of transistors and other electronic components.

Circuit board: The plastic board on which electronic components are mounted.

Clock: A device, usually based on a quartz crystal, that gives off regular pulses used to co-ordinate a computer's operations.

Command: A statement, such as PRINT or COPY, that sets in motion a preprogrammed sequence of instructions to a computer.

Compuserve: National network of bulletin boards, e-mail, travel agencies, airlines, national store chains, banking.

Computer: A programmable machine that accepts, processes, and displays data.

Control key: A key that, when pressed in combination with other keys, generates control characters.

Copy protection: To reduce unauthorized copying of their programs, software publishers often resort to tricks to make their disks difficult to copy. This is a great annoyance to legitimate users, who can't make backups. And, unfortunately, some people find the breaking of copy-protection schemes an intellectual challenge.

CPU: Central processing unit—the part of a computer that interprets and executes instructions. It is composed of an arithmetic logic unit, a control unit, and a small amount of memory.

Crash: A computer system is said to crash when it stops working for some reason and must be restarted by the operator.

CRT: Cathode-ray tube—a television-like display device with a screen that lights up where it is struck from the inside by a beam of electrons.

Cursor: The movable spot of light that indicates a point of action or attention on a computer screen.

Daisy wheel: A printer type element resembling a flower. The end of each "petal" carries a different symbol. In use, the wheel spins rapidly until the desired character is in position. Then a hammer strikes the type, forcing it against the ribbon and paper and imprinting the character.

DEC: Digital Equipment Company.

Digital: Pertaining to the representation or transmission of data by discrete signals.

Digitize: To convert analog information into binary-coded on-off signals that can represent the information within a digital computer.

Disk drive: The mechanism that rotates a storage disk and reads or records data.

Disk: A round magnetized plate, usually made of plastic or metal, organized into concentric tracks and pie-shaped sectors of storing data. Some are internally or externally mounted with large memory capacities and are referred to as hard disks.

DOS: Disk operating system. System developed by IBM to perform basic disk functions, allowing the computer to accept and read the disk and move from one function to another.

Dot-matrix printer: An impact printer that uses a pattern of dots arranged in rows and columns to print text or graphics.

Download: The process of copying a file (document or application) from an on-line service to your computer or disk.

E-mail: Electronic mail. Messages delivered via local area network or through a modem to a large-scale network.

Electrostatic printer (laser printer): A nonimpact printer that employs particles of dry ink, which cling in the desired pattern to electrically charged paper.

Escape key: Key found on some keyboards. When pressed, it redefines all the other keys, giving them new meanings. This allows the use of special characters or codes not normally found on the keyboard. May also be called "alternate."

Fiber optics: The technology of encoding data as pulses of laser light beamed through ultrathin strands of glass.

Floppy disk: A small, flexible disk used to store information or instructions.

Font: The configuration (size and style) of characters (a, b, c, etc).

Function keys: Extra keys on a keyboard used to initiate operations that would otherwise require several keystrokes. Often they are programmable and have different meanings according to what program is being run.

Hacker: Someone who loves to experiment with computers.

Hard copy: Printed computer output, usually on paper.

Hardware: The physical apparatus of a computer system.

IBM: International business machine.

Icon: A symbol that represents a command or an object on a display screen.

Initialize: The process of preparing a volume so that you can get information from or save information to the volume. In the case of a floppy disk, it eliminates any chance of recovering data because the disk is completely cleared of information.

Input: Information fed into a computer or any part of a computer.

IS: Information science.

Kilobyte (K byte): 1,024 bytes (1,024 being 1 K, or 2 to the 10th power); often used as a measure of memory capacity.

LAN: Local area network—a network of communication cables that physically links personal computers together. It usually includes cabling, network software, and application software.

Language: A set of rules or conventions to describe a process to a computer.

LCD: Liquid crystal display—a digital display mechanism made up of character-forming segments of a liquid crystal material sandwiched between polarizing and reflecting pieces of glass.

Light pen: Looks like a bulky pen with a cable attached; it can detect the presence of light when held to a video screen. Depending on the program, a light pen can be used to draw things, point to things, or move things around on the screen.

Logon: Command to enter appropriate prompts to identify disk and program to be used.

Mainframe computer: The largest type of computer, usually capable of serving many users simultaneously, with a processing speed about 100 times faster than that of a microcomputer.

Memory: The storage facilities of a computer; the term is applied only to internal storage as opposed to external storage, such as disks or tapes.

Microprocessor: A single chip containing all the elements of a computer's central processing unit; sometimes called a computer on a chip.

Microsoft: International software company.

Minicomputer: A midsized computer smaller than a mainframe and usually with much more memory than a microcomputer.

Modem: A device (modulator; demodulator) that enables data to be transmitted between computers, generally over telephone lines but sometimes on fiber optic cable or radio frequencies.

Number crunching: The rapid processing of large quantities of numbers.

Optical disk: A storage medium that holds information in the form of a pattern of marks on a rigid platter; an optical-disk drive reads, erases, or writes data on the disk with a laser beam.

Output: The data returned by a computer either directly to the user or to some form of storage.

Password: In multiple user systems, users are often asked to identify themselves with a password, unique to each user, before the computer will let them use the system.

Plotter: An output device that produces charts, graphs, and other artwork in the form of line drawings on paper or film.

Ports: Connectors for attaching peripherals to a computer's main board.

Program: A sequence of detailed instructions for performing some operation or solving some problem by computer.

Pull-down menus: Menus activated with mouse or F (function) keys that resemble a window shade and can be activated by pulling down the cursor.

Purging: In a computer's memory, the automatic erasure of stale information to create more storage space.

Queue: A data structure that in some ways resembles a stack. In a stack items are added and removed only from one end, whereas in a queue items are added at one end and removed from the other. This resembles a line queue waiting at a ticket window, hence the name.

RAM: Random-access memory—a form of temporary internal storage in which contents can be retrieved and altered by the user; also called read-and-write memory.

ROM: Read-only memory—permanent internal memory containing data or operating instructions that can be read but not altered by the user.

Scrolling: The motion of lines on a video terminal. As new lines appear on the bottom of the screen, the existing lines move upward, eventually disappearing off the top of the screen.

SCSI: Small computer system interface—an industry standard, high-speed interface that transfers data from one device to another.

Semiconductor: A solid crystalline substance whose electrical conductivity falls between that of a metal and an insulator.

Silicon Valley: An area in California south of San Francisco that is a center of the semiconductor industry in the United States.

Software: Instruction or programs that enable a computer to do useful work; contrasted with hardware, or the actual computer apparatus.

Time-sharing: It enables many people to use the computer at once. Each user sits before a terminal that is used to type in his or her program or changes. The computer does a small part of one user's program, then quickly shifts to the next user. The computer can do this so quickly that each user has the feeling of having sole use of the computer. The biggest advantage of time-sharing is immediate response from the computer and a chance to change the program immediately if it doesn't work right the first time.

Trojan Horse: A seemingly innocuous program with a hidden purpose. The Trojan Horse presents itself as a useful, normal application. But once resident on the system, hidden routines are unleashed to inflict damage.

Vaccine: A program that is meant to provide virus protection.

Virus inhibitors: One or more resources added to a file that prevents infection by a specific, known virus.

Virus: A program designed to infect and modify data, altering your computer's behavior, and often meant for destruction. Examples: Trojan Horse, WORM, SCORES, NVIR, ANTI, MAG, ZUC, INIT29, WDEF, Joshi, Francie.

WORM: A malicious program that, once resident on the computer system, inflicts damage by burrowing through the files to corrupt the data.

References

1. Beninger J: Information society and the control revolution. *Computerworld,* 1986, p 86.
2. Walter J: Information management: The technological revolution, in Mathews J: *Practice Issues in Physical Therapy.* Thorofare, NJ, Slack Publishers, 1989.
3. Cougar JD: New books aid managers in organizing information systems. *Computerworld,* June 23, 1986, p 87.
4. Moreau R: *The Computer Comes of Age.* Cambridge, Mass, The Massachusetts Institute of Technology Press, 1984.

5. Provenzo EF Jr: *Beyond the Gutenberg Galaxy: Microcomputers and the Emergence of Post-Typographic Culture*. New York, NY, Teacher's College, Columbia University, 1986.

6. The computer age. *Computerworld*, 1986, pp 20–32.

7. Baldridge JV, Roberts JW, Weiner TA: *The Campus and the Microcomputer Revolution*. New York, NY, MacMillan Publishing Co, 1984.

8. Toffler A: *The Third Wave*. New York, NY, William Morrow and Company, Inc, 1980.

9. Naisbitt J: *Megatrends*. New York, NY, Warner Books, 1982.

10. Lasch C: *Culture of Narcissism*. New York, NY, WW Norton Co, p 37.

11. Gogia PP, Braatz JH: Computers and the physical therapist: A survey. *Clin Manag Phys Ther* 1986; 6:30–31.

12. Martin JA: San Francisco man found guilty in software piracy case. *Computerworld*, Feb 10, 1986, p 14.

13. Martin R: Lawsuits may choke US software industry. *Computerworld*, March 13, 1986, pp 63–64.

14. Maginnis NB: Market for hot computer goods keeps thieves in business. *Computerworld*, Oct 13, 1986, p 141.

15. Betts M: Congress accelerates action on computer crime legislation. *Computerworld*, April 28, 1986, p 12.

16. Betts M: House Judiciary Committee passes electronics privacy bill. *Computerworld*, 1986, p 2.

17. Bloombecker JJB: New federal law bolsters computer security efforts. *Computerworld*, Oct 27, 1986, pp 53–65.

18. Alfano S: The ethic of hacking. *Psychol Today,* 1984, p. 66.

19. Newquist H: Vendors, users just can't see eye to eye on copy protection. *Computerworld*, June 23, 1986, p 17.

20. Hays C: A golden rule for software. *New York Times* April 12, 1987, p 9.

21. Christensen WW, Stearns EI: *Microcomputers in Health Care Management: Strategies and Applications for the 1990s*. Rockville, Md, Aspen, 1990.

CHAPTER 7

Managing the Work: Management Systems

INTRODUCTION

The management literature has reported a myriad of systems of managing the work of an organization. In an earlier chapter the organizational chart of the pyramid builders was depicted (Fig 7–1). In fact, ancient "managers," people who were assigned the task of performing work, used span of control, division of labor (specialization), and delegation as the first management systems to accomplish that work.

These ancient systems grew out of and were a part of the military system where hierarchical organizational structures, battle strategies, absolute obedience, and the promise of social advancement for exemplary performance were the hallmarks of the system. Even today, some managers in hospital administration speak of the management system as a feudal system of knights and serfs, kings and queens, and jousts and battles.

The model of management that the physical therapy manager adopts will affect the outcome of the system. The manager must first determine the desired outcome and assess the environment and then choose a management model that will produce that outcome. If the outcome is only product and service oriented, the manager may choose an autocratic model. If, on the other hand, the outcome also involves building a cohesive professional team or incorporating continuous quality improvement concepts in a production model, the manager may choose a more humanistic

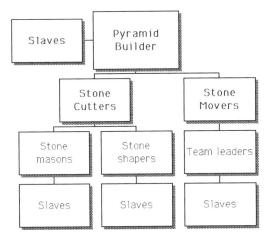

FIG 7–1.
Span of control, delegation, and division of labor.

model. The premise is that no management model works in all situations all of the time. Certain tasks, projects, or outcomes require certain approaches, whereas other tasks, projects, and outcomes require other approaches.

The earliest examples of the hierarchical system in which strict rules of obedience governed relationships were the apprenticeship models of the 18th and 19th centuries, in which masters took on apprentices for long periods of time. These apprentices were expected to work long hours for little financial remuneration, most often only for room and board. The masters were the experts, and they revealed their "secrets" gradually to the apprentice. The apprentice had no understanding of the process of becoming a master. He simply engaged in the process. The master knew the secrets of becoming a master, monitored the apprentice's progress, and at some point would declare the apprentice as a journeyman or assistant. The apprentice would then be declared a master or, more likely, upon the death of the master, would assume that role.

The early factories of the industrial revolution were characterized by "bosses" who were the supreme authority. They were often seen as cruel and as taking advantage of the individual. The work was paramount, the individual was treated as property, and the manager was expected to produce at all costs.

During this period new machines were invented, and materials began to be mass produced for the first time. Individual craftsmen found that their skills were not needed in the factories of the early 20th century, and managers were able to replace more highly paid craftsmen with women and children. The manager relied on his own knowledge and intuition and trial and error to manage the work. Workers themselves were thought of as a part of the machinery, a tool necessary to monitor the work of the machine and appropriately feed raw materials into the system.

• • • • • • • • • •
SCIENTIFIC APPROACH TO MANAGEMENT

During the early 1900s the scientific approach to management was introduced as a method of increasing productivity. Among the outstanding contributors to this phase of evolution of management thought were Frederick W. Taylor, Henri Fayol, and Frank and Lillian Gilbreth.

Taylor's main contribution to the field of management theory was his emphasis on observation of worker performance and the rational analysis of productivity problems. Taylor had thought that if managers used the scientific approach to management and increased productivity that they would want to share the results of those gains by improving working conditions. Unfortunately, the managers and other management theorists focused on the increased efficiency of the system and did not share the gains in productivity with the workers.

Fayol developed specific management principles to guide the work of the managers. As an engineer and a scientist, he felt that there was a body of knowledge related to management that could be taught to perspective managers. In addition to his principles of management, he postulated that there was a theory of management that could be applied to any management situation. Many of Fayol's management principles were not only applicable to a variety of settings, they have also stood the test of time and are still applicable today (Box 7–1).

Frank and Lillian Gilbreth* made their primary contributions to work efficiency. Frank Gilbreth was "a pioneer in developing time and motion studies. . . . He was interested in efficiency, especially in finding the 'one best way to do the work.' "[2(p63)] Lillian Gilbreth continued her husband's work after his untimely death. She "was most interested in the human aspects of work, such as the selection, placement, and training of personnel."[2(p63)] Her interest in the worker lead to the first book on management psychology. Many companies began to look at Gilbreth's work as critical to the success of their company and developed special offices of personnel management that focused on hiring and training of personnel. Taylor, Fayol, and the Gilbreths represented the scientific approach to management. Their focus was on the work and methods of increasing the quality or quantity of the work.

Although management theory was evolving, most managers continued to manage the factories by trial and error and intuition. Therefore, working conditions in factories during this time were abysmal and were to remain that way until the 1920s.

BUREAUCRACY APPROACH TO MANAGEMENT

Max Weber advanced the concept of bureaucracy in management and concentrated on the structure of the organization. His theory stated that tasks were divided into specialized jobs, success could be predicted by following a rigorous set of rules, there were clear relationships between authority and responsibility that must be maintained, superiors dealt with subordinates in an impersonal manner, employment and promotions were based on merit, and that lifelong employment was accepted by all citizens.

By rigidly following Weber's theory of bureaucracy, organizations became unyielding places to work, adhering to rules and treating all employees in an impersonal manner. Weber's theory provided a model for organizations during the transition from the psychoanalytic to the behavioral approach to work and workers. Successful employees were those who were highly productive and adhered to the rules. The worker saw himself as the "company man," a person who strove for inanimate recognition and a sense of belonging to an institution.

---

*Frank and Lillian Gilbreth are the main characters in the book and movie entitled *Cheaper by the Dozen,* which was written by 2 of their 12 children.

. . . .
BOX 7–1   FAYOL'S PRINCIPLES OF MANAGEMENT*

1. Division of work. By performing only one part of the job, a worker can produce more and better work for the same effort. Specialization is the most efficient way to use human effort.
2. Authority and responsibility. Authority is the right to give orders and obtain obedience, and responsibility is a corollary of authority.
3. Discipline. Obedience to organizational rules is necessary. The best way to have good superiors and clear and fair rules and agreements is to apply sanctions and penalties judiciously.
4. Unity of command. There should be one and only one superior for each individual employee.
5. Unity of direction. All units in the organization should be moving toward the same objectives through coordinated and focused effort.
6. Subordination of individual interest to general interest. The interests of the organization should take priority over the interests of an individual employee.
7. Remuneration of employees. The overall pay and compensation for employees should be fair to both the employees and the organization.
8. Centralization. There should be a balance between subordinate involvement through decentralization and managers' retention of final authority through centralization.
9. Scalar chain. Organizations should have a chain of authority and communication that runs from the top to the bottom and should be followed by managers and subordinates.
10. Order. People and materials must be in suitable places at the appropriate time for maximum efficiency—that is, a place for everything and everything in its place.
11. Equity. Good sense and experience are needed to ensure fairness to all employees, who should be treated as equally as possible.
12. Stability of personnel. Employee turnover should be minimized to maintain organizational efficiency.
13. Initiative. Workers should be encouraged to develop and carry out plans for improvements.
14. Esprit de corps. Management should promote a team spirit of unity and harmony among employees.

*From Fayol H: *General and Industrial Management.* Cited by: Megginson L, Mosley DC, Pietri PH: *Management Concepts and Applications,* ed 3. New York, NY, Harper and Row, 1989, p 62.

. . . .
BEHAVIORAL APPROACH TO MANAGEMENT

In the 1920s, behaviorism gained significant recognition as an approach to maximize the individual's output by the use of rewards and punishments. John Watson, the founder of behaviorism, introduced the concepts of stimulus-response behavior, which demonstrated that behavior could be shaped with rewards and punishments that were delivered to individuals at key points in time to reinforce the positive behaviors and to extinguish the negative behaviors. In management situations, these rewards and punishments were in the control of the manager, and the theory focused on the relationship between the manager and the worker and those factors that influenced the worker's output.

The behavioral approach to management began with the Hawthorne experiments at the Hawthorne plant of the Western Electric Company near Chicago. During these experiments, the investigators intended to look at the relationship of the intensity of lighting to productivity. What they found was that regardless of whether the lighting was raised or lowered, productivity increased. The simple fact was that the workers had been chosen for the experiment and that any attention, whether increased or decreased lighting, had a positive effect on the worker's output.

The behavioral approach in management focuses on the individual rather than the product or productivity, assuming that if worker morale and participation are high then output will also be high.

· · · · · · · · · · ·
MANAGEMENT SCIENCE APPROACH TO MANAGEMENT

Management by Objectives (MBO)

Peter Drucker, who has been called the founding father of management science, developed a system of management by objectives (MBO), which is based on the fact that each job within an organization must be directed toward specific objectives of the business as a whole. This system assumes that each layer of manager is responsible for connecting each job to specific objectives. "Objectives are needed in every area where performance and results directly and vitally affect the survival and prosperity of the business."[3(p63)] If these objectives are met, the organization will succeed.

This system is very clearly tied to the hierarchical system. The objectives of lower levels of the hierarchy are tied to those at the next highest level of the heirarchy until the mission of the organization is fully defined by objectives throughout the organization. The system appears to work because the managers are committed to the objectives of the organization that relate to their specific functions due to their active involvement in the creation of those objectives and because in setting them they have predicted a specific outcome that they will strive to accomplish.

When Drucker first described MBO, he also described the use of this system as a means of self-control. By self-control, he meant a system that would allow individual managers to assess their own performance and the outcome of that performance. It was not his intent that MBO be used as a system to control managers through the hierarchical system, but as a system that can be continually assessed by the manager.

These management process theories focus on the manager and improving the manager's functions through scientifically based management theories.

Systems Approach

The systems approach to management was introduced by Richard Johnson, Fremont Kast, and James Rosenzweig, and in more modern times has been propelled by systems engineers Jay Forrester at Massachusetts Institute of Technology and Dennis and Donella Meadows and Barry Richmond at Dartmouth College. A system is represented by an input, throughput, output, and feedback loop set within a specific environment (Fig 7–2).

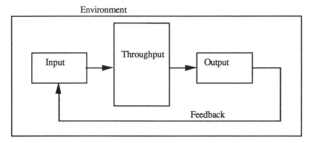

FIG 7–2.
System design.

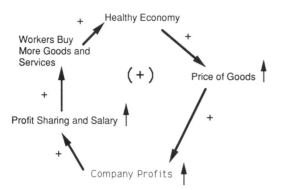

FIG 7−3.
Positive causal loop.

The systems engineer develops a complex model of the system or subsystems by looking at causal loops in which the interrelationship of all of the component parts of the system is clearly articulated. A positive causal loop leads to success, negative causal loops lead to decay of the system.

From a macro perspective, if the economy is healthy, the price of goods goes up; if the price of goods goes up, company profits go up; if company profits go up, profit sharing and salaries go up; if salaries go up, workers will buy more goods and services; if more goods and services are sold, the economy is stimulated. This is a positive causal loop (Fig 7−3).

In a negative causal loop the overall effect of the relationships of the causal factors is negative, and the system will tend to decay over time. For example, if insurance costs go up, insurance benefits go down; if insurance benefits go down, elective medical procedures go down; if elective medical procedures go down, overhead costs of medical facilities and personnel go up; if overhead costs of medical facilities and personnel go up, medical costs go up; if medical costs go up, insurance costs go up (Fig 7−4).

By developing and analyzing causal loops, the system engineer is able to determine where the system problems are, how to stimulate the system, and how to correct system problems by altering specific components. This approach focuses on the organization and its component parts.

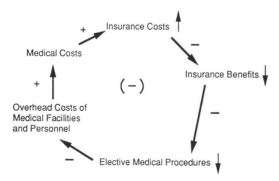

FIG 7−4.
Negative causal loop.

Total Quality Management

Although many authors refer to the behavioral approach as a humanistic approach, the humanistic approach maximizes human potential by focusing on the individual. In the behavioral approach, the focus is at times on the individual, but always with an eye toward the productivity of the individual.

W. Edwards Deming developed a manufacturing discipline in the 1930s that focused on the process of continuous improvements, in which the role of management is to coordinate and facilitate the process of work and the role of the worker is to take responsibility for the output of the system and to generate new ideas about how the process can improve. Deming has had a tremendous affect on the world economy. He first presented his management theories to Japanese manufacturers after World War II. The success of Japan's production of quality products and its leadership role in the world economy are often credited to Deming's work. Prior to World War II Japanese products were considered to be cheap, shoddy, and of cottage industry quality. When we think of Japanese products today, we think of electronics and cars of high quality, durability, and cost. This transition is not a result of new production techniques, it is the result of continuous quality improvement.

Deming presented 14 basic points to continually improve the products and processes of management (Box 7–2).[4(pp23–24)]

Deming and his followers assert that none of these 14 points can stand by themselves. The Deming approach to quality improvement is a holistic approach. The key to success in producing quality products is to control and reduce variability and maintain continuous quality improvement.

· · · · · · · · · ·
CONTINGENCY THEORY OF MANAGEMENT

The contingency theory of management recognizes all of the approaches to management that have been developed throughout the history of work. Although many of these theories have major strengths, they also have major weaknesses. The manager who identifies and uses the best of each of these approaches is following a contingency or eclectic approach to management. When managers practice the contingency theory of management, they are also said to be practicing style flexibility.

No approach works all the time in every situation. Modern managers understand that managing the work involves managing people and that situations may call for situational solutions. Eclectic managers use the best and most appropriate aspects of each theory to manage the work—trial and error approach, scientific approach, bureaucratic approach, behavioral approach, and management science approach, which includes MBO, systems theory, and total quality management.

Contigency managers are perhaps the most successful managers in the most successful companies in the United States. The review of books, tapes, and films in the area of management again and again reveals examples of the full gamut of managerial theories being practiced by Ford Motor Co, General Motors, IBM, and Delta Airlines. The fact that these companies remain not only viable, but leaders in American business attest to the fact that the managers of those companies adjust to a constantly changing environment, including the environment of management theories.

Rosabeth Moss Kanter,* in her latest book, *When Giants Learn to Dance,*[5] speaks

---

*As the Chairperson of the Department of Sociology at Yale University, Dr. Kanter was one of the first women chairpersons of an academic department in an ivy league school. She is currently the editor of the *Harvard Business Review* and a professor of business at Harvard. Dr. Kanter has made a significant contribution to the field of management science with her sociological studies of business and the publications of a trilogy of management science books entitled *Men and Women of the Corporation, The Change Masters,* and *When Giants Learn to Dance.*

· ·
BOX 7-2 DEMING'S 14 POINTS FOR MANAGEMENT*

1. Create constancy of purpose toward improvement of product and service, with the aim to become competitive and to stay in business and to provide jobs.
2. Adopt the new philosophy. We are in a new economic age. Western management must awaken to the challenge, must learn their responsibilities, and take on leadership for change.
3. Cease dependence on inspection to achieve quality. Eliminate the need for inspection on a mass basis by building quality into the product in the first place.
4. End the practice of awarding business on the basis of price tag. Instead, minimize total cost. Move toward a single supplier for any one item, forming a long-term relationship of loyalty and trust.
5. Improve constantly and forever the system of production and service to improve quality and productivity, and thus constantly decrease costs.
6. Institute training on the job.
7. Institute leadership. The aim of supervision should be to help people and machines and gadgets to do a better job. Supervision of management is in need of overhaul, as well as supervision of production workers.
8. Drive out fear, so that everyone may work effectively for the company.
9. Break down barriers between departments. People in research, design, sales, and production must work as a team to forsee problems of production and in use that may be encountered with the product or service.
10. Eliminate slogans, exhortations, and targets for the work force asking for zero defects and new levels of productivity. Such exhortations only create adversarial relationships, as the bulk of the causes of low quality and low productivity belong to the system and thus lie beyond the power of the work force.
11. a. Eliminate work standards (quotas) on the factory floor. Substitute leadership.
    b. Eliminate management by objective. Eliminate management by numbers, numerical goals. Substitute leadership.
12. a. Remove barriers that rob the hourly worker of his right to pride of workmanship. The responsibility of supervisors must be changed from sheer numbers to quality.
    b. Remove barriers that rob people in management and in engineering of their right to pride of workmanship. This means, inter alia, abolishment of the annual or merit rating and of management by objective.
13. Institute a vigorous program of education and self-improvement.
14. Put everybody in the company to work to accomplish the transformation. The transformation is everybody's job.

*From Deming WE: *Out of Crisis.* Cambridge, Mass, Massachusetts Institute of Technology, pp 23-24.

of the metaphorical games that big businesses are playing. As Dr. Kanter has traveled around the world, she has asked business leaders to think about the game that best represents their business in today's environment. Computer companies have likened business to the roller derby, in which they are constantly jamming to keep up with the competition, blocking the competition, sometimes finding themselves being thrown out of the ring, and all of this in a fast-paced and time-limited environment. Other companies have used the metaphor of water polo in which they have assembled the best possible team and the best net and ball; they know the rules of the game and are well prepared to win the game; however, they find themselves in a totally fluid environment that greatly reduces their ability to predict the outcomes of individual plays or the outcome of the game.

It is this fluid, dynamic, changing environment that Kanter reflects on in terms of the game she envisions when she thinks of today's businesses. Kanter likens the business process to the croquet game in *Alice in Wonderland,* in which nothing is as it appears to be. The croquet mallet is really a flamingo that turns its head just as the ball is to be hit. The ball is a hedgehog that begins to roll, but then uncurls and scampers away. The only thing that is constant in today's business is change—the same is true of the health care business.

This dynamic, constantly changing environment is calling for not only an eclectic management approach, but one that is sensitive to change and can assist the manager in predicting change and predicting outcomes. Managers must become change agents who are able to effect changes in both the people in the organization and the structure of the organization. Given the rapidly changing environment, these managers must also effect changes relatively quickly, which means employing both long-term planning strategies as well as incremental decision-making strategies.*

POPULAR† APPROACH TO MANAGEMENT

Among the most popular management theorists at this time are Thomas J. Peters and Robert Waterman, the authors of *In Search of Excellence: Lessons from America's Best-Run Companies.*[8] Their research on some of the best companies in America has resulted in the identification of eight characteristics that distinguish these excellent companies (Box 7–3).

Although some authors claim that elements of success are missing from the list of eight characteristics, there is no question that Peters and Waterman have had an affect on management, not only from the perspective of managers, CEOs, Boards of Trustees, and owners, but from the perspective of the consumer as well.

In 1985, Naisbitt and Aburdene[9] posed ten considerations in reinventing the corporation (Box 7–4).

These authors are heralding the emergence of the humanistic approach to organizational management. The most successful corporation is that business which stresses quality, constantly scans the environment testing product success and consumer satisfaction, and builds worker cohesion and commitment to the organization.

Peters and Waterman may be the most successful and influential of the popular theorists, but there are many others who are producing scores of books and other media in the area of management. As well as new theories, old theories are being

---

*Incremental decision making is decision making that occurs over a short time span one step at a time. The second decision in the process will then be made on the success of the first decision; the third decision will be based on the success of the second decision, and so forth.

†Popular in this context means the management theories that have attracted a great deal of popular attention. The proponents of the theories are in high demand as consultants and lecturers; the theories are published and marketed broadly and the theories are written about in the mass media. Audiotapes and videotapes are widely marketed on the theories, and managers at all levels of the organization are familiar with the concepts.

BOX 7–3 CHARACTERISTICS OF EXCELLENT COMPANIES*

1. A bias for action
2. Closeness to the customer
3. Autonomy and entrepreneurship
4. Productivity through people
5. Hands-on, value-driven
6. "Stick to the knitting"
7. Lean staff, simple form
8. Simultaneous loose-tight properties

*Adapted from Peters TJ, Waterman R: *In Search of Excellence: Lessons From America's Best-Run Companies.* New York, NY, Harper and Row, 1982.

· ·
BOX 7–4 CONSIDERATIONS IN REINVENTING THE CORPORATION*

1. The best and brightest people will gravitate toward those corporations that foster personal growth
2. The manager's new role is that of coach, teacher, and mentor
3. The best people want ownership—psychic and literal—in a company; the best companies are providing it
4. Companies will increasingly turn to third-party contractors, shifting from hired labor to contract labor
5. Authoritarian management is yielding to a networking, people style of management

6. Entrepreneurship within the corporations—intrapreneurship—is creating new products and new markets and revitalizing companies inside out
7. Quality will be paramount
8. Intuition and creativity are challenging the "it's all in the numbers" business school philosophy
9. Large corporations are emulating the positive and productive qualities of small business
10. The dawn of the information economy has fostered a massive shift from infrastructure to quality of life

*Adapted from Naisbitt J, Aburdene P: *Re- Inventing the Corporation.* New York, NY, Warner Books, 1985, pp 45–46.

resurrected. Innovators such as Deming are being rediscovered, and their theories are being applied to new situations.

The physical therapy manager must understand that management and business have come a long way since the industrial revolution and management by trial and error. Management is not a skill that can be learned on the job, through disjointed continuing education programs, or from the popular literature. The manager must be well grounded in management theory, understand and contribute to management science research, and be a skilled manager of people and organizational structures.

References

1. Fayol H: *General and Industrial Management.* Belmont, Calif, David S. Lake Publishers, 1987.
2. Megginson LC, Mosley DC, Pietri PH: *Management Concepts and Applications,* ed 3. New York, NY, Harper and Row, 1989.
3. Drucker PF: *The Practice of Management.* New York, NY, Harper and Row, 1982.
4. Deming WE: *Out of Crisis.* Cambridge, Mass, Massachusetts Institute of Technology, 1986.
5. Kanter RM: *When Giants Learn to Dance.* New York, NY, Simon and Schuster, 1989.
6. Kanter RM: *The Change Masters.* New York, NY, Simon and Schuster, 1983.
7. Kanter RM: *Men and Women of the Corporation.* New York, NY, Basic Books, Inc, 1977.
8. Peters TJ, Waterman R: *In Search of Excellence: Lessons From America's Best-Run Companies.* New York, NY, Harper and Row, 1982.
9. Naisbitt J, Aburdene P: *Re-inventing the Corporation.* New York, NY, Warner Books, 1985.

Managing People: Organizational Behavior

· · · · · · · · · · ·
THE CHANGING PHYSICAL THERAPY ENVIRONMENT

Managing individuals is perhaps one of the most challenging functions within an institution. Physical therapy managers are responsible for a number of different categories of workers, including professional staff, support staff, students, and volunteers.

In an organization, professionals behave differently from the traditional "worker" and therefore require different management strategies to maximize their contribution to the organization. Groups of professionals who are expected to exercise judgment and act in creative or innovative ways are best managed in a loosely coupled system. This is a system that recognizes that the individuals are autonomous and will perform their responsibilities most effectively if that autonomy is supported. It is therefore the responsibility of the manager to develop creative strategies to allow professional autonomy while maintaining a clear set of expectations regarding organizational behavior among all workers—including the professional staff. The successful manager of autonomous units is a manager who builds a structure that is maximally supportive to the professional staff and runs the business of the institution in such a way that the goals and missions of the institution are met.

The environment within the physical therapy service and the health care system in general is highly charged. Professionals are driven to maintain a high level of competence. This drive comes primarily from an internal need to provide the best possible care and to, above all else, maintain a high enough level of competence that the professional will do no harm. When the drive to maintain competence is not present, the manager is challenged to establish an environment that will encourage the individual to upgrade skills and increase knowledge in specific practice areas.

In addition to this drive for professional competence, the staff physical therapist is also driven to deliver quality care and to provide each patient with the best possible care. Although admirable and understandable, this drive for quality at times comes in conflict with the manager's desire for a service that is both efficient and effective.

Given the shortage of physical therapists, there is a considerable amount of pressure placed on the system to accept more patients than the individual or the service can adequately manage. For the most part, physical therapy managers as well as physical therapist staff members understand that they must maintain a reasonable schedule of patients in order to deliver quality care. Effectively managing the waiting list for the physical therapy service will reduce the pressure to move patients through the system too quickly.

Human Resource Shortages in Physical Therapy

Physical therapists are in great demand, and the percentage of the physical therapy population working in hospitals has declined (Table 8–1) from over 40% in the early 1980s, although the number of hospitals is increasing. In addition, relatively few new physical therapists are available each year when compared with other disciplines in health care (Table 8–2). As the profession of physical therapy becomes more autonomous, the physical therapist is seeking practice situations in which independence of practice and autonomy are valued. Those values are found more often in private practice, home health practice, nursing home practice, and school system practice than in traditional hospital practice. Therefore, all hospital settings are faced with developing creative employment opportunities in order to attract physical therapists to these settings as the demand dictates. The human resource shortage in physical therapy has resulted in a number of changes that are critical to the physical

TABLE 8–1. Percentage of Physical Therapists Employed by Setting*

Employer	1990
Hospitals	38.3†
Rehabilitation center	15.0
Private practice	33.9
Home health	19.3

*From *1990 Membership Survey*. American Physical Therapy Association, 1111 N Fairfax St, Alexandria, Va 22314. It is tempting to compare these data to the 1983 and 1987 membership survey data. However, the surveys were dissimilar enough that practice settings cannot be perfectly matched. There has been a shift away from hospital settings and toward private practice and home health settings, but that shift cannot be accurately documented.
†29.6% primary setting.

therapy manager. Significant increases in salary at the entry level and increasing pay scales to counteract compression and increase retention are some of the most obvious results of the shortage of physical therapists (Box 8–1).

The staff physical therapist is also driven toward autonomy. Increasingly, educational programs and the professional association are preparing physical therapists to function as autonomous professionals. Autonomy of decision making, alternative organizational structures that encourage participatory management, and concepts such as practice privileges that free the therapist of the traditional organizational structure contribute to the therapist's presumption that the individual professional within the organization is not bound by rules, policies, and procedures. Most importantly, the physical therapists may not see that they are a part of an organization or that they have responsibilities to that organization.

Physical therapists are often motivated by what the organization expects, but also by what other professionals and the professional organization expects.[1] Organizational objectives are always, to some degree, colliding with related professional objectives, and professional objectives often provide greater rewards for the physical therapist than organizational objectives (Box 8–2).[1]

TABLE 8–2. Human Resource Data

Profession	No. of Persons
Nursing*	
Licensed	2,118,900
Graduates (1989–1990)	61,060
No. of nursing education programs	
Associate degree	829
Diploma	152
BS	489
MS	231
Doctoral	50
Total	1,751
Physician†	
Licensed	615,421
Graduates (1990)	15,499
No. of medical schools	126
Physical therapy‡	
Licensed physical therapists	66,030
Physical therapist graduates (1990)	4200
No. of physical therapist educational programs (1990)	123
No. of physical therapist assistant educational programs (1990)	112

*Verbally reported by the American Nurses Association, March 1992.
†Verbally reported by the American Medical Association, March 1992.
‡Verbally reported by the American Physical Therapy Association, March 1992.

···

BOX 8–1   IMPACT OF HUMAN RESOURCE SHORTAGES
IN PHYSICAL THERAPY

Increased salaries
Increased resources for recruitment and retention
Increased resources for academia
Increased burnout
Movement away from institutions
Encroachment
Aggressive intervention

Establishing and Maintaining a Motivational Environment

Most of the popular literature in management admonishes the manager to change the traditional roles of the manager to roles that facilitate and coach the employee. The traditional roles of the manager include those of decision maker, referee, advocate, "devil's advocate," analyst, announcer, pronouncer, prognosticator, and futurist. These roles are still critical to run a department, service, or business. However, managers must not only run the department, they must also build it. Building a department involves developing a positive environment in which the employee meets personal needs while also meeting the needs of the organization. This means that the manager must develop leadership roles such as facilitator, mentor, coach, builder, nurturer of winners, enthusiast, cheerleader, and representative of others.

In order to be an effective leader, the manager must first of all know himself and then commit himself to being the leader of the department as well as the manager. Professionals (and probably most workers) are less productive when they are managed in the traditional sense because management strategies applied to people feel more like manipulation than management. Managers talk about the bottom line, productivity, quotas, resource allocation, insurance mix, budgets, and quality improvement processes. Leaders talk about building trust, open atmospheres, listening, setting professional goals, providing positive feedback, and representing and supporting the professional to the rest of management.

Physical therapists who are managers most often represent a mix of the qualities and roles of both managers and leaders. They most often function along a contin-

··

BOX 8–2   POINTS TO PONDER REGARDING PROFESSIONAL BEHAVIOR*

1. The professional is trained to operate independently
2. Power rests with the professionals
3. Professionals join organizations to obtain shared resources and skill enhancement
4. Work is coordinated and enhanced primarily through *standard* routines, communication, and common knowledge
5. Control is extremely difficult when it comes to professionals
6. The bureaucracy is set up to serve the professionals
7. Innovation and change are difficult to achieve
8. The successful professional bureaucracy gives preference to professional goals over bureaucratic goals
9. Selection of professionals is the most important organizational process

*Adapted from Feitelberg SB: Product/Service Line Management [audio tape]. Orlando, Fla, Combined Sections Meeting, American Physical Therapy Association, 1991. Produced by Infomedix, 12800 Garden Grove Blvd, Suite F, Garden Grove, CA 92643.

uum of leadership ranging from boss-centered leadership to subordinate-centered leadership (Fig 8–1).

Leadership represents a series of situational behaviors. There are situations in which workers have little to offer a particular management decision, and it is perfectly appropriate for the manager to make the decision and inform the workers of that decision. In other instances, where the worker has special knowledge or skills that will be critical to a decision, the manager will be most wise to utilize the skills of the worker in making the best decision. Continuous quality improvement focuses on subordinate-centered leadership styles, since quality improvement is predicated on the fact that the worker has significant involvement in the quality of the product or service. In addition, individuals mature within an organization or profession. As they gain maturity, they will need fewer directives from the manager and will seek more participation in organizational decision making.

It is important to separate the roles the manager plays, understand the individual manager's strengths and weaknesses in each of these roles, and then build skills that will meet both the needs of the organization and the individual worker. Given the changing needs of organizations and the opportunities outside of institutions for physical therapists and physical therapist assistants, the role of the manager is becoming increasingly complex. There is a need to master more complex management skills to compete in the rapidly changing health care environment and a need to develop leadership skills to build departments that are positive environments and enhance recruitment and retention of personnel.

Motivation is an internal process. A manager (leader) cannot motivate another person, but can establish a positive environment that enables individuals to maximize their potential. There are several personal development and management theories that should be considered by the manager in meeting the needs of the employee.

HUMAN DEVELOPMENT THEORIES

Maslow's Hierarchy of Needs

In the 1940s Abraham Maslow postulated that there was a hierarchy of needs which underlay human motivation.[2] Maslow constructed a basic hierarchy in which the most basic needs were represented at the base of a pyramid (Fig 8–2).

Physiological needs

The most basic of human needs are physiological needs that represent physical needs such as warmth, breathing, elimination, shelter, and food. These needs motivate the employee to work for a wage that will satisfy his physiological needs and those of his family. In an organization, these physiological needs are met by providing adequate wages and benefits, rest rooms, clean air and environment, and work breaks. Managers cannot make assumptions about the degree to which an individual feels that a given salary and benefit package meets that individual's physiological needs. Family size, number of working members of the family, educational loans, financial commitments, and life-style will vary from one worker to another. Once these needs are satisfied, then the next level of needs becomes the major motivator.

Safety needs

Safety needs are manifested in as many ways as there are individuals. They arise from the normal anxieties associated with the individual's personality. Fear may arise from the safety of the work environment, the location of the business, the dynamic

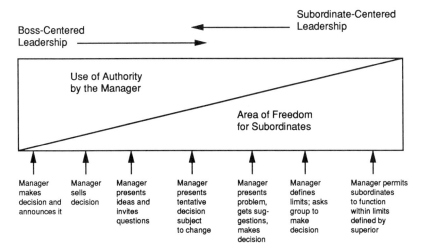

FIG 8–1.
Continuum of leadership behavior. (From Tannenbaum R, Schmidt WH: *Harvard Business Rev* 1958; 36:96–101.)

nature of the business or environment, economic security of the job, the degree of risk taking involved in the job, or even generalized fears of the shifting economy and its affect on the business and, ultimately, on the individual. Sometimes managers either do not take these fears seriously or they discount them. It is important to recognize that fears and anxieties may prevent the employee from excelling in the work environment. It is often within the power of the manager to reduce or eliminate the source of the fear or to help the individual understand and control the fear so that he can move on to higher level motivators. For example, a woman physical therapist working in an inner city hospital for the first time may have fears regarding the commute to work, parking, walking from the parking lot, and worries about the security of her car. This individual's manager may be able to institute security measures that will significantly reduce fears related to the parking lot, which will then alleviate worries that interfere with the physical therapist maximizing her potential on the job. In health care and the physical therapy environment, the constant state of change may cause many individuals to spend an extraordinary amount of energy trying to stabilize the environment.

Belonging needs

Belonging needs, which have also been referred to as social needs, loving, and affiliation, are very strong among physical therapists and physical therapist assistants, es-

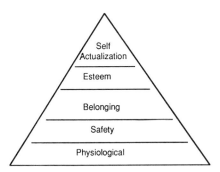

FIG 8–2.
Maslow's hierarchy of needs, physiological needs dominating.

pecially at the level of the new graduate. It is important for these individuals to feel acceptance from a professional peer group. It is this early group experience that socializes the physical therapist to clinical physical therapy and begins to establish an internal sense of both being a professional and belonging to a profession. The mere presence of other workers during intense periods of work as well as periods of relaxation add to the sense of belonging. Group work, such as special projects, inservices, conferences, and other kinds of meetings, encourages the sharing of professional experiences and the use of language and concepts that provide the framework for the profession. Managers can help structure this experience by organizing regular group meetings. However, the informal networking of the group may be equally rewarding for the individual. Managers often worry about informal groups and the informal power they gain within the department. Informal relationships allow the individual to see and experience the informal structure of the profession and to ask all of the questions that cannot be asked in a formal setting. Informal groups and relationships within the physical therapy department can be important in meeting the belonging needs of the individual. Once this sense of belonging is established, it is easier to move into more isolated work situations and still feel affiliated with a group of peers through independent activities, such as reading professional journals, attending professional meetings, representing the profession on institutional and community committees and boards, and reinforcing the roles and rules of physical therapy through peer review and continuous quality improvement activities.

Self-esteem needs

Paradoxically, once the professional or employee feels comfortable with the organization and feels a part of the group, the need to be recognized for a unique or special contribution to the group or organization motivates the employee to specialize or excel within the group. Individuals may seek a variety of specialty tracts within the physical therapy department. These tracks include management, in which the individual may become a senior physical therapist (senior physical therapist assistant), assistant manager, and manager of a department. Educational tracks begin with supervising students (physical therapy and physical therapist assistant students) as a clinical instructor, assisting the coordinator of clinical education (CCE), becoming a CCE, and eventually becoming an assistant manager responsible for all educational activities. Increasingly, with the establishment of formal clinical specialization processes through the American Board of Physical Therapy Specialities, staff physical therapists are seeking board certification as a clinical specialist. The clinical specialization not only gives therapists recognition for a specialized body of knowledge and skills, it also exposes them to other opportunities such as becoming involved in service line management in their area of specialization. The development of a variety of career ladders within the department provides individuals with avenues to build self-esteem through professional accomplishments. Once they feel competent and accomplished in their area of specialization, the need for self- actualization motivates the individual.

Self-actualization

When self-actualization is the dominant need, Maslow's pyramid may be thought of as turned upside-down (Fig 8–3). That is, each level below self-actualization has been met, and the individual is least driven by physiological needs and most driven by self-esteem and self-actualization needs. Self- actualization needs are individual and cannot be easily grouped. The individual will decide the appropriate mix of activities that will continue to reinforce self-esteem and lead to a sense of self-fulfillment and achievement. This drive appears to be similar to Erik Erikson's concept of integrity as a psychological motivator. The individual strives to feel complete, whole,

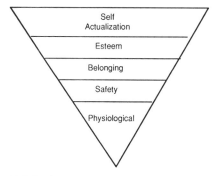

FIG 8–3.
Maslow's hierarchy of needs, self-actualization needs dominating.

accomplished, recognized, highly regarded, as if he has "arrived." This individual is least motivated by those around him or by the organization and most motivated by an internal sense of completeness. Managers sometimes assume that only CEOs achieve this level of need satisfaction. Individuals can (and do) find satisfaction and self-actualization within every employment track and every kind of work. They take pride in their work and their accomplishments. They seek challenging assignments and creative work and are committed to continuing to develop their skills. Although these individuals are sometimes perceived as a threat to the manager, they do not want the manager's job. They want to contribute and can be a powerful source of creative ideas and a work force to carry out special projects.

Locus of Control

The concept of locus of control relates to the degree to which individuals believe they have the power to control or change a given situation. Control can be seen as external to the individual or internal. When applied to patients, locus of control means the degree to which they see the control of the disease to be within or outside of their control. When asked to draw "arthritis," children who feel unable to control the disease often draw a monster much larger than themselves. They draw themselves as very small and passive. Children who feel that they have some control of the disease often draw a more realistic picture of themselves, with red, hot, swollen joints and show themselves taking their medications or doing their exercises.

Many individuals perceive organizations as monoliths that are beyond their control. They feel that they have little to contribute and that the organization is too big or intimidating to approach through management systems. Rewards and punishments are seen as being in the control of the managers and as being delivered without a clear relationship to individual performance. Although there may be innovations that these employees could suggest to increase efficiency or effectiveness of the system, they are too intimidated to contribute. Instead, they may make suggestions to their work group or, worse, will assume that nothing can change and will miss opportunities to make an impact on the operation of the organization.

When employees have a sense of internal control, they see the organization as a series of interconnected parts and perceive that they can influence the organization by making changes or suggestions related to the parts of the organization. These individuals understand that rewards or the lack of rewards is directly related to their performance and that they can influence the delivery of those rewards by their performance. These employees will make contributions and suggestions to management to increase efficiency and effectiveness of the organization. They are often the "employee of the month" because they go out of their way to try new approaches, develop innovations, and work extra hours because they see that innovations in the workplace will positively affect themselves and the organization.

Forces of Psychological Theory

Maslow has developed a schema of psychological forces at work in American society (Box 8–3). These forces have driven society to treat individuals in certain ways in its institutions (e.g., industry, health care). During the late 1800s and early 1900s, Freud's psychoanalytic theories predominated. In this force, there is a dominant authority figure who is all-knowing. The authority figure (boss, doctor) engages the individual (worker, patient) in activities that the individual may have little true appreciation for or understanding of (in industry, working machines in factories; in health care, submitting oneself to batteries of tests). In this model, the factory worker was never aware of the manufacturing process or the outcome of the work. The worker was instructed in the job and, through a series of punishments, was expected to perform that function without question.

The Hawthorne experiments were the first experiments in industry in which management gained some insight regarding behavioral theories. The Hawthorne experiments indicated that workers responded to stimuli that were representative of attention by management. It lead to the development of a broad array of reward systems related to productivity. Many of these techniques are still in existence today. Some of these rewards appeal to the individual's need for recognition and included employee of the month and other incentives for productivity. Other strategies appeal to the need for increased salaries and self-esteem and included piecemeal work in which the employee is paid for the number of pieces of products produced in a given time period. These strategies rely on a stimulus-response reaction by individuals. The employer provides a stimulus and the employee responds in a predictable way.

Current management theories rely more on maximizing the potential of the individual and in maximizing that potential, turning out the best quality product. American business is turning the corner from a mindset on producing the most to a commitment to producing the best. Continuous quality improvement, quality assessment, and quality circles are now the key to production lines rather than quotas. American management understands that if a quality product is to be produced, the worker has to be committed to quality and must have some input into the ways in which quality is measured and produced. This move toward quality is also affecting health care and health care management. The continuous quality assessment concepts have been adopted by the Joint Commission on the Accreditation of Healthcare Organizations as well as many individual health care organizations. The individual worker is now being rewarded for the outcome of the work rather than the volume. Physical therapy managers have to find creative ways to measure productivity with a quality measure incorporated into the productivity standard.

· ·

BOX 8–3 SCHEMA OF PSYCHOLOGICAL THEORIES IN AMERICAN SOCIETY*

1850s	1920s	1960s	1970s
Psychoanalytic	Behavioral	Humanistic	Self- determination

*Adapted from Goble FG: *The Third Force: The Psychology of Abraham Maslow.* New York, NY, Simon and Schuster, 1970.

Adult Development

One of the landmark studies in adult development was conducted by Daniel Levinson, a social psychologist at Yale. Levinson followed 40 men (aged 35 to 45 years), representing blue collar, white collar, professional (academicians), and artistic (novelists) occupational groups, for 5 years. Teams of evaluators interviewed the men regularly regarding personal, professional, and work activities, fears, anxieties, hopes, and other psychological reactions to changes occurring in their lives. The analysis of the research data lead to the book *Seasons of a Man's Life,* which details the study and the results. Basically, Levinson found that men went through several periods of development during their adult lives that could be organized into stable periods and transition periods (Fig 8–4).

The transition periods are periods of unrest, during which Levinson feels adults must make decisions regarding issues such as accepting a new identity as an adult during early adult transition. When decisions are made, even provisional ones, the individual moves into a more stable period of life and solidifies changes that result from the decisions.

Erikson had earlier identified eight levels of development from birth to old age, which he called the eight ages of man. He characterized these stages of development according to certain psychological tensions between opposing forces (dialectics), in which provisional decisions were called for before the person could successfully move to the next stage of development (Box 8–4).

When individuals do not make decisions related to the dialectics or when those decisions are on the negative side (mistrust, inferiority, or identity confusion), the individual must still confront these tensions in later stages of development and come to some resolution. Leaving many stages incomplete causes the individual to arrive at major transition points in life in which the work of sorting out decisions regarding life choices must be accomplished for many stages at once. This added burden of work undone can cause many transition points in development to become traumatic periods of time.

Levinson connects Erikson's dialectics to adult development and the transition periods that move the adult from early to late adulthood (Table 8–3). Levinson's study was conducted entirely on men. Similar studies are now being conducted on groups of women. Levinson's stages of development may be similar for women. It is possible, however, that rather than a mid-life transition in the fourth decade of life, women experience a major transition period in the third decade of life, when they are faced with decisions regarding bearing children (biological clock) or continuing to pursue career opportunities.

Managers must realize that individuals continue to grow as adults. As adults, they

· ·

BOX 8–4   ERIKSON'S STAGES OF DEVELOPMENT*

Dialectics	Developmental Phase
Trust vs. mistrust	Infancy
Initiative vs. guilt	Early childhood
Autonomy vs. shame	Early childhood
Industry vs. inferiority	Childhood and adolescence
Identity vs. identity confusion	Adolescence
Intimacy vs. isolation	Young adulthood
Generativity vs. stagnation	Adulthood and middle age
Integrity vs. despair	Old age

*From Erikson EH: *Identity and the Life Cycle.* New York, NY, WW Norton Co, 1980.

TABLE 8–3. Adult Development*

Age (yr)	Stage	Erikson's Dialectics	Characteristics
17–22	Early adult transition	Identity vs. identity confusion	Moving out of pre–adult world; modify or terminate existing relationships with important people, groups, institutions
22–28	Entering the adult world	Intimacy vs. isolation	Fashion a provisional structure that provides a workable link between the valued self and the adult society; makes and tests choices in occupation, love, and peer relationships, values, and life-style
28–33	Age 30 transition		Work out flaws and limitations of the first adult structure; create the basis for a more satisfactory structure
33–40	Settling down		Invest self in major components of the structure (work, family, friendships, leisure, community) and realize youthful aspirations and goals
40–45	Mid-life transition		Life structure comes into question; yearning for a life in which actual desires, values, talents, and aspirations can be expressed
45–50	Entering middle adulthood	Generativity vs. stagnation	Make choices and form a new life structure
50–55	Age 50 transition		Work further on the tasks of the mid-life transition. May be time of crisis for those who changed little in mid-life transition
55–60	Culmination of middle adulthood		Stable period—building a second middle adult structure
60–65	Late adult transition	Integrity vs. despair	Terminates middle adulthood; forms a basis for starting late adulthood; major turning point in the life cycle; conclude efforts of middle adulthood and prepare for the era to come

*Adapted from Levinson D: *Seasons of a Man's Life.* New York, NY, Ballantine Books, 1978.

will have long stable periods in that development and dramatic transition periods. The transition periods are times when workers examine work along with many other aspects of life and make employment decisions that are in line with overall decisions during these periods of time.

In a master's project, Maggie Everett, P.T., M.S., described the physical therapist's drives toward autonomy of practice based on levels of psychological development. This project was a pilot study of a small number of physical therapists who practiced in geriatrics. It was speculated that the therapist would make predicable practice decisions based on stages of adult development and professional experiences and professional growth (Fig 8–5).

Through interviews with physical therapists at varying levels of development professionally and personally, Everett found that there was a relationship between the psychological needs of therapists and their practice setting decisions. Younger therapists seemed to make practice decisions guided by the need to forge a new identity as a professional. That identity was reinforced by working with peer groups. New graduates most often choose to work in an institution with a large staff in a position, which gives them exposure to the broad spectrum of practice.

As therapists become more experienced in the general practice of physical therapy and approaches the intimacy vs. isolation dialectic, they will be prepared to make specialty decisions that will isolate them from their peers.

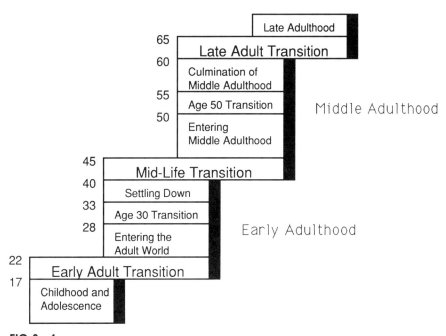

FIG 8—4.
Levinson's stages of adult development. (From Levinson D: *The Seasons of a Man's Life.* New York, NY, Ballantine Books, p 57.)

Career Choices and Personality Type

Many studies have been conducted of personality types and work. The most common inventories used to study personality types is the Myers-Briggs Personality Inventory, an inventory based on jungian psychology focusing on degrees of introversion and extroversion.

Personality types of physical therapists have been studied and demonstrate physical therapists to be predominantly ISFJ (introverted, sensing, feeling, judging), ESFJ (extroverted, sensing, feeling, judging), and ISTJ (introverted, sensing, thinking, judging) personality types. ISFJ personality types are practical and adapt easily to routine. In addition, they value loyalty, consideration, and the common welfare of others. People who are ESFJ personality type usually choose an occupation that provides them with an opportunity to help others. They are practical, matter-of-fact, and the most adaptable to routine of all the 16 types. People who are ISTJ personality type enjoy responsibility and lend stability to situations through their use of past and present experiences. They emphasize logic, analysis, decisiveness, and are painstakingly thorough. A high number of ISTJs is not common for health care workers since they usually seek administrative and executive positions.

Among the health care workers Js (judging types) are more prominent, but generally by only 10% to 15% more. Several recent studies of physical therapist personality types have demonstrated a predominant number of people demonstrating judging as a personality characteristic. This would suggest that physical therapists work best when they can organize/plan their activities and follow that plan. They dislike ambiguity and prefer a regular routine rather than a less time-oriented setting.

Knowing the personality characteristics of the physical therapist has important implications for self-evaluation and self-counseling within individual career paths. Managers can use these tools to better understand themselves and to assist individuals in understanding their choices and work behaviors. From a management per-

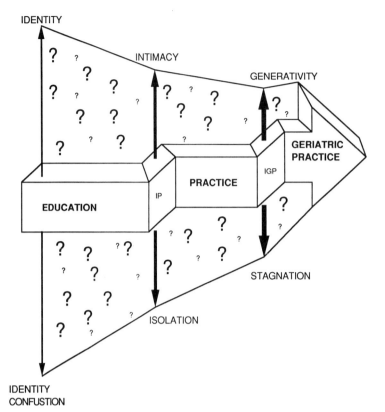

FIG 8–5.
Physical therapist practice and specialty choices. *IP* = initial practice; *IGP* = initial geriatric practice.

spective, it is important to know that diversity exists in the profession, that some personality types are more common in physical therapy, and that there is a relationship between work behaviors and personality type.

Transactional Analysis

Among the popular psychological theories are those developed by Eric Berne and reported in popular psychology books such as *I'm OK, You're OK.* Berne presents a theory of interaction using the ego states of parent, adult, and child. Basically, Berne states that open communication exists when there is complementary communication between two parties. For example, if a person speaks to another (transaction) from an adult-to-adult perspective, the expected result will be an adult-to-adult response. If the individual receiving the first communication responds in an unexpected manner such as parent-to-child (defensiveness), that transaction is crossed and communication will stop (Fig 8–6).

These are only two of the many kinds of transactions that Berne discusses. Concentrating on transactions between individuals and within groups will lead to more open and productive communication.

Many individuals are hampered by poor communication role models. Concepts such as transactional analysis provide individuals with a common framework with which to work on communication. They learn a language related to transactions which they can share with their peers and use in a nonthreatening way to improve communications with coworkers and supervisors.

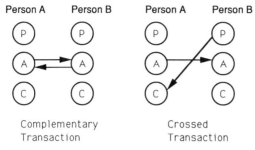

FIG 8−6.
Open and closed transactions.

Dealing With Defenses

Everyone uses defense mechanisms to protect themselves from threats. Some people become very quiet, some cry, some strike out, some joke, and others dig their heels in and do not move. It is important that managers understand they are not psychologists. It is not appropriate to confront the individual about their defense mechanisms. When a worker feels threatened, normal defense mechanisms will emerge. The worker will be able to control these defenses and move on if the manager focuses on the work behavior under question, not on the individual, and gives the individual enough time to cope with the facts that are presented. Although managers often feel that workers must have known that their work was deficient, or that a particular act would put the organization at risk, that is often not the case. Therefore, when the worker is confronted it is often a surprise, which causes defensiveness. Time allows the individual to cope with the facts or the issues and reduces the need to react defensively.

• • • • • • • • • • •
MANAGEMENT THEORIES RELATED TO MANAGING PEOPLE

Herzberg's Theory of Motivation

The two-factor management theory of work motivation is most often attributed to Frederick Herzberg (Box 8−5). Many managers do not feel that the theory has held up to the scrutiny of management research and have dismissed it as a valid theory of motivation. However, it remains popular as a management theory among many managers, including health care managers. The theory is based on two sets of factors, those that motivate the individual to work and those that, if absent, would lead to dissatisfaction with the job (hygiene/maintenance factors). The factors related to as motivators cause the individual to be excited about the work. If motivators are not present, people will not necessarily leave the job, or even complain. However, they will not feel that their talents are being fully utilized, and they will not excel.

When hygiene or maintenance factors are absent, employees are dissatisfied. Again, they will not leave the job, but morale will be low and absenteeism and turnover will be high.

McGregor's Theory X and Theory Y

In the early 1960s, Douglas McGregor introduced Theory X and Theory Y of motivation (Box 8−6). He speculated that the traditional employers of the time perceived

. . . .
BOX 8–5 HERZBERG'S THEORY OF MOTIVATION

Motivating factors
  Achievement
  Responsibility and power
  Recognition and utilization of abilities
  Advancement and visibility within the organization
  Creative and challenging work
  Possibilities for growth on the job
  Tasks that lead to improvement of knowledge or skills
  Autonomy
  Involvement in the "big picture"
Hygiene (maintenance) factors
  Company policies and administration
  Quality of technical supervision
  Interpersonal relationships; supervisors treating employees well; time to
    relate to other employees
  Salary and fringe benefits
  Job security, seniority rules, and promotion system
  System of recognition of diligence and loyalty
  Physical working conditions
  Good orientation program
  Open communications

the worker as basically lazy, unmotivated to work, seek security above all else, and are in need of close supervision in order to accomplish tasks (Theory X). McGregor felt that modern managers had to change their perception of workers to be more in line with maximizing the worker's human potential. That meant that employers should perceive the worker as a person who likes work, is motivated at all levels of need toward excellence in work, and needs supervisors who can facilitate the work and worker (Theory Y).

. . . .
RECRUITMENT AND RETENTION

Recruitment and retention of physical therapists is one of the major problems facing managers in the hospital setting. Reflecting on many of the motivational theories that have been introduced in this chapter, several programs have been instituted in hospital physical therapy programs to enhance the individual's motivation to remain in this setting.

The shortage of physical therapists has caused starting salaries to increase dramatically. At the same time, compression of salaries for more experienced physical therapists is leading to low morale. Incentive plans are being developed throughout the health care system to encourage individuals to remain in the institution. Incentives have become an important tool for physical therapy managers to improve retention. When financial incentive programs are being planned, it is important to build a quality measure into the system so that individuals are not simply rewarded for an increase in numbers (patients treated, dollars collected). Many incentive programs are attractive to workers because they can pace themselves and know the financial rewards that they will earn with specific levels of output on their part. Some incentive programs such as career laddering will also give physical therapists the opportunity to enrich their professional credentials and their work environment. The

· ·
BOX 8–6 MCGREGOR'S THEORY*

Theory X	Theory Y
1. Most people do not want to work	1. Work is a natural activity, if the conditions are favorable
2. Most people are lazy, have little desire for responsibility, and prefer to be directed	2. Self-control is valued in achieving organizational goals
3. Most people have little capacity for creativity in solving organizational problems	3. The capacity for creativity in solving organizational problems is widely distributed among the workers
4. Motivation occurs only at the physiological and safety levels	4. Motivation occurs at the belonging, esteem, and self-actualization levels, as well as physiological and safety levels
5. Most people must be closely controlled and often coerced to achieve organizational objectives	5. People can be self-directed and creative at work if properly motivated

*From McGregor D: *The Human Side of Enterprise.* New York, NY, Harper and Row, 1959.

incentive programs are also valuable to the manager because it enhances worker commitment to the department, it gives the manager definitive tools to measure individual productivity and contribution, and it links the salary program to definitive results of work.

Variable pay incentive programs support the humanistic culture and reduce the worker's sense of entitlement to specific salary, promotions, and seniority benefits. They also increase the therapist's role as a stakeholder in the department and the institution and they communicate a set of values related to the relationship between the productivity and quality of the product/services.

There are several kinds of financial incentive programs. Some will focus on the *individual worker* and productivity. In these systems target productivity levels within a set of quality guidelines are established and the individual worker is paid predetermined variable amounts of money for achieving specific targets. These are perhaps the most easily assessed and fairly administered incentive programs. Individual systems are also sometimes built on the management by objectives principles, and the individual manager is financially rewarded for meeting objectives at a specific quality level. These programs are fraut with bias similar to the bias of a performance appraisal system.

Profit sharing is determined by a pre-arranged formula. It does not focus on productivity, but on the bottom line. Individuals will receive a specified share of the profits after all expenses are paid and the profit for the year is determined.

Group incentive plans are sometimes developed for groups of workers and are based on a framework of what people are to achieve and the rewards that will be paid for achieving specific targets. This system is similar to the piecemeal incentive programs used in American industry.

Wherever possible, physical therapy managers are increasing salary steps to decrease salary compression. Bonuses or lump sum incentive pay is being instituted based on creativity and quality performance. The bonus concept provides a financial reward to the therapist without increasing base salary, which often appeals to upper management.

In addition to salary considerations, physical therapy managers are concentrating on the self-esteem and self-actualizational needs to provide incentives for staff. These incentives include expanded educational leaves and sabbaticals, the development of educational loan programs for individuals who are seeking certification or advanced degrees, and cultural exchange programs with other countries such as England, Japan, and India. Although licensure has not been worked out with these exchange programs, the therapists have a significant opportunity to learn about health care in the exchange community and to learn another language and culture.

Clinical ladders and mentoring programs have also been developed for all levels of staff to recognize special contributions and to help individuals to refine skills and gain new skills. These programs can be seen as incentive programs that reward knowledge and skills.

The shortage of physical therapists has increased the need to keep more experienced physical therapists in institutions and devoted to clinical practice. Clinical ladders provide opportunities for advancement in the area of practice. The goals of the ladder are to serve the patients, staff, and department.

Physical therapy managers should first determine the departmental values related to clinical practice and the mission of the department in relation to the institution and determine the clinical goals of the department. These goals might include quality patient care, professional growth and development for department staff, and engaging in quality clinical research. Clinical ladders can help to meet those goals and provide for advancement and recognition of individual therapists.

Many departments have created clinical ladders with a variety of levels of therapists. Most of these models focus on clinical practice, staff development, clinical research, and community outreach activities (Box 8–7).

These clinical ladders should also consider the need to retain experienced physical therapist assistants and their developmental needs and develop similar depart-

. . . .

BOX 8–7 CLINICAL LADDER MODEL*

1. Entry level
   Staff therapist at entry level (new graduate or returning to the field)
      Develop expertise
      Build skills
      Develop a specialty
2. Demonstrated clinical expertise
   Two years' experience
      Define specialty
      Act as a resource
      Develop clinical skills
      Share clinical skills with patients and staff
3. Clinical specialist
   Five years' experience
      Teach staff and community
      Facilitate professional growth in the department
      Develop clinical skills for themselves and others
      Conduct clinical research
      Take part in community outreach
4. Senior
   Four years' experience
      Bridge the gap between the administrative levels
      Assume responsibility for special projects
      Participates in day-to-day management of department
      Continue own skill development
      Focus on overall departmental growth

*From Edwards A: Clinical Ladder [audiotape]. San Francisco, Calif, Combined Sections Meeting, American Physical Therapy Association, 1992.

mental levels for them. In very large departments physical therapy aides are also included in a clinical laddering program.

A wide variety of staff recognition programs also meet self-esteem needs of the staff. These programs vary from employee-of-the-month awards to award dinners where staff members are recognized for a variety of contributions. In addition, the establishment of awards for people associated with the department provide an avenue for them to recommend professionals or staff members from other departments who have been particularly helpful to individual therapists or the department. For example, one department developed a Physical Therapy Service Award, which was given once a year to a person in another hospital department who provided exceptional services to the physical therapy department. The award was given at a lunch hosted by the physical therapy department for the awardee, his/her guests, supervisors from his/her department, and selected hospital administrators. The first award was given to a carpenter who had gone out of his way to work with a number of the therapists to modify and build equipment. Several of the innovations developed jointly by this person and the therapists had been published in the physical therapy literature and one was being considered for mass production by an equipment company. The head table consisted of the guest of honor and his wife, his supervisor and hospital administrator, and the therapists he had worked with over the past several years (even some therapists who had left the department returned for the event). Pictures of the innovative equipment were blown up and displayed around the room. The event was covered by both the hospital and local press and received a great deal of local coverage. These kinds of activities meet the needs of the therapists for recognition as well as those of the awardee.

SUPERVISORY RELATIONSHIPS

Physical Therapist: Physical Therapist Assistant

Physical therapist assistants have been in existence since the 1950s, when the first educational program was established and the first licensing law was passed that defined their role. The American Physical Therapy Association (APTA) recognized the assistant and made provisions for a special category of membership in the association in 1971, when the House of Delegates created the Affiliate Member category. Physical therapist assistants are technical health care workers who perform certain physical therapy procedures under the supervision of the physical therapist. It is critical to remember that this worker is called a physical *therapist* assistant, not a physical *therapy* assistant. The intent is that, in states where the assistant is licensed, the licensing laws should reflect that this category of worker is directly responsible to a physical therapist and should not work independently or under the supervision of a health care provider other than a physical therapist.

Although the intent of the supervisory requirement is not always adhered to in state laws or in practice, it is incumbent upon the manager and the physical therapist assistant to support the supervisory intent that was established in the creation of this category of worker.

Physical therapist assistants are not qualified to conduct initial patient evaluations, plan programs, or perform some complex therapeutic procedures. The reality of practice is that no health care worker can—or should—apply a procedure without evaluating the patient's response and taking some action based on that response. Therefore, in order to work safely and competently, the physical therapist assistant is called upon to perform some evaluative functions. This kind of evaluation is called a formative evaluation. It is the process of evaluation in action. As physical therapist assistants conduct these evaluations of immediate response to treatment, the information is both recorded and called to the attention of the physical therapist. Initial evaluations and evaluations conducted at specific follow-up points are called summative evaluations. *Physical therapist assistants should not conduct summative evaluations.* The supervisory relationships and scope of practice of the physical therapist and the work of the physical therapist assistant should be clearly stated in written policy and procedure documents within the department.

Given the shortage of physical therapists in the United States, it is very tempting for the individual therapist as well as the manager to extend the responsibilities of the physical therapist assistant. It is equally tempting for physicians and facility administrators to hire physical therapist assistants to provide physical therapy services without the supervision of a physical therapist. In states where physical therapist assistants are licensed, careful attention must be paid to the points of law, administrative rules, and the intent of the legislation regarding supervision and scope of work. When there is no law governing physical therapist assistants, physical therapy managers should continue to be guided by the APTA's policies and procedures related to this category of worker. For instance, since the Commission for the Accreditation of Physical Therapy Education Programs has standards and criteria related to educational programs for physical therapist assistants, managers must not develop short-term, institutionally based educational programs for the training of individuals whom the institution then calls physical therapist assistants. Individuals who work in the physical therapy environment, are not physical therapist or physical therapist assistant students, and have not graduated from an accredited educational program for physical therapist assistants *must* not be called physical therapist assistants. Even if these individuals have been specially trained by the institution, they are still physical therapy aides—not physical therapist assistants. Unless physical therapists and physical therapy managers respect the standards of training and practice for this category of worker, there will be great confusion throughout the United States regarding the training and responsibilities of such workers.

On the other hand, physical therapist assistants have the same self-esteem and self-actualization needs as any other worker. In the department, career ladders should be considered which promote, where appropriate, the development of a senior physical therapist assistant position or physical therapist assistant clinical instructor position. Physical therapist assistants have a traditionally technical degree (associate arts) from a community or technical college. Many of these individuals are continuing their education to obtain advanced degrees in management, education, and the behavioral sciences. They are satisfying their entrepreneurial needs by establishing businesses such as contract services in which they provide physical therapist and physical therapist assistant services to home health agencies and nursing homes. Physical therapy managers, along with the profession in general, must examine the alternative paths available to physical therapist assistants and the potential impact these paths will have on the physical therapist assistant and the profession. Each department must clearly articulate through its policies and procedures both the rights and the limitations of responsibilities for all categories of workers.

Professions and Professionals

There is an ongoing debate between physical therapist assistants and physical therapists regarding the designation of the physical therapist assistant as a professional. Physical therapist assistants feel that they have the same values, traditions, and commitment as the physical therapist. Furthermore, society uses the term professional loosely, assigning it to the professional cosmetologist, barber, plumber, and maintenance worker.

The process of becoming a profession and the definition of a profession have become the topic of many sociological studies. The only true professions, according to many authors, are law, medicine, and the clergy. Other professions such as physical therapy are considered to be semiprofessions, since they have not met all of the criteria of a profession, which include autonomy, the existence of a unique body of knowledge, a code of ethics, responsibility for life and death decisions, and public recognition. Forsythe has studied the process of development as a profession (Box 8–8). During phase I of development, the profession must examine if it is "essential (of serious importance to clients), exclusive (the occupational practitioners have a monopoly on the service-task), and complex (the service-task is not routine and typically involves the individual and discretionary application of a specialized body of knowledge)."[3] In addition, the profession must demonstrate in phase I that it is engaged in image-building activities that are usually carried out by a professional organization.

In phase II of the development process, the public defers to the "expert skill and knowledge of the individual professional practicing that service-task. The deference shown by the public and the uncertainty of the service-task may singly, or in combination, limit the control of the employing organization over individual professionals and their tasks."[3] It is this level of autonomy that is in question in physical therapy. In many states, physical therapists may not practice autonomously, and in most institutions they are considered to be employees, not independent professionals.

Phase III is concerned with stabilizing and maintaining the status of the profession and assuring that it continues to meet the criteria of a profession. This is the phase in which standards are applied to the educational and practice processes.

If we adhere to the strict definitions and scholarly concepts of professions and professionals, then physical therapist assistants are not professionals, and in that light are not considered to be professionals by the national association. However, if we consider the popular view and existence of mimic professions, which take on the appearance of professions but are not, then we may consider the physical therapist assistant a professional. If the profession is to move to a true profession with the degree of autonomy dictated by such a designation, then we cannot consider the physical therapist assistant as a professional from a public policy perspective.

The key to recruiting and retaining physical therapist assistants is the relationship between the physical therapists and the physical therapist assistants and the de-

. . . .

BOX 8–8 DEVELOPMENT OF A PROFESSION*

Phase I
    Service is essential, exclusive, and complex
    Image-building activities are in place
Phase II
    If successful public recognition, there is
        Autonomy from the client
        Autonomy from the employing organization
    If unsuccessful public recognition, profession is identified as a mimic profession
Phase III
    Client autonomous: semiprofessions
    Organizational autonomy: semiprofessions
    Full autonomy: true professions

*From Forsyth PB, Danisiewicz TJ: *Work Occup* 1985; 12:59–76.

gree of understanding and respect for the role of the physical therapist assistant by the department and facility administration. The physical therapist assistant has a need (as all workers) to belong. They are still struggling to achieve this sense of belonging in the APTA and within the state and facility in which they work. There are many facilities in which the administration is still proud to announce that they have not hired one physical therapist assistant. Physical therapist assistants cannot begin to meet their self-esteem and self-actualization needs until they feel a part of the profession, the association, and the facility in which they work. Once this is accomplished there will be a greater need to look at career laddering, educational leaves, and recognition.

The primary goal of the physical therapy manager is to include the physical therapist assistant in appropriate levels of decision making and department activities and clearly articulate with that person the role of the physical therapist assistant in the profession and the facility. These discussions should be followed by the development of procedures and policies that will reinforce the involvement of the physical therapist assistant.

Physical Therapist: Physical Therapist Assistant: Physical Therapy Aide

Physical therapy aides are unlicensed workers who are trained on the job to perform basic tasks that are related to the operation of the physical therapy department. Traditionally, the physical therapy aide is supervised by the physical therapist who is present at the same site as the physical therapy aide. In some states where physical therapist assistants are licensed, those licensing laws allow the physical therapist assistant to supervise physical therapy aides, physical therapist assistant students, and volunteers. In states other than those governed by licensing laws for the physical therapist assistant, it may also be the customary practice of the physical therapy service to allow the physical therapist assistant to supervise physical therapist assistant students and physical therapy aides. When physical therapist assistants do supervise other workers, there should be written policies regarding the conditions of this supervision and the responsibilities of the physical therapist assistant in this situation.

Physical therapy aides traditionally perform non–patient related duties without direct supervision.* These activities include cleaning and repair of equipment and facilities, transportation of patients, equipment preparation (filling of whirlpools), and preparation of patients for treatment (transfers, dressing activities, draping). The physical therapy aide may also perform some direct patient care with little supervision when that patient is at the point in the treatment process where the patient or a family member could be taught to perform the treatment. Activities such as ambulation, doning of splints and braces, transfers, and wheelchair mobility may be included in direct patient care responsibilities of the physical therapy aide.

Physical therapy aides may be restricted by laws and administrative rules from engaging in specific patient care activities. For instance, in some states wound debridement is considered a medical procedure and may be delegated by the physician only to health care professionals who are licensed.

Physical therapy managers should also consider standards of supervision and practice that are supported by the profession. These standards can be discerned by reviewing policies and procedures of the APTA and by engaging in discussions and debates regarding the appropriate use of support personnel. Physical therapy aides should not engage in either formative or summative evaluations of patients, program

---

*Physical therapy aides should be supervised on site on a continuous basis. However, there are many instances in which on-sight supervision is not necessary. This on-sight supervision is referred to here as direct supervision.

planning or modification, documentation, or the performance of advanced therapeutic procedures.

Under no circumstances should a physical therapy aide act in such a manner as to be represented as a physical therapist or a physical therapist assistant.

Again, it is tempting during this period of human resource shortage to overutilize the physical therapy aide. Physical therapy managers should carefully monitor the use of aides and the volume of patients and make adjustments in patient volume whenever the quality of care is significantly threatened by overutilization of technical personnel.

Volunteers

Many volunteers are interested in working in physical therapy environments for a variety of reasons. Some of these people have received or have had a relative receive a significant course of physical therapy and they have become interested in helping other people through the process. These volunteers are often motivated by a need to help other people as a patient model. The role of the manager is to fully understand the volunteer's motivation for offering services. If it is to provide a patient perspective, the volunteer must be carefully interviewed and supervised regarding the quality of the interaction with patients and families. Volunteers are more apt to impose their personal values on others if those values/beliefs have helped them through similar experiences. If persons volunteer for such an assignment, they will be most comfortable in jobs in which they are able to speak to patients and families and will usually volunteer to transport patients, sit with patients during modalities, or sit with waiting patients and families.

Other volunteers may have little interest in patient-related activities, but would like to provide a variety of services to the department. Some of these include sewing sandbags for weights, building equipment, crocheting wheelchair lap robes, and making small exercise equipment.

The growing number of physical therapist and physical therapist assistant applicants to educational programs provides another ready source of volunteers in physical therapy departments. Although these students are willing to take part in all activities, it will be most helpful to the student in deciding on physical therapy as a career or solidifying that decision, to take part in a number of patient/therapist interactions even if the role of that volunteer is to observe. These volunteers may be willing to work in isolated environments or to perform a variety of cleaning tasks, but those tasks may not be of most benefit to the student at this early stage of decision making.

The physical therapy manager must closely screen volunteers and only accept volunteers when there is a match between the needs of the volunteer and the needs of the department. If volunteers are accepted as extra hands or simply because they want to volunteer, there is a great potential of increased supervisory time managing the volunteer.

The manager should also take an active part in seeking volunteers for specific activities by speaking to community service organizations. Volunteer efforts can reduce the costs of running the department, and community members will often volunteer when they know that there will be a direct savings or increased services for ill or disabled members of the community. Women's clubs are often anxious to produce small handmade items, organize activities for outpatients such as swimming outings or trips to the flower show, and to transport patients to appointments. Men's clubs are often interested in assisting with major redecorating or moving activities, organizing handicapped sporting events, and producing large equipment such as mats or exercise tables. Many community service organizations have taken on major projects to assist the visually and hearing impaired, and they are anxious to get involved in other health-related activities that will benefit their community.

SOCIAL AND MORAL NORMS

The workplace is changing, and the health care workplace is changing dramatically. Daniel Yankelovich, in his book *New Rules,* presented national norms related to work from decades of public opinion research conducted in the 1930s, 1940s, 1970s, and 1980s. These norms are important to consider because the health care professional and support staff do not come to the work environment devoid of any opinions or values related to work. If the physical therapy manager is going to establish a motivating environment, it is important to understand the values and attitudes of the American workers. Max Weber has stated that "man is an animal suspended in webs of significance he himself has spun."[4(p12)] Yankelovich has applied Weber's philosophical statement to Americans and states that "the webs of significance Americans have spun revolve around the shared meaning of self-fulfillment."[4(p13)] Yankelovich states that "in our preoccupation with self-fulfillment we have also grown recklessly unrealistic in our demands on our institutions."[4(p3)] Although Yankelovich's work covers a wide variety of social and moral norms, only a few of those norms are considered that may have an impact on the health care worker (Box 8–9).

The roles of men and women are changing in American society. Although many women have worked in the past, such as during the industrial revolution when they worked for much cheaper wages than men and during wars when men were not available, more women work today out of choice in more responsible positions than ever before. As women have found work to be rewarding and the state of the economy has increasingly made two salaries a necessity, the American family has changed also. Workers no longer believe, for instance, that child care is strictly the responsibility of women. Men are taking more time off to care for children. Men and women usually share responsibility for caring for unexpected illnesses, absence of a babysitter, or doctor/dentist appointment keeping. Physical therapy managers must be prepared to deal with the changing roles of men and women without bias.

At one time in our history, work was the center of the individual's life and the family was organized around that work. Meals were scheduled at convenient times for the worker, family outings were deferred to nonworking hours, and family vacations became a function of the work vacation. Most workers no longer see the job to be the center of either their life or that of their family. Although workers continue to plan most activities around work hours, they will often erode work hours for health care appointments, car repairs, home services appointments, and many other activities. In addition, it is less common for workers to put in overtime with or without compensation or to rearrange vacations or holidays for work-related activities. Phys-

BOX 8–9 SOCIAL ATTITUDES RELATED TO WORK

Disapprove of a married woman earning money if she has a husband capable of supporting her	1938 = 75%; 1978 = 26%
Agree that both sexes have the responsibility to care for small children	1970 = 33%; 1980 = 56%
Agree that hard work always pays off	1969 = 58%; 1976 = 43%
Agree that work is at the center of my life	1970 = 34%; 1978 = 13%
Would go on working for pay even if they didn't have to	1957 = 58%; 1976 = 77%

ical therapy managers should understand that some of these values will require rules to assist the worker in planning time and activities. In addition, because workers are less likely to make short-term changes in life-style, managers must try to plan ahead and notify workers of changes in schedules or expectations.

· · · · · · · · · · ·
MEN AND WOMEN IN ORGANIZATIONS

Most of the information we have about workers either relate directly to male workers or are conceptualized and analyzed by men using predominantly masculine constructs related to organizations, managing the work, and motivating the worker. Many of the management theories presented in this book and used extensively in management are grounded in information and conceptual frameworks related to work and workers in a traditional society in which men are the primary breadwinners and women are the primary caregivers. Many of these societal constructs are changing, and with those changes there are significant changes in work and workers.

A recent study by Raz and coworkers examined the needs of women physical therapists in the profession (Box 8–10). Although this was a limited study, it poses many questions regarding the work experiences of women physical therapists and the values which they bring to the work environment.

· ·
BOX 8–10 VALUES AND EXPERIENCES OF WOMEN PHYSICAL THERAPISTS*

Relationship and caring	Interpersonal relationships with patients and colleagues are highly valued
Context	Patients are viewed in the context of home, family, and community
Empowerment	Foster independence and individual growth in patients
Family role	Family responsibilities have both limitations and enhancements and have a significant impact on the work lives of women physical therapists
Enhancements	Single mothers have an increased incentive to develop and maintain their professional identity
	Reproductive, nurturing, and caregiving roles may increase the appeal of pediatric, obstetric, and geriatric physical therapy for some women
Limitations	Time and energy constraints from family responsibilities
	Impact of constraints on full participation in professional activities, continuing education, and administrative opportunities
	Commitment to work is in conflict with commitment to family; the degree of this conflict varies among individuals
	Women still take primary responsibility in rearing children
	Women must make compromises
Coping strategies	Choose to work part time
	Limitations on hours worked
	Job sharing
	Flex hours
Leadership	Limited time to pursue positions
	Sense of powerlessness without leadership positions
	Some experience sexism in pursuit of leadership positions

*Adapted from Raz P, Jensen GM, Walter JM: *Physical Therapy* 1991; 71:530–540.

This study did not suggest that women hold these values or have these experiences exclusively. Men may also share these values and experiences to some degree.

Rosabeth Moss Kanter was one of the first leading sociologists to conduct scholarly work in organizations related to the differing roles of men and women.

Among the many differences between men and women in an organization is the manner in which they are mentored within the organization. In a practice environment in physical therapy, most people who could serve as mentors are women. Several researchers who have looked at women as mentors have discovered that many women see mentoring as a burden and are less likely to do it. Most women do not realize that mentoring younger generations will enhance their own skills and enrich their career. Men are more naturally drawn to the mentoring process by virtue of hundreds of years of work behavior that has focused on guiding young men into skilled work. The early craftsmen served as masters to young apprentices, colonial college teachers lived in student living/learning centers and guided the young man's learning, and early professionals took on young clerks in medicine and the law to teach professions that were not yet grounded in professional education. Women have come to the work force and to professional careers much later in the evolution of work in the United States. They are not socialized to guiding, sponsoring, and mentoring younger generations from a work perspective. The mentoring skills of women are often grounded in their family and community oriented nurturing skills and are not easily adapted to the work environment.

Within the corporate health care environment most mentors are men, but women are becoming more visible in this role as they emerge in the corporate structure as managers and executives. In addition to the traditional role of sponsors to teach and open doors, Kanter describes three other important functions.

1. To fight for the person in question.

2. Provide opportunity to bypass the hierarchy.

3. Provide a signal to others, a form of reflected power (Kanter, 1977, pp. 182–183). As important as sponsors are to men, Kanter points out that they are even more important to women—and more difficult to find (Kanter, 1977, p. 184).

Corporate executives (managers) must conscientiously groom new executives (managers). Jennings describes four different sets of superiors who can sponsor individuals in an organization. Evaluators have the necessary visibility to evaluate the manager's performance. Nominators are evaluators who stand well enough with their peers and superiors to be asked to nominate men for promotions. Sponsors are nominators who stand so well with the authority that the latter will think twice before the sponsor's recommendations are rejected. Promoters have the authority to place people.[5]

From a developmental perspective, Levinson, whose studies have focused on men's adult development, describes the mentor as a man who is several years older than the novice and as having greater experience and sensitivity. The mentor is a teacher, advisor, and sponsor. Levinson has dealt briefly with the issue of women in a mentoring relationship, indicating that "cross-gender mentoring . . . is often limited by the tendency frequently operating in both of them (man and woman) to make her less than she is, to regard her as attractive but not gifted. . . , as an intelligent but impersonal pseudo male or as a charming little girl who cannot be taken seriously."[6(p98)] Levinson describes the mentor's characteristics with great similarity to the descriptions that emerge from the management literature. The mentor functions as a teacher, sponsor, host, exemplar, counselor, and parent (Box 8–11).[6(p98)]

Levinson's research suggests that mentoring relationships for men last 2 to 3 years and may last as many as 10 years. It usually ends when one man moves,

· ·
BOX 8–11   MENTOR'S FUNCTIONS ACCORDING TO LEVINSON*

Teacher	To enhance the person's skills and intellectual development
Sponsor	To facilitate the person's entry and advancement by using his influence
Host and guide	To welcome the initiate into a new occupational, social world and acquaint him with the values, customs, resources, and cast of characters
Exemplar	To model through his own virtues, achievements, and way of living
Counselor	To provide moral support in time of stress
Parent analogue	To support and facilitate the realization of the dream; in this role, to believe in the novice, share the dream, bestow his blessing, help to define the emerging self, and create a base on which to build a life structure that contains the dreams

*From Levinson D: *Seasons of a Man's Life*. New York, NY, Ballantine Books, 1978, pp 98–99.

changes jobs, or dies. Sometimes it comes to a natural end, and after a "cooling off period" the two form a warm but modest friendship. It may end totally with a gradual loss of involvement. Most often, however, an intense mentor relationship ends with strong conflict and bad feelings on both sides. The young man may have powerful feeling such as bitterness, rancor, grief, abandonment, liberation, and rejuvenation. The mentor finds the young man touchy, unreceptive to even the best counsel, irrationally rebellious, and ungrateful.[6(p100)]

The termination of the mentor relationship often occurs when a man is in his late 30s and feels the drive to move toward becoming a senior adult and having authority. Levinson also feels that men are most capable to giving themselves fully to the role of mentor in their 40s, when competition with the younger man is diminished and the man is able to display more caring toward the younger man.

The woman who makes a decision to pursue a career embarks on a course that will make strategic people available to her. As an achiever she understands her non–work related skills and capitalizes on them. She brings a variety of resources and talents to her position. Colleagues or peers allow her to experiment with relationships, and she begins to appreciate how to mobilize multiple resources to her advantage. Colleagues most effectively serve as guides. However, competition will limit their effectiveness as sponsors. Supervisors, bosses, teachers, and group leaders can serve in the position of evaluator. They must be perceived by the individual as having a level of expertise that makes their evaluation valuable. Evaluators will focus on the individual, assessing her in relation to her productivity as well as her peer relationships and use of resources. This traditional hierarchy is understandable to women in the work force. Evaluators are not always in a position to promote or sponsor a person within the organization. They may be relatively invisible to those people the individual wants to be exposed to, or they may be so consumed by competition that they do not open doors. Throughout her work experience a woman will gather perceptions from role models and will try to incorporate certain of their attributes into her work-related personality.

In an unpublished master's thesis, Walter describes the characteristics of the mentoring relationships in women (Box 8–12).

Women need someone to test the emerging self on, someone who does not threaten her existence in the workplace. This person will advise, tutor, and sponsor her at critical points in her career development. This mentor also has the power to catapult her in the organization because the mentor endows her with power by sponsoring her. She and the mentor are bound by tradition which neither may be able to articulate. She learns to manage power under this person's guidance while respecting the hierarchical nature of their relationship.

· ·

BOX 8–12   CHARACTERISTICS* OF THE MENTORING RELATIONSHIP FOR WOMEN

Mentor characteristics	Personal
	Sensitivity/genuineness
	Honesty
	Trustworthiness
	Charisma
	Respectability
	Professional prestige
	Reliability
	Professional skills
	Counseling/knowledge
	Knowledge/leadership
	Counseling/leadership
	Credibility
How acquired	Mentor serves as one's boss
	Novice seeks out
	Mentor seeks out
	Personal relationship
	Assigned
Age	Mentor in 40s
	Novice in 20s
Protege characteristics	Intelligent
	Willing to work hard
	Not confined by time or other constraints
	Professional
	Career oriented
Measure of success	Equality with mentor
	Relationship becomes friendship or collegial relationship
Formalization	Organizations should promote concept but not practice
	Organizations should not structure
	Relationship needs to be better understood before it is structured
Availability	Women average 2.7 mentors
	73.9% of women studied have mentored more than four proteges
	Still a sense of too few women in powerful positions
Long-term outcomes	Networks
	Relationships
	Stronger organizations
	Reduction of societal barriers related to women in the work force
Trends	More women in middle management
	More women in top management
	Less extraneous pressure on women in power, making them more accessible to proteges
	Move toward andragogical educational approach (education encouraging student to capitalize on experiences of others)
Barriers	Sexual stereotyping
	Sexually charged society
	Societal myths
Role of mentor	Facilitate career planning
	Facilitate personal growth
	Assist with research/publications

(Continued.)

· ·
BOX 8–12   (cont.).

	Teacher
	Advisor
	Sounding board
	Critic
	Promoter
Settings where mentors are found	Education
	Employment
	Personal lives
	Community
Sex of mentor	Male most often
Sex of novice	Female most often

*All characteristics are presented in order of importance according to statistical analysis of questionnaire results in a study of 33 nationally recognized women in education, business, government, and the professions.

She still relies heavily on the work structure to advance her through nomination to committees and task forces, in which she cannot only demonstrate her talents, but also work more closely with or be visible to higher levels of management. These individuals may then be willing to sponsor her for promotions or new levels of responsibility. Since exposure to this level of management may be fleeting, power that is reflected from the sponsorship of her mentor will be crucial to her success.

It appears that the mentoring relationship grows out of mutual respect and appreciation for each other's talents and attributes. There is a power that derives from the relationship that may be best described as reflections of self. The mentor sees in the novice himself at an earlier age, perhaps an age when the time was not right for him to do all that he was capable of doing, or perhaps a self that lacked confidence to aggressively pursue dreams and goals. The novice sees in the mentor a reflection of her future self. She strives to emulate the mentor, to possess the same level of expertise, self-confidence, and ability.

References

1. Feitelberg SB: Product/Service Line Management [Audiotape]. Orlando, Fla, Combined Sections Meeting, American Physical Therapy Association, 1991. Produced by Infomedix, 12800 Garden Grove Blvd, Suite F, Garden Grove, CA 92643.
2. Maslow A: A theory of human motivation. *Psych Rev* 1943;50:370–396.
3. Forsyth PB, Danisiewicz TJ: Toward a theory of professionalization. *Work Occup* 1985; 12:59–76.
4. Yankelovich D: *New Rules.* New York, NY, Bantam Books, 1981.
5. Jennings E: *Routes to the Executive Suite.* New York, NY, McGraw Hill Book Co, Inc, 1971.
6. Levinson D: *Seasons of a Man's Life.* New York, NY, Ballantine Books, pp 98–99.
7. Harris M: *America Now.* New York, NY, Simon and Schuster, 1981.
8. Harvey JB: *The Abilene Paradox.* Lexington, Mass, Lexington Books, 1988.
9. Hersey P, Blanchard K: *Management of Organizational Behavior,* ed 4. Englewood Cliffs, NJ, Prentice-Hall, 1982.
10. Hickok R: *Physical Therapy Administration.* Baltimore, Md, Williams and Wilkins, 1979

Suggested Readings

Kanter RM: *Men and Women of the Corporation.* New York, NY, Basic Books, 1977.
Kanter RM: *The Change Masters.* New York, NY, Simon and Schuster, 1983.

Kanter RM: *When Giants Learn to Dance.* New York, NY, Simon and Schuster, 1989.

Leavitt HJ: *Managerial Psychology.* Chicago, University of Chicago Press, 1978.

Naisbitt J, Aburdene P: *Re-inventing the Corporation.* New York, NY, Warner Books, 1985.

Peters TJ, Austin N: *A Passion for Excellence.* New York, NY, Random House, 1985.

Peters TJ, Waterman RH: *In Search of Excellence.* New York, NY, Warner Books, 1985.

Scott WR: *Organizations, Rational, Natural, and Open Systems.* Englewood Cliffs, NJ, Prentice-Hall, 1981.

Webber RA: *Management: Basic Elements of Managing Organizations.* Homewood, Ill, Richard D. Irwin, Inc, 1979.

CASE 8.1:

Motivation Case: The New Director

Peter Kovacek, P.T., M.S.A.

John Doe has been director of physical therapy and rehabilitation at St. Issac Hospital for 6 weeks. He has 10 years' experience as a manager and 15 years' experience as a physical therapist. Prior to John accepting this position, it had been vacant for 12 months after the previous director was terminated. John is not completely aware of all the circumstances leading to the dismissal.

St. Issac Hospital is a 250-bed community hospital in suburban Chicago. Physical therapists at St. Issac are involved in treating patients on the medical/surgical units, the 20-bed adult rehabilitation unit, and in the outpatient department.

Suburban Chicago has been a very difficult recruitment environment for quite some time. There are many physical therapy positions available and not enough physical therapists to fill them. Currently St. Issac has eight full-time physical therapists, but four additional positions are open and have been for over 8 months.

John reports to Jane Smith, Vice President of Professional Services, who hired him. She believes that physical therapy, like all of the services under her, should be productive, growing, and fully staffed. She often considers physical therapists as technicians in the same category as housekeeping and maintenance personnel. John has repeatedly explained that physical therapists are much more like medical staff members in terms of their autonomy and ability to produce revenue and positive patient relationships for the hospital. He is sure, however, that Jane is unswayed by his arguments.

Upon his arrival, John decided to be sure he knew what was going on in the department before he changed anything. He found no managerial hierarchy within the department. Each staff member reported directly to him. There were no differentiated duties or expertise recognized within the department. Volume within the department was increasing steadily, but so was staff frustration, complaints, and use of sick time. Staff members were treating 12 to 15 patients each day, including at least 2 rehabilitation patients. He was also seeing a full load of patients to help keep up. Staff morale was low, and there were rumors of a possible staff "mass exodus" if the new director "did not fix things quickly."

One morning, after 6 weeks on the job, John was called to Jane's office because members of the staff had written a letter to the administration to complain.

During the brief meeting Jane would not show John the letter, but told him that it came from most but not all of his staff. The complaints that Jane related to him included the following (in the order that she mentioned them).

1. The work load is too high for quality treatment.

2. Things are no better with the new director than they were when the position was open.

3. There is no program development occurring.

4. Morale is terrible.

5. The director is not available to staff because he spends too much of his time on unimportant "political" issues.

6. No new staff has been hired to help.

7. When problems are brought to the new director, he "doesn't solve them for us" but says "let's work this through together." Then he expects the staff to solve the problem.

8. No one knows how they are performing. No one says thanks.

9. Rumors are out of control.

10. If things don't get better, a large percentage of the staff will leave very soon.

Jane told John to fix the situation immediately, and that she didn't want any more letters of this kind.

When John asked for suggestions, Jane suggested that the problem was his to solve, but to keep her informed in writing.

In this case, consider where the real problems are and the reason for the staff's reaction. Consider the administrator's style of management compared with the manager of physical therapy. Why is this called a case in motivation? Consider the solutions to the problems that are brought out in this case.

⋮⋮⋮⋮⋮ CASE 8.2 ⋮

Changing Roles of the Physical Therapist Assistant

Jane Walter, P.T., Ed.D.

Physical therapist assistants are changing their roles with increased experience and with the attainment of advanced degrees. Just as any individual may choose to pursue a degree in management, education, or anatomy, the physical therapist assistant will also pursue advanced degrees. These individuals will then be in a position to hire and supervise physical therapists in a variety of roles, including clinical practice, education, and research. Consider the following scenarios.*

Home health facility. A physical therapist assistant is working in a home health facility and is recognized and compensated for overseeing medicare documentation. This individual has attended medicare documentation workshops and is now responsible for training all new staff in medicare documentation.

Private practice. John Doe, P.T.A., works for a private practice, receives profit sharing, works as a senior physical therapist assistant, supervises physical therapist assistant students, and has been trained in joint mobilization.

---

*Many of these scenarios are paraphrased from examples of physical therapist assistant job responsibilities given by Janet Rogers, P.T.A., M.A., at the 1992 Combined Sections Meeting at the Directors Forum of the Section for Administration in San Francisco. Ms. Rogers is herself currently on a physical therapist assistant faculty and is pursuing a doctoral degree in education.

Work hardening.   Steve Smith, P.T.A., schedules all work hardening clients after the physical therapist's evaluation. He also delivers work hardening care following the program established by the physical therapist. He has worked in a local work hardening clinic and has also worked with clients directly at the work site.

Rehabilitation facility.   Bill Jones, P.T.A., manages a physical therapy department in a rehabilitation facility. He has a management degree in addition to an associate arts degree in physical therapy assisting. He hires physical therapists as consultants to do patient evaluations and hires physical therapist assistants and aides to carry out a wide variety of patient care activities following the programs established by the physical therapist.

Physical therapist assistant as owner.   Jane Anderson, P.T.A., owns a private practice that is focused on home care. She hires physical therapists to perform evaluations and establish programs and also hires physical therapist assistants to carry out programs. She supervises documentation by the physical therapist to assure that it meets all regulatory guidelines and submits all patient billing to the appropriate agency.

School-based practices.   Sue Cook, P.T.A., coordinates a 0- to 3-year-old program in a local school district. She is responsible for submitting charges, setting up schedules, and following through on programs established by the physical therapist.

Consider the laws, regulations, and professional standards governing the work of physical therapist assistants. What dilemmas are posed by the changing roles of the physical therapist assistant? Who is responsible for monitoring the changing role of the physical therapist assistant? How will the profession of physical therapy change in the future to accommodate these roles?

CHAPTER 9

Controlling Organizational Behavior

INTRODUCTION

The physical therapy manager is responsible for controlling many aspects of the work environment. The American worker today, whether a professional or not, would like to work in an institution that does not attempt to control behavior. Control is seen as a management concept left over from the behavioral approach to the individual, in which rewards and punishment were used to modify behavior. It would truly be a utopian society if we could depend on every worker to be motivated by an internal sense of commitment and pride to perform at the highest possible level of ability and if that highest level of ability matched the needs of the job. In addition to financial control and quality control mechanisms that are discussed in other sections of this book, the physical therapy manager is responsible for controlling organizational behavior.

DEPARTMENT MISSION AND GOALS

The foundation of the physical therapy practice or service comes from the mission and goals of the institution. In addition to an institutional mission, it is important for the physical therapy department to establish its own goals even if those goals only reinforce the goals of the institution. These goals may be broadly stated and will reflect the commitment to the community, the kind of patients/clients treated, the relationship to the referral community, and the range of services provided to referral sources, the institution, the community, the staff, and the professionals represented in the department. The goal-setting process should be shared with the staff to receive both their input and their commitment. As departmental policies and procedures are developed, they will be tied to the goals and mission of the institution.

POLICIES AND PROCEDURES

Policies and procedures guide and to some degree standardize certain behaviors within the organization. Policies are broad statements that guide the physical therapy manager in decision making. A salary policy, for instance, might state that salaries shall be established consistent with salaries within the physical therapy community and maintained at a level that allows physical therapy managers to recruit for positions without undue delays. Procedures are specific guides to job behaviors for managers, staff, volunteers, visitors, and patients. Most managers are particularly interested in specifying or standardizing activities that hold a high degree of risk. Risk can come from inherent dangers of equipment, procedures, and the level of training of departmental staff. The Joint Commission on the Accreditation of Healthcare Organizations and other regulatory agencies require the physical therapy manager to maintain an up-to-date policy and procedure manual. Each department and each manager will focus on different areas within the policy and procedure manual depending on the needs of the institution. An example of the table of contents of a hospital-based physical therapy department can be seen in Box 9–1.

Clearly defining the policies and procedures within the facility and giving employees a good orientation to these procedures will greatly reduce errors and risk of injury within the department. The policy and procedure manual should be readily available to all staff. Although maintaining several manuals is more difficult for the clerical staff, a policy and procedure manual that remains on the office shelf is of little use to the employee or the manager. Many of the issues addressed in a well-

BOX 9–1 TABLE OF CONTENTS: POLICY AND PROCEDURE MANUAL

Physical Therapy Department

Orientation schedule
General hospital information
   Mission of the institution
   Organizational chart of the institution
Philosophy of the physical therapy department
Organizational chart of the physical therapy department
Committee structure of the physical therapy department
Department meetings
   Dates
   Purposes of meetings
   Roles and responsibilities of department staff at meetings
Job descriptions
Performance appraisal procedures
   Performance appraisal forms
   Timetable for performance appraisal
   Corrective actions
   Promotions, raises, bonuses, and other performance-based rewards
Rotations
Weekend and holiday procedures and scheduling
Time off, leaves of absence, sabbaticals
Supervision of support staff
Seminars and inservices
Scheduling procedures
   Inpatients
   Outpatients
   Special patients (rehabilitation unit)
Documentation procedures
   Inpatients
   Outpatients
Billing procedures
Procedures and policies regarding patient family visits in physical therapy
Discharge planning
   Discharge summaries
   Discharge conferences
   Discharge follow-up
Third-party reimbursement
   Coding procedures
   Billing procedures
   Forms
   Computer access
   Faxing reports
Safety procedures
Emergency procedures (cardiopulmonary resuscitation, codes)
Equipment procedures
   Cleaning
   Maintaining
   Requisitioning
   Scheduling
   Training requirements
Telephone system
Computer system
Hazardous waste management

(Continued.)

· ·
BOX 9–1   (cont.).

Precaution procedures
    Sterile techniques
    Notice of patient precautions
    Bloodborne pathogens
Patient information and photography releases
Specific guidelines from referral sources
    Hand surgeons
    Orthopedic surgeons
    Pediatrics
    Dentists
    Others

designed manual are covered in other chapters in this book. This chapter concentrates on job descriptions, job analysis, and the performance appraisal system as mechanisms for controlling organizational behavior.

· · · · · · · · · · ·
DEFINING THE JOB AND MEASURING JOB PERFORMANCE

Those managers who subscribe to continuous quality improvement and the concepts of making the employee more personally responsible for the produce believe that job satisfaction is very clearly tied to worker involvement in decision making and pride in producing a quality product. These individuals point to the industrialization of Japan and the writings of W. Edwards Deming as examples of the importance of employees who are commited to the institution. The United States may never achieve this level of commitment, not because of the workers, but because of the many ways in which the United States differs from Japan in freedom of choice and equal opportunities for workers.*

The physical therapy manager may be obligated by the institution to measure performance. Whether performance appraisal systems are in place or the physical therapy manager is faced with the task of developing such systems, the first question which must be asked is who the appraisal system is intended to serve. Most often

---

*For more information, there are numerous books and articles written on Japanese culture and the work of W. Edwards Deming, who introduced the concepts of total quality management to Japanese industrialists after World War II (WWII). Because of the very large population, Japan was limited in its ability to educate all of its citizens after WWII. Therefore, an educational system developed that is highly competitive and not equally available to all citizens. Children must compete for admission to all levels of education for quality programs and then must compete for the relatively few university programs available for preparation for the professions. The future of children is often determined early by virtue of the educational opportunities available to them. This leaves a very large population seeking jobs in industry. Again, because of the very large population, there is a high level of competition for these jobs as well. The average factory worker in Japan does not have the choices available that the American worker has in terms of education and employment. The American culture, despite a variable unemployment rate, leads the individual to believe that if he/she is a good worker that there are a number of opportunities available in the work force (especially in the most productive work years—20 to 55 years of age). Although the American worker values the benefits of working in a single industry for a long period of time, the average worker does not feel that a single job is the only chance for meaningful work. There are many cultural pressures on the worker that differ between Japan and the United States. A management system that works in one country cannot be simply transplanted to another country and be expected to meet with the same degree of success.

such a system purports to serve the administration, the department, the client, and the employee. If that is the case, the system must reflect areas of importance to each of these groups or individuals. The administration wants a system that measures and monitors productivity and turnover; the physical therapy manager is seeking to measure the success of the department; the client is interested in the outcomes of the services; and the individual is interested in obtaining feedback from supervisors and peers and to be appropriately compensated for the job performance.

The performance appraisal system may be formal or informal. Managers have a tendency to formalize the process for technical and clerical staff using a specific form and providing feedback on a fixed schedule. The more autonomous the worker, as in the case of the physical therapist specialist or the physical therapy manager, the less formal and structured the process and the more difficulty the employee has assessing his/her position in the organization. Physical therapy managers have the opportunity to explore the use of self-directed performance appraisal systems for the more autonomous employees. Appraisal systems traditionally use rating scales, ranking of skills, comparisons with other employees, and narratives as methods of ranking objectives or performance standards. The trend today is to use performance standards from the job description as the foundation for the appraisal system and to use both rating scales and narratives to describe performance within these standards.

It is the responsibility of the manager to control organizational behavior without the worker being controlled in a personal sense. The control is over the worker's work behavior in the organization. Few people argue with reward systems (although they may be as manipulative as any other system), and managers make no attempt to help the employee see that the work behavior is being rewarded, not the individual. However, when a worker fails to discharge his duties as an employee, any system of reprimand or limitations on responsibilities is seen as manipulative and is often taken as a personal assault. The message that the employee receives when reprimanded is that the individual is being reprimanded as a person, not that his organizational behavior is being questioned or controlled.

Even in this time of significant shortages of physical therapists, physical therapist assistants, and support staff, there are times when an employee's behavior is so inconsistent or so out of synch with the institution that the employee must be asked to leave. Of all of the duties managers face, monitoring, controlling, and modifying behavior as well as terminating an employee are among the most difficult.

There is a systematic approach to controlling organizational behavior that begins with determining the types of jobs and skills that are needed by the organization, establishing performance standards, establishing a system of measuring performance, and developing a system of review and corrective actions (Box 9–2).

- -

BOX 9–2 CONTROLLING ORGANIZATIONAL BEHAVIOR

1. Determine types of jobs and skills needed
2. Determine nonskill job requirements
3. Establish performance standards
4. Establish system of measuring performance
5. Develop system of review
6. Determine corrective action
7. Monitor performance and provide feedback

Determine Types of Jobs and Skills

Determining the type of jobs needed within an organization or an individual department begins with an analysis of the mission of the organization, the clients served, and the outcome of the system. If, for example, a physical therapy satellite facility is to be established to concentrate on the rehabilitation of sports injuries, specific physical therapy skills will be needed to work with this population. In addition, there will be nonskill requirements such as some lifting of limbs, individual clients, and equipment weighing 50 to 100 lb. It is also probable that the clients will be able to participate in certain aspects of their rehabilitation with minimal guidance and some assistance in setting up equipment, suggesting the need for physical therapist assistants or aides as adjuncts to the physical therapy staff.

Case example

When a gait analysis laboratory is set up in an academic health center next door to the outpatient physical therapy clinic a rough sketch of skills needed to establish and run the laboratory was determined by the Director of Physical Therapy. These skills included biomechanical analysis, maintenance of gait equipment, maintenance of computer equipment, scheduling of patients, reporting results to appropriate parties, triage of referrals, developing and carrying out research projects, working closely with other disciplines (orthopedics) in the establishment of policies and procedures of the laboratory and purchasing equipment.

The physical therapy manager then determined the category of worker who could best accomplish the tasks. She considered both current categories of workers available on staff as well as new positions (new skills not represented in the department are indicated with an asterisk) as follows: *physical therapist with advanced degree to perform biomechanical analysis, physical therapist assistant to maintain gait equipment, *computer science student to maintain computer equipment, receptionist to schedule patients, physical therapist to report results to appropriate parties, physical therapist to triage referrals, physical therapist with others to develop and carry out research projects, physical therapist manager to work closely with other disciplines (orthopedics) in the establishment of policies and procedures of the laboratory, and a physical therapist manager to purchase equipment.

Nonskill requirements were determined to be the following: minimal to moderate assistance lifting 50 to 200 lb, moving heavy equipment of 200 to 250 lb, mounting cameras on tripods and overhead platforms, focusing on computer output for 15 to 30 minutes at a time, patience in setting up the environment, ability to stand or sit for 30 minutes during setup times, and the ability to move rapidly to protect compromised patients.

From this information, it became obvious that, depending on the volume of patients using the laboratory and the cooperation of other disciplines, the laboratory would need a physical therapist with an advanced degree in biomechanics, a physical therapist assistant with knowledge of computers and an interest in learning about the maintenance of computers and camera equipment (instead of a computer science student who would be available through the college, but would not be a stable employee and would have somewhat unpredictable skills), and a part-time receptionist who, for the time being, would not be hired. The receptionist duties would be incorporated into the physical therapy outpatient department, which is next door to the space planned for the gait laboratory. The manager further decided that after an initial period of working closely with the manager, this position would have a degree of supervisory responsibility in order to work effectively with other disciplines and maintain the lab.

This is a simplistic example of determining the skill requirements of a job. The most complete analysis is accomplished when the physical therapy manager works with the personnel and industrial relations (PAIR) professionals in the organization to conduct an in-depth analysis of each job. PAIR professionals analyze the services provided, the worker activities and behaviors, equipment used, the work environment, and the personal characteristics of the workers. The job analysis is done through interviews, direct observation, critical incident analysis, and functional job analysis methods.

Although a physical therapy manager with advanced coursework or continuing education in personnel management may feel prepared to engage in the job analysis, it is a very time-consuming process for the professional who does not regularly engage in this work. Consultants from the personnel (human resources) department should be considered as partners in this endeavor. In addition to the job analysis skills of the personnel professionals, these individuals can also provide the physical therapy manager with a significant amount of insight into the job analysis process. For example, the personnel professionals are most familiar with the supervisory requirements for supervisory level jobs, the kinds of skills that will distinguish a specialist from a nonspecialist from an institutional perspective and the percentage of time in which employees must be engaged in particular activities in order for certain jobs to qualify for specific categories. The actual rating of the job and the salary levels attached to the job will be determined by the human services division of the institution. It is politically wise to involve this group in analyzing jobs prior to the rating process so that the PAIR professionals are able to be advocates for the job and for the physical therapy manager during the process.

Determine Nonskill Job Requirements

The nonskill job requirements have often been overlooked when planning a job. However, with the advent of the Americans With Disabilities Act, it has become increasingly important to specify the nonskill requirements (physical, mental, and emotional) of all jobs. The articulation of these requirements is both important to the employee and the employer in selecting the right person for the job and in preparing the individual for the job. In a physical therapy environment, understanding the lifting requirements, the postural positions that the employee may have to assume, the quick response to patients who become compromised, and the emotional aspects of dealing with people with disabilities are the primary areas of nonskill job requirements to be considered when analyzing a job.

As was discussed in an earlier section of the book, discriminating against a worker because of age, sex, disability, or race is unlawful in most institutions. It is therefore critical that the job specifications (the nonskill areas) are clearly spelled out to all applicants. It is then the responsibility of the individual to assure the employer that he/she can perform each of the job specifications and, if not, what assistance will be needed to accomplish the task. If a person accepts a job indicating that he/she can perform all of the job specifications and then tells the employer that he/she cannot perform those items specified in the job description after being hired, the employer is justified in terminating the individual. The Americans With Disabilities Act is meant to provide equal opportunity to individuals with disabilities, not to burden employers with employees who cannot perform the specifications of the job.

Once both the skills and nonskill requirements of a job are determined, it is possible to establish the job description. Examples of physical therapy department job descriptions can be found in Appendix 9.1.

Establish Performance Standards

A performance appraisal system must begin with a job analysis, development of a job description, and the establishment of performance standards. Performance standards are units of measurement related to the outcomes of the specific jobs within the physical therapy environment. The institution's objectives for the physical therapy manager may include meeting the goals of the department in concert with the mission of the institution; establishing and monitoring a realistic budget; hiring, monitoring, evaluating, and firing personnel; setting quality standards, monitoring quality, and providing feedback appropriately; coordinating billing procedures and monitoring appropriate billing; coordinating planned growth of physical therapy services; and maintaining a high level of visibility within the institution and the community. Although these objectives are broadly stated, there are more specific performance standards that relate to each area (Box 9–3).

The performance standards for the physical therapist and physical therapist assistant may include units of time, number of patients treated, quality measurement standards, accurate and timely documentation, level of professionalism, attendance at conferences, and units of continuing professional development. Support staff may be held to standards of hours worked, quality of work produced, ability to maintain assigned area, and ability to work cooperatively in meeting the goals of the department.

· ·

BOX 9–3 PERFORMANCE STANDARDS FOR THE MANAGER OF PHYSICAL THERAPY

Objective	Performance Standard
Meet the goals of the department	Number of units billed or the number of patient visits per year
Establishing and monitoring budget	Budget is realistic, reflecting planning for short- and long-term objectives; budget projections are accurate
Hiring, monitoring, evaluating, employees	Quality of the evaluation systems established for employees; total staff turnover and the fiscal implications of turnover
Setting quality standards	Realistic system of monitoring quality; actual numbers of citations of quality improvement committees; trends related to eroding quality identified over time within the quality improvement system of the facility
Coordinating billing	Billing reflects an insurance mix consistent with the mission of the institution; there is balance between insured and uninsured and a minimal number of denied bills
Coordinating planned growth	Unit of growth (i.e., industrial physical therapy satellite unit) is built, staffed, and managed in a timely and cost- effective manner
Maintaining high level of visibility	Number of committees served on within institution and community; involvement in community service organizations. Number of community-related services provided by the department

Establish a System of Measuring Performance

A single performance measurement tool will not adequately measure performance for all employees. The physical therapy manager must develop a system that focuses on each standard of performance for *each job* and the appropriate timetable for measuring that particular standard. The key here is to develop an appraisal tool for the JOB, not for the individual. Although it is often difficult to separate individuals from jobs in a small organization, it is critical to set job standards for the job and expect the individual to perform within those job standards. For instance, measuring productivity on an annual basis is inappropriate. Productivity must be measured on a daily or weekly timetable so that feedback can be offered and productivity can be enhanced on a timely basis. The following guidelines will assist the manager in developing a meaningful appraisal system for individual positions within the department.

Guiding Principles

Develop a valid process
When a system for measuring performance is developed, it is critical to ask questions that will truly measure the item which is intended to be measured. Validity is assured when you can answer the question, am I measuring what I intended to measure? Each performance standard derived from the job description should have a measurable behavioral component that, when measured, will truly assess that standard.

Develop a reliable process
The appraisal system should be able to be used by numerous evaluators over time and continue to measure the performance consistently.

Develop an acceptable process
If all parties who have a stake in the appraisal system do not accept the process, there will be resistance in the administration of the system and barriers to interpreting and using the results. If administration and other managers have expectations from the process, the physical therapy manager should make sure that they play a role in designing the process—the appraisal tool as well as the process of interpreting the assessment.

Develop a fair process
The process should focus on the job, including job behavior, not on the individual. Employees should have an active role in the assessment, such as developing a concurrent self-evaluation or developing goals based on the evaluation. Many managers only allow the employee to comment at the end of the process and then only as a measure of agreement or disagreement with the supervisor's assessment. Managers should be careful of the "halo effect," in which a positive or negative characteristic of an employee influences the rating of the employee in all other areas of the appraisal system.

Develop a meaningful process
The performance appraisal must have real impact on the organization, the department, the client, or the individual. A system that has only perfunctory functions will never be embraced by the key players in the evaluation process. Actual performance standards must be measured and that measurement must result in remedial action or the appropriate rewards.

The process must begin with a description of performance discrepancy, an assessment of the importance of the discrepancy, and a determination of the specific skills that are deficient. From that point, the manager must determine why the skill is deficient and proceed to develop a plan to reinforce or remediate the skill. A performance appraisal process that leaves the employee to solve the problems without adequate support will lead to unsatisfactory results.

Develop a system that incorporates assessments from all parties served by the employee

In many instances the employee is responsible to a single supervisor in a hierarchical organizational structure. However, as physical therapists and physical therapist assistants become more involved in alternative organizational structures such as service line management, the physical therapists and physical therapists assistants will work for a variety of individuals inside and outside the traditional organizational lines of the department. The appraisal system should accommodate the thoughtful assessment of the individual by all people who are in a position to supervise or receive services from the individual. Since many of these people are not traditional supervisors, the physical therapy manager may have to be creative in designing a system (along with the individuals involved) that collects observations from these consumers of services.

Build an appraisal system that fits the needs of the department

A number of appraisal systems and tools are available on the market. It is sometimes tempting to try to fit these tools to the appraisal needs of the department. In many cases, most of these systems will not work by themselves and have to be supplemented either by additional materials that the manager must develop or by resorting to using a battery of tools in order to evaluate all of the performance standards that must be measured. More is not better! If you cannot use the data, do not collect them. Desk drawers are full of data that managers think they may need or use some day. Streamline the process and the tools used to collect just the right amount of data. Do not be enticed by companies that advertise appraisal systems that they will analyze, submitting a report to you, and promising more satisfied employers and employees.

Performance appraisal tools do not assess job performance in its totality

There are many aspects of work that result in observable actions, e.g., the number of patients treated, units of care delivered and billed, insurance mix of clients, and collectible units of care that are regularly recorded within a physical therapy department. These work results must be used to assess work on a regular basis. In some cases the physical therapy manager may want to attach such data to the appraisal form to discuss with the employee in a formal, summative evaluation. If that is the case, the physical therapy manager should establish a system with the clerical and billing staff to separate the work results of individual employees so that this information is easily retrievable. In most cases these kind of data are discussed with the entire unit on a regular basis, since allowing discrepancies to slide will have serious financial implications for the department. If the work of one employee is particularly divergent from the group, the manager must deal with this employee in a timely manner.

Develop a tool that works

There are many options to developing the performance appraisal tool and its measurement component. It must be remembered that the tool actually started with the analysis of the job and the development of performance standards. Without these basic building blocks, the performance appraisal tool may not be truly integrated with the job. The measurement options include ranking systems, rating scales, and weighted rating scales. The most common approach to performance appraisal is the use of rating scales. The best of these scales identifies each behavior, characteristic, or job result, and the specific job performance at each ranking. For example, when quantity of work is assessed, a scale of 1 to 5 can be used, with 5 indicating highest possible while maintaining high level of quality; 4, above most workers; 3, average; 2, below department standard; and 1, unacceptable—below minimal standard.

Another approach to building an appraisal form is to develop a rating system that is then applied to a number of characteristics, behaviors, or job results. For example, the following scale was developed for use by the educational specialist in the physical therapy department of a large academic health center, where 5 indicates almost always does this, is consistently good at this, ranks high; 4, usually does this, is usually good at this, ranks above average; 3, sometimes does this, is occasionally good at this, ranks average; 2, seldom does this, rarely good at this, ranks fair; 1, never does this, is not good at this, ranks poor; and 0, does not apply, do not know.

This scale is then applied to a number of standards, such as the following.

1. Assess the overall educational needs of the staff in both patient and nonpatient areas. Recommend educational objectives and programs to the administrative director.

- ___ • Seeks advice of the department supervisory staff
- ___ • Takes part in the performance appraisal process for staff
- ___ • Assesses the impact of educational programs
- ___ • Considers individual needs and interests of the staff
- ___ • Considers rotation/service assignments when assessing educational needs
- ___ • Has contributed to the development and assessment of audit criteria that reflect the quality of education in the department

2. Another approach to appraisal forms is to use peer assessment. This is particularly important for the more autonomous employee who is interested in receiving feedback from peers. The physical therapist specialist will usually welcome such an assessment in areas such as clinical research, education, and supervision of staff. Peers in this case may be considered as other physical therapist specialists and supervisors who might be on the same organizational line and use the services of the specialist in their division. An example of the rating scale used for a clinical specialist in cardiopulmonary physical therapy follows.

- ___ • 5=Consistently excellent; independent in all respects
- ___ • 4=Excellent performance, seeks some supervision appropriately
- ___ • 3=Good performance, may need occasional supervision
- ___ • 2=Performance acceptable, but needs to be reminded to follow through
- ___ • 1=Performance unacceptable, needs constant guidance and reminders
- ___ • 0=Cannot rate; have not observed

This rating scale is applied to clinical performance standards, educational activities, and clinical research.

3. Clinical research:
   A. Organizes clinical research with staff:
      ___ (1.) Assists staff in identifying researchable problems.
      ___ (2.) Refines the problem.
      ___ (3.) Guides staff in conducting literature reviews.
      ___ (4.) Designs research project.

    __ (5.) Guides the staff in collaborating with evaluators.

    __ (6.) Writes an effective proposal with staff input.

    __ (7.) Identifies funding sources.

    __ (8.) Collaborates with colleagues.

B. Implements clinical research:

    __ (1.) Effectively organizes resources.

    __ (2.) Follows research protocol.

    __ (3.) Understands research design and data collection system.

    __ (4.) Is meticulous about details of study.

    __ (5.) Completes research in a timely fashion.

    __ (6.) Keeps all parties well informed regarding progress.

    __ (7.) Accurately reports findings.

    __ (8.) Writes in clear, understandable language.

    __ (9.) Successfully publishes findings.

Although the rating scales are the most common performance appraisal tools, the physical therapy manager may also choose to use a totally narrative approach to evaluation. The primary weakness of this approach to performance appraisal is that it is highly dependent on the manager's ability to write and develop points of view. Such an approach may also be unreproducible by other evaluators, since it is not clearly organized around specific standards using a specific rating scale.

A growing trend in health care organizational performance appraisal systems is the use of weighted rating scales. These scales still use the rating scales above, but the performance standards are weighted by a certain factor to denote the degree of importance of this performance standard to the job. When weighted scales are used the rating scale is given a number, such as 5 indicates consistently excellent, independent in all respects; 4, excellent performance, seeks some supervision appropriately; 3, good performance, may need occasional supervision; 2, performance acceptable, but needs to be reminded to follow through; 1, performance unacceptable, needs constant guidance and reminders; and 0, cannot rate, have not observed.

These numbers are then multiplied by the weighting factor of the performance standard. For example, the following standards from the physical therapist performance appraisal form have been weighted and rated (Box 9–4).

The danger of weighting systems is that the numbers are often turned into compensation scales. In Box 9–4 the weighting scale ranges from 1 to 5, with the most important job standards weighted most heavily. The assessment points earned reflect good performance according to the rating scale (3), but that one average rating on a highly weighted performance standard has had a significant impact on the overall performance rating. In this example, the manager linked the assessment points to the annual raises. Because the overall rating up to this point on the appraisal form represents approximately an 80% rating, the employee will receive an average raise for what appears to be an overall above-average performance (Table 9–1).

An even more serious problem with weighted performance appraisal systems is that financial considerations are often fixed by cash flow, the economy, status of the institution, and a number of other factors. This can cause administrative dictates re-

TABLE 9–1. Raise Scales for Physical Therapy

	Scale							
Raises	95–100	90–94	85–89	80–84	75–79	70–74	65–69	<65
%	5	4.5	4	3.5	3	2.5	2	0

· ·

BOX 9–4 PERFORMANCE RATINGS

Self	**Supervisor**	
<u>4</u>	<u>4</u>	1. Maintain and upgrade evaluation and treatment skills (factor=4)

Assessment points = 4 × 4 = 16

| <u>4.5</u> | <u>5</u> | 2. Evaluate patient's problems subjectively and objectively and document data via SOAP format (factor=5) |

Assessment points = 5 × 5 = 25

| <u>5</u> | <u>5</u> | 3. Assess patient's problems and formulate appropriate treatment plan (factor=5) |

Assessment points = 5 × 5 = 25

| <u>5</u> | <u>4.5</u> | 4. Assess patient progress and alter treatment plan as needed (factor = 5) |

Assessment points = 4.5 × 5 = 22.5

| <u>4</u> | <u>3</u> | 5. Provide accurate and professional documentation as required by departmental policy (factor = 5) |

Assessment points = 3 × 5 = 15

| <u>5</u> | <u>5</u> | 6. Initiate physical therapy services upon physician referral with applicable diagnosis and orders, which must be renewed for continued physical therapy services beyond 30 days of the referral date (factor = 5) |

Assessment points = 5 × 5 = 25
Total assessment points possible on six items = 145*
Assessment points earned = 118.5

* Commonly weighted performance appraisal systems allow approximately 400 total assessment points.

garding raise percentage scales. When these fixed scales are then applied to the performance appraisal system, it may cause the dollars to drive the system and not allow the manager to give a fair appraisal of the individual's performance.

The benefits of this system are that the performance standards that contribute the most to the job are duly recognized as being the most important standards. The employee should be held accountable for performance standards that are most important to the job.

There are pitfalls in performance assessment

When a five-point rating scale is used, a great tendency exists to move toward the middle of the scale and rate the employee as average. Managers must make every effort to use the full scale or develop a four-point scale so that the temptation of giving average ratings is reduced. Managers, like everyone else, are also susceptible to using the system to rate personality rather than job performance. Although managers will always have some employees who are more difficult to manage than others, it is important to use the appraisal system to rate job performance. If the individual's personality causes problems for the organization or the manager, then that issue should be addressed independent of the job performance assessment.

Everyone has weaknesses

Criticism is difficult to give and receive. The sensitive manager will anticipate the employee's reactions and defensiveness and allow the individual the time necessary to work through the process. All individuals have weaknesses, and most employees can make specific changes to improve the quality of their work. However, appraisal systems are not intended only to point out weaknesses. If the weaknesses are unimportant to the work, they should not be brought up. Many managers feel that they have to say something negative in an appraisal session. Employees should also be rewarded for good work, and appraisal sessions can be pleasant experiences of reinforcing good work behaviors and discussing further development and the ways in which the manager can help the individual to continue growing and increasing the contributions to the institution.

Be creative

The majority of performance appraisal systems are developed for hierarchical systems in which the employee engages in a restricted job environment. In physical therapy, where autonomy and professional development are keys to employee satisfaction, measuring job performance requires a creative process. The tendency will be to move away from structured and formal appraisal systems, but the manager should not abandon all attempts at measuring autonomous practice and professional development. Autonomous workers should be encouraged to work with the physical therapy manager to develop self-directed performance appraisal systems. The self-directed nature of this kind of evaluation process supports the autonomy and life-long learning and self-evaluation goals of the physical therapist. An experimental process of evaluating the specialist has been developed for the educational specialist within a physical therapy department.[1(p702)] In this model various consumers of the specialist's services are asked to evaluate performance using the rating scale that was described earlier. It is the responsibility of the specialist to develop the appraisal tool in coordination with the physical therapy manager, administer the tool, and collect and analyze the responses. In the analysis of the responses, the specialist accounts for variances between the scores of the consumers and his own assessment of performance. This variance becomes the focus for a discussion with the physical therapy manager. The manager's responsibility is to assess the development of the specialist in relation to both the perception of the consumers and the role of the specialist in evaluating his performance and assessing the needs of the consumers and developing a plan for further professional development. The performance appraisal system therefore becomes more collegial and developmental and less disciplinary and reward oriented.

Conducting the appraisal interview

This is a very important event for the manager, the employee, and the institution and should be conducted professionally. The employee should be given adequate notice of the meeting date and time and a completed assessment form should be given to the employee prior to the interview. This allows the individual to think about the assessment, work through any emotional responses to critical sections of the assessment, and to formulate comments regarding performance. At the time of the interview, the employee should not be kept waiting and should be made to feel as comfortable as possible. Conducting the interview at a table with pens, pencils, extra paper, something to drink, and tissues nearby prepares the employee and the manager for all possible contingencies and will reduce interruptions. The manager should not take any phone calls or other interruptions during the interview and should ask the secretarial staff to hold all interruptions for either the manager or the employee. Some managers even find it easier to meet outside of the department in a conference room where there is more assurance of no interruptions.

Once the interview starts, the manager should concentrate on job performance and the facts that have led to the assessment. If the employee is extremely upset about the assessment, it is important to reinforce the fact that the performance is being assessed, not the individual's worth. The interview should be a discussion with free exchange between the employee and the evaluator, not a lecture or one-sided discussion. Many managers provide coffee, soft drinks, or even water at the interview and as a rule of thumb feel that if their cup is full, they are doing too much talking.

Whether the assessment is basically positive or negative, the employee should leave the interview with a provisional plan of further development to be embellished and finalized at a scheduled follow-up meeting.

Determine Corrective Action

Completing the formal, informal, or creative performance appraisal often uncovers deficiencies in worker characteristics, work behaviors, or work results. It is then the responsibility of the physical therapy manager to determine the corrective action and a timetable for that action. In order to determine the corrective action, it may be necessary to break performance standards down into their component parts. For example, if the performance standard is to complete billing forms accurately and a physical therapist consistently makes errors in billing, particularly in identifying the ICDA-9-CM code on the billing form, the physical therapy manager will have to understand the task well enough to determine where in the process (Fig 9–1) a breakdown of the task may lead to a consistently poor performance rating in this standard. In this case, by building a task flow chart, the manager can more discretely analyze the problem and help the employee understand where the breakdown in performance occurs and therefore the best corrective action. If, for example, the problem is that the therapist never schedules a quiet time to complete billing, the scheduling of dedicated time for billing may solve the problem; if the problem is that the ICDA codes are not on the patient paperwork and the therapist does not take the time to look them up, then corrective action may be for the therapist to record the ICDA

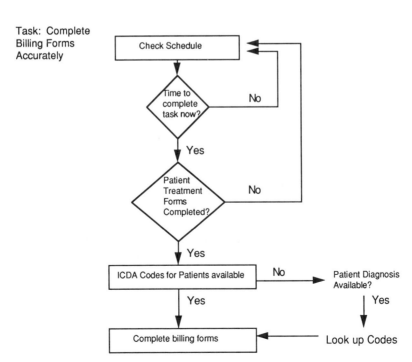

FIG 9–1.
Task analysis for completing billing forms accurately.

code on referrals as soon as they are received or create a filing system for active patient containing all relevant information, including codes. This kind of training or retraining is best done on the job, with feedback being provided on a continuing basis as close to the performance discrepancy as possible. It may be necessary to take the employee out of the environment for corrective action. For example, the above example could also occur with a foreign trained physical therapist who does not understand the US health care system and the issues of third-party reimbursement, which leads to some sloppiness in the billing procedures. In this case, it may also be helpful to send the therapist to an educational program (or to the training department) for a thorough review of the US health care system while feedback and training continue within the clinic.

The timetable for corrective action is also critical in this process. In the billing example above, immediate action must be taken by the manager and the therapist to correct the problem or significant loss of reimbursement will result. Therefore, the remedial steps must be clearly established and monitored on a daily basis with an expectation of immediate change.

The immediacy of action relates to the degree to which the employee's problem is a problem for the institution. If the employee's deficiency causes a financial burden to the instituion that increases every day, that problem becomes not only the employee's problem, but the physical therapy manager's problem as well. When problems become the manager's problems, the manager must act more swiftly and with less understanding than if the problem belonged to the employee and had relatively little effect on the institution. For example, if the therapist needs to enhance skills in manual therapy to provide better quality care and there are three other therapists who are working on the same goal within the department, the physical therapy manager can be more patient with the speed with which the therapists move to correct their deficiencies as long as they progress in that direction.

Monitor Performance and Provide Feedback

Once a plan for corrective action is in place, it is the role of the physical therapy manager to monitor the employee performance and provide feedback regarding progress toward correcting the deficiencies. It should be made clear to the employee the degree of severity of the deficiencies and the impact of those deficiencies on the organization. With that understanding, the employee should then be informed of the timetable over which the deficiency must be corrected and the next disciplinary step that will be taken if sufficient progress in not made to correct the problem.

Monitoring performance and providing feedback are also important for those employees who are making significant contributions to the department. This feedback will often support the continuation of the positive influences the good employee is having in the department and may serve as its own reward.

The best job is one in which the employee experiences some control over the work and resources, personal accountability, feedback from supervisors, opportunities for learning, and in which skills are both required and maximally utilized. Employees want to know where they stand in the organization and the manner in which their work is contributing to the overall goals of the organization. At the same time, the institution wants to identify the best workers and develop mechanisms to reward and maintain those employees who will reinforce the institutional work standards. A well thought out and administered performance appraisal system and related policies and procedures can help ensure that the goals of both the workers and the institution are met.

References

1. Emery M, Walter J: Self-assessment: Performance appraisal system in a time of increasing specialization. *Phys Ther* 1981; 61:702.

Selected Readings

Bohannon RW: The performance appraisal: Considerations for supervisors and staff. *Clin Management* 1987; 7:10–13.

Davis GL, Bordieri JE: Perceived autonomy and job satisfaction in occupational therapists. *Am J Occup Ther* 1988; 42:591–595.

Egan A: Peer review: One department's experience. *Phys Ther* 1979; 59:000.

Hamric A, et al: Staff evaluation of clinical leaders. *J Nurs Admin* 1978, pp. 18–26.

Leavitt HJ: *Managerial Psychology.* Chicago, Ill, University of Chicago Press, 1978.

McConnell CR: An integrated view of performance appraisal. *Health Care Superv* 1987; 5:61–78.

Megginson LC, et al: *Management Concepts and Applications.* Cambridge, Mass, Harper and Row, 1989.

Smith DM: Organizational socialization of physical therapists. *Phys Ther* 1989; 69:000.

Stevens BJ: Accountability of the clinical specialist: The administrator's viewpoint. *J Nurs Admin* 1976; 6:30–32.

Stone TH: *Understanding Personnel Management.* Chicago, Ill, Dryden Press, 1982.

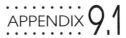

APPENDIX 9.1

Job Descriptions

(These job descriptions are adapted from job descriptions in a variety of facilities and therefore vary in style and content)

Job title.   Director of Physical Therapy (this is the job description of a person often referred to as a working chief physical therapist; the person is both responsible for managing the department and engaging in patient care).

Department.   Physical Therapy

Immediate Supervisor.   Assistant Administrator of Patient Services

I. General Summary of Responsibilities: Coordinates and supervises operation of the department of physical therapy

II. Specific Job Responsibilities:

A. Management

1. Supervision of the work of the staff physical therapists, physical therapist assistants, aides, orderlies, technicians, and secretary.

2. Care of the physical plant and machinery related to the Physical Therapy Department.

3. Preparation of and operation within an annual budget for personnel and equipment.

4. Maintain records pertinent to personnel and operation of the department:
   a. Record data of new employees and all information relative to work performance of all employees of the department.
   b. Complete an annual performance review on each of the employees in the department.
   c. Responsible for the completion of the daily attendance record and payroll attendance record.
   d. Prepare an annual budget for equipment and personnel.
   e. Assess needs and completes forms for weekly purchase supply order and Central Supply.
   f. Complete a job analysis for each job classification and updates same each year.
5. Maintain standards as established by the American Physical Therapy Association regarding physical therapy treatment and professional ethics.
6. Complete daily schedule of patient treatments.
   a. Assigns new patients to respective physical therapist.
   b. Tranfers patient's name from outpatient schedule book to the daily treatment schedule board.
7. Maintain the highest possible level of department cleanliness and safety.
8. Interview prospective employees for hire.
9. Train personnel:
   a. Utilize on-the-job training for nurse, physical therapist assistant, physical therapy aide, and orderly according to the training breakdown established for the groups.
   b. Assist director of inservice training by conducting educational programs for graduate registered and licensed practical nurses relative to physical therapy and rehabilitation procedures.
B. Clinical
   1. Administer physical therapy per referral:
      a. Interpret and further develop diagnosis of patient and take all precautions for observing indications and contraindications.
      b. Complete evaluation of patient in a timely fashion.
      c. Develop treatment plan.
      d. Prepare patient for treatment. Schedule equipment.
      e. Apply physical agents and modalities according to departmental procedures.
      f. Direct physical therapist assistants and aides in preparation of patient and application of treatment modalities and techniques.
      g. Consult with physicians and other referral sources.
   2. Observes and evaluates treatment effect:
      a. Recommend change to referral source if indicated.
      b. Discuss condition and treatment course of patient with staff physical therapist and referral source.
      c. Analyze patient's psychological and physical needs and deal with them accordingly.

   3. Maintain records pertinent to patient treatments:
     a. Provide accurate and professional documentation.
     b. Submit patient discharge summary in a timely fashion.
   4. Maintain and upgrade evaluation and treatment skills.

III. Job Specifications:
   1. Graduate of accredited entry-level degree physical therapy program.
   2. Advanced courses in management desirable.
   3. State physical therapy licensure mandatory.
   4. Must be familiar with and practice techniques which reduce the transmission of communicable diseases.
   5. In management capacity, must be able to direct others and be perceived as a leader.
   6. Emotionally able to listen to others and react appropriately.
   7. In capacity as a physical therapist practicing patient care, must meet job specifications in PHYSICAL THERAPIST Job Description.

Job title.   Senior Physical Therapist

Department.   Physical Therapy

Immediate Supervisor.   Director of Physical Therapy

I. General Summary of Responsibilities: Under the general direction of the manager of physical therapy, is responsible for educating the staff, physicians, and other health care personnel regarding physical therapy services and issues. Responsible for program development, staff recruitment and retention. Contributes to the development of the budget and represents the physical therapy department on hospital committees.

II. Specific Job Responsibilities:
   1. Management
     a. Works as part of the physical therapy management team to assign and direct physical therapy staff and the distribution of work loads, inter/intra-departmental relationships, and compliance with department policies and procedures.
     b. Contributes to regularly scheduled meetings with physical therapy staff to keep them abreast of pertinent information, and to receive their concerns/suggestions.
     c. Responsible for recruiting and interviewing for physical therapy department positions.
     d. Contributes to preparation and presentation of performance evaluations for all departmental members.
     e. Contributes to creation/maintenance of current job descriptions for physical therapy department staff and makes changes as deemed necessary.
     f. Promotes physical therapy services to hospital personnel, community programs, and other agencies.
     g. Assists in planning and preparation, assist with monitoring expense, revenue, and capital budgets for physical therapy manager.

    h. Contributes to developing and enforcing departmental policies and procedures.

    i. Contributes to development and implementation of quality assurance program to monitor the efficiency and effectiveness of physical therapy services.

    j. Coordinates cohesiveness between physical therapy and all other health care disciplines in attempts to promote a team-oriented approach.

    k. Performs other management duties as assigned by the physical therapy manager.

2. Clinical

    a. Maintains and upgrades evaluation and treatment skills.

    b. Evaluates patient's problems subjectively and objectively and documents data via SOAP format.

    c. Assesses patient's problems and formulates appropriate treatment plan.

    d. Assesses patient progress and alters treatment plan as needed.

    e. Provides accurate and professional documentation as required by departmental policy.

    f. Initiates physical therapy services requiring physician prescription with applicable diagnosis and orders, which must be renewed for continued physical therapy services beyond 30 days of the referral date.

    g. Submits progress/discharge reports to referral source on a regular and timely basis.

    h. Attends and contributes to team conferences and rounds.

    i. Directs and follows through on treatment responsibilities delegated to appropriate personnel.

    j. Respects the dignity and confidentiality of patients, hospital employees, and hospital.

    k. Reports on time or notifies the physical therapy manager of absence in a timely manner according to hospital policy.

    l. Keeps current on department/hospital standards and policy/procedures.

    m. Maintains cardiopulmonary resuscitation certification.

    n. Performs other duties as required.

    o. Reports any pertinent or unusual information to the appropriate personnel (may include special precautions for specific patients and information related to total unit safety).

    p. Supervises students involved in professional programs and provides a positive clinical experience for these students.

III. Job Specifications

1. Graduate of an accredited physical therapist educational program.
2. State physical therapist licensure.
3. Three years' experience; advanced degree in management or an area of clinical specialization desired; advanced courses in management or an area of clinical specialization required.
4. Will be required to travel as a representative of the department.

5. Must possess problem-solving skills and tact in resolving difficult issues.
6. Demonstrates ability to plan and organize time.
7. Displays courtesy and tact when dealing with staff, hospital personnel, visitors, and the public.
8. Lift 100 lb and support up to 250 lb.
9. Transfer adult patients up to 250 lb and 6 ft tall.
10. Bend over equipment such as hubbard tank and whirlpool for extended periods of time (15 to 30 minutes) to deliver patient care.
11. Maintain static postures for several minutes while applying therapeutic procedures.
12. Respond quickly to compromised patients.
13. Work as part of the health care team, cooperating with a variety of health care professionals.
14. Appreciate the emotional aspects of illness and effectively apply appropriate strategies to work with a variety of patients and family members experiencing loss, disability, or disease processes.

Job title.   Physical Therapist

Department.   Physical Therapy

Immediate supervisor.   Director of Physical Therapy

I. General Summary of Responsibilities: Under the general direction of the department supervisor, is responsible for providing physical therapy services as determined by medical direction, therapist judgment, patient needs and desires, and available facilities.

II. Specific Job Responsibilities:
   a. Maintain and upgrade evaluation and treatment skills.
   b. Evaluate patient's problems subjectively and objectively and document data via SOAP format.
   c. Assess patient's problems and formulate appropriate treatment plan.
   d. Assess patient progress and alter treatment plan as needed.
   e. Provide accurate and professional documentation as required by departmental policy.
   f. Initiate physical therapy services upon physician referral with applicable diagnosis and orders, which must be renewed for continued physical therapy services beyond 30 days of the referral date.
   g. Must submit progress/discharge reports to physicians and other referral sources on a regular basis.
   h. Attend and contribute to team conferences and rounds.
   i. Direct and follow through on treatment responsibilities delegated to other personnel.
   j. Instruct families in home program prior to patient discharge.
   k. Assist the department supervisor with the orientation and training of new personnel.

l. Keep up to date in the profession through literature, workshops, seminars, etc.

m. May function as clinical instructor for physical therapy students.

n. Maintain cardiopulmonary resuscitation certification.

o. Perform other related duties as required.

p. Report any pertinent or unusual information to the appropriate personnel (may include special precautions for specific patients and information related to total unit safety).

III. Job Specification:

1. Graduate of an accredited entry-level degree program in physical therapy.
2. State physical therapy licensure.
3. No prior experience necessary.
4. Function with a minimum of supervision.
5. Must be adept at making appropriate decisions in order to plan and carry out treatment program to meet the individual needs of the patient.
6. Lift 100 lb and support up to 250 lb.
7. Transfer adult patients up to 250 lb and 6 ft tall.
8. Bend over equipment such as hubbard tank and whirlpool for extended periods of time (15 to 30 minutes) to deliver patient care.
9. Maintain static postures for several minutes while applying therapeutic procedures.
10. Respond quickly to compromised patients.
11. Work as part of the health care team, cooperating with a variety of health care professionals.
12. Appreciate the emotional aspects of physical therapy and effectively apply appropriate strategies to work with a variety of patients and family members experiencing loss, disability, or disease processes.

Job title. Physical Therapist Assistant

Department. Physical Therapy

Immediate supervisor. Physical Therapist(s)

I. General Summary of Responsibilities: The physical therapist assistant works under the direct supervision of the physical therapist in the delivery of physical therapy services. The role of the physical therapist assistant includes delivery of care in accordance with the plan of care determined by the physical therapist. Physical therapist assistants may evaluate patient responses during treatment, but may not conduct initial patient evaluations.

II. Specific Job Responsibilities:

1. Review the patient's evaluation with the referring therapist.
2. Deliver physical agents, therapeutic exercise, gait training, and other modalities of care in accordance with the policies of the department following the plan of care determined by the physical therapist.
3. Collect and document evidence of patient's response to treatment.
4. Report any untoward responses to treatment to the physical therapist.

5. Supervise physical therapist assistant students under the direction of the clinical coordinator of education.
6. Supervise physical therapy aides in the preparation of patients and equipment.
7. Work under the direction of up to three physical therapists.
8. Assume responsibility for delegated activities such as the production of lifts and other small equipment in the department workshop.
9. Supervise volunteers in the department workshop.
10. Maintain and upgrade treatment skills.
11. Provide accurate documentation of patient progress using SOAP format.
12. Attend rounds and conferences as directed.
13. Maintain cardiopulmonary resuscitation certification.
14. Perform other duties as required.

III. Job Specifications:
1. Graduate of an accredited physical therapist assistant educational program.
2. State physical therapist assistant licensure.
3. No prior experience necessary.
4. Work closely and cooperatively with supervising therapist(s).
5. Lift 100 lb and support up to 250 lb.
6. Transfer adult patients up to 250 lb and 6 ft tall.
7. Bend over equipment such as hubbard tank and whirlpool for extended periods of time (15 to 30 minutes) to deliver patient care.
8. Maintain static postures for several minutes while applying therapeutic procedures.
9. Respond quickly to compromised patients.
10. Work as part of the health care team, cooperating with a variety of health care professionals.
11. Appreciate the emotional aspects of illness and effectively apply appropriate strategies to work with a variety of patients and family members experiencing loss, disability, or disease processes.

Job title.   Physical Therapy Aide

Department.   Physical Therapy

Immediate supervisor.   Physical Therapists and Physical Therapist Assistants

I. General Summary of Responsibilities: Primarily responsible for preparing patients and equipment for treatment, transportation of patients, and tasks related to maintaining a tidy department. Under the supervision of the physical therapist or physical therapist assistant, may assist in the treatment of the patient.

II. Specific Job Responsibilities:
1. Departmental.
   a. Requisition and dispense linen.
   b. Change linen on treatment tables/mats.
   c. Clean equipment as needed following department protocols.
   d. Use mop to dry around hydrotherapy tanks as needed.

     e. Clean storage shelves and furniture as needed.

     f. Take inventory and order supplies following department procedures.

     g. Photocopy.

     h. Perform receptionist duties at times.

     i. Orient volunteer aides.

     j. Maintain tidiness of department.

     k. Other duties as assigned.

2. Under the direct supervision of the physical therapist or physical therapist assistant.

     a. Transports patients to/from department.

     b. Prepares equipment and patient for physical therapy.

     c. Assists physical therapist and physical therapist assistant in treatment procedures as directed.

     d. Stops equipment/treatment and notifies physical therapist or physical therapist assistant at completion of treatment period.

     e. Observes patients during treatment and notifies supervising therapist or assistant of any distress or malfunctioning equipment.

     f. Monitors patient vital signs.

     g. Maintains cardiopulmonary resuscitation certification.

III. Job Specifications:

1. High school graduate.
2. Completion of department aide training program.
3. No prior experience necessary.
4. Work under a minimum of supervision for tasks involving cleaning, patient transport, and linen duties.
5. Lift 100 lb and support up to 250 lb.
6. Prolonged stooping, squatting, sitting, standing, and walking.
7. Bend over equipment such as hubbard tank and whirlpool for extended periods of time (15 to 30 minutes) to clean or assist with patient care.
8. Organize time. Adapt schedule as needs arise.
9. Respond quickly to compromised patients.
10. Display qualities of tact, empathy, gentleness, and emotional stability when dealing with various patients.
11. Work from written and oral instructions.

APPENDIX 9.2

Sample Performance Appraisal Forms

PHYSICAL THERAPIST ASSESSMENT FORM

XYZ Hospital
Physical Therapy Department
Performance Appraisal
Physical Therapist

Note: Allows for application of a rating scale, use of self-evaluation, and narrative supporting statements.
O=Outstanding. Consistently performs at the highest level
G=Good. Consistently performs at or above expected level
I=Needs Improvement. Inconsistent performance
U=Unacceptable. Consistently performs below expected level

Self   **Supervisor**   1. Maintain and upgrade evaluation and treatment skills.

_____   _____   _____
_____   _____   _____
_____   _____

2. Evaluate patient's problems subjectively and objectively and document data via SOAP format.

_____   _____   _____
_____   _____   _____
_____   _____

3. Assess patient's problems and formulate appropriate treatment plan.

_____   _____   _____
_____   _____   _____
_____   _____

4. Assess patient progress and alter treatment plan as needed.

_____   _____   _____
_____   _____   _____
_____   _____

5. Provide accurate and professional documentation as required by departmental policy.

_____   _____   _____
_____   _____   _____
_____   _____

6. Initiate physical therapy services upon physician referral with applicable diagnosis and orders, which must be renewed for continued physical therapy services beyond 30 days of the referral date.

_____   _____   _____
_____   _____   _____
_____   _____   _____

p. 2

XYZ Hospital
Physical Therapy Department
Performance Appraisal
Physical Therapist

7. Must submit progress/discharge reports to physicians and other referral sources on a regular basis.

8. Attend and contribute to team conferences and rounds.

9. Direct and follow through on treatment responsibilities delegated to other personnel.

10. Instruct families in home program prior to patient discharge.

11. Assist the department supervisor with the orientation and training of new personnel.

12. Keep up to date in the profession through literature, workshops, seminars, etc.

13. May function as clinical instructor for physical therapy students.

14. Maintain cardiopulmonary resuscitation certification.

15. Perform other related duties as required.

16. Report any pertinent or unusual information to the appropriate personnel (may include special precautions for specific patients and information related to total unit safety).

Comments:

. . . .
PHYSICAL THERAPIST ASSISTANT ASSESSMENT FORM

XYZ Hospital
Physical Therapy Department
Performance Appraisal
Physical Therapist Assistant

Note: Allows for application of a rating scale, use of self-evaluation, and narrative supporting
statements.
O=Outstanding. Consistently performs at the highest level
G=Good. Consistently performs at or above expected level
I=Needs Improvement. Inconsistent performance
U=Unacceptable. Consistently performs below expected level

Self   **Supervisor**

1. Review the patient's evaluation with the referring therapist.

   _____
   _____
   _____

2. Deliver physical agents, therapeutic exercise, gait
   training, and other modalities of care in accordance
   with the policies of the department following the plan
   of care determined by the physical therapist.

   _____
   _____
   _____

3. Collect and document evidence of patient's response to treatment.

   _____
   _____
   _____

4. Report any untoward responses to treatment to the
   physical therapist.

   _____
   _____
   _____

5. Supervise physical therapist assistant students under
   the direction of the clinical coordinator of education .

   _____
   _____
   _____

6. Supervise physical therapy aides in the preparation
   of patients and equipment.

   _____
   _____
   _____

7. Work under the direction of up to three physical therapists.

   _____
   _____
   _____

p.2

XYZ Hospital
Physical Therapy Department
Performance Appraisal
Physical Therapist

Self   **Supervisor**

8. Assuume responsibility for delegated activities such as the production of lifts and other small equipment in the department workshop.

_____   _____

_____   _____

_____   _____

9. Supervise volunteers in the department workshop.

_____   _____

_____   _____

_____   _____

10. Maintain and upgrade treatment skills.

_____   _____

_____   _____

_____   _____

11. Provide accurate documentation of patient progress using SOAP format.

_____   _____

_____   _____

_____   _____

12. Attend rounds and conferences as directed.

_____   _____

_____   _____

_____   _____

13. Maintain cardiopulmonary resuscitation certification.

_____   _____

_____   _____

_____   _____

14. Perform other duties as required.

_____   _____

_____   _____

_____   _____

Comments:

. . . .
PHYSICAL THERAPY AIDE ASSESSMENT FORM

XYZ Hospital
Physical Therapy Department
Performance Appraisal
PT Aide Evaluation

Note: Allows for application of a rating scale, use of self-evaluation, and narrative supporting statements.

O=Outstanding. Consistently performs at the highest level
G=Good. Consistently performs at or above expected level
I=Needs Improvement. Inconsistent performance
U=Unacceptable. Consistently performs below expected level

Self	**Staff**	**Chief**	
___	___	___	1. Requisition and dispense linen.
___	___	___	
___	___	___	
			2. Change linen on treatment tables/mats.
___	___	___	
___	___	___	
___	___	___	
			3. Clean equipment as needed following department protocols.
___	___	___	
___	___	___	
___	___	___	
			4. Use mop to dry around hydrotherapy tanks as needed.
___	___	___	
___	___	___	
___	___	___	
			5. Clean storage shelves and furniture as needed.
___	___	___	
___	___	___	
___	___	___	
			6. Take inventory and order supplies following department procedures.
___	___	___	
___	___	___	
___	___	___	
			7. Photocopy.
___	___	___	
___	___	___	
___	___	___	
			8. Perform receptionist duties at times.
___	___	___	
___	___	___	
___	___	___	
			9. Orient volunteer aides.
___	___	___	
___	___	___	
___	___	___	
			10. Maintain tidiness of department.
___	___	___	
___	___	___	
___	___	___	

p.2

XYZ Hospital
Physical Therapy Department
Performance Appraisal
PT Aide Evaluation

Self	**Staff**	**Chief**	
‒‒	‒‒	‒‒	11. Other duties as assigned.
‒‒	‒‒	‒‒	
‒‒	‒‒	‒‒	
‒‒	‒‒	‒‒	12. Transports patients to/from department.
‒‒	‒‒	‒‒	
‒‒	‒‒	‒‒	
‒‒	‒‒	‒‒	13. Prepares equipment and patient for physical therapy.
‒‒	‒‒	‒‒	
‒‒	‒‒	‒‒	
			14. Assist physical therapist and physical therapist assistant in treatment procedures as directed.
‒‒	‒‒	‒‒	
‒‒	‒‒	‒‒	
‒‒	‒‒	‒‒	
			15. Stops equipment/treatment and notifies physical therapist or physical therapist assistant at completion of treatment.
‒‒	‒‒	‒‒	
‒‒	‒‒	‒‒	
‒‒	‒‒	‒‒	
			16. Observe patients during treatment and notify supervising therapist or assistant of any distress or malfunctioning equipment.
‒‒	‒‒	‒‒	
‒‒	‒‒	‒‒	
			17. Monitor patient vital signs.
‒‒	‒‒	‒‒	
‒‒	‒‒	‒‒	
‒‒	‒‒	‒‒	18. Maintain cardiopulmonary resuscitation certification.
‒‒	‒‒	‒‒	
‒‒	‒‒	‒‒	
‒‒	‒‒	‒‒	

Comments:

CHAPTER 10

Ethical Aspects of Physical Therapy Management

INTRODUCTION

Whenever a manager deals with resources such as money, machines, or personnel, that manager will encounter ethical issues and be placed in a position of making decisions that have ethical implications. Organizations represent specific cultures. The physical therapy culture in most institutions today is characterized by human resource shortages, a growing public awareness of physical therapy as a professional entity within health care, and increasing autonomy of decision making and action.

Cultural changes within American society have brought with them changes in cultural traditions within organizations. American business and organizations of the turn of the century supported and valued individual initiative and the entrepreneurial spirit among the higher echelons of management and new independent entrepreneurs (founders of the automobile, airline, and computer industries). Within the worker's ranks conformity and commitment to a rigorous work ethic were highly valued. These values and cultural components were discussed in earlier chapters.

The individual *leader* in the modern American business culture is being replaced by the *manager,* who models what is expected and is concerned primarily with technique and measurable outcomes and less concerned with innovation, individualism, entrepreneurial skills, moral debate, and moral decisions. There is a loss of the sense of duty and virtue and a separateness from tradition and community.

Because of the human service nature of the business of health care, physical therapy managers must not lose sight of their responsibilities to explore the culture and the dilemmas that arise on a daily basis and engage the staff, referral sources, and other members of the community in ethical debates. The physical therapy manager must understand and engage in ethical debates in the manager's role in order to encourage a moral environment in which too many managers have a tendency to manipulate resources in order to meet the goals and mission of the institution.

MORAL DILEMMAS

The physical therapy service provides a rich environment for ethical debate and deliberation. There are many moral dilemmas that the manager and the staff face every day (Box 10–1). A moral dilemma is a situation in which two or more goods are in conflict and occurs when an individual can rely on moral considerations for taking each of two opposing courses of action. For example, in the moral dilemma of abortion, some individuals appeal to the moral consideration of the right to life and define life at some point of gestation, while others debate the rights of the mother to self-determination and freedom of choice. Both arguments are grounded in the ethical principle of autonomy and focus on the duty of society to, on one hand, protect the rights of the fetus, and, on the other hand, to protect the freedom of choice and self-determination of the mother.

The abortion debate also points out the role of laws in ethical debates. Traditionally, a law is an ethical minimum. It is the minimal behavioral requirement that a society has decided upon for the governance of that society. The fact that the laws related to abortion have appeared to be built on "shifting sands" suggests that the American society has not yet agreed upon an ethical minimum in this area.

MORAL PRINCIPLES

This chapter focuses on obligations and rights, the correlativity thesis and the process of ethical debate. Moral principles are fundamental rules or codes of conduct. They serve as the foundation for moral rules and a source of justification for actions

BOX 10–1 EXAMPLES OF MORAL DILEMMAS

Issue:	Moral principles in conflict
Documentation:	Therapist's obligation to tell the truth vs. therapist's obligation to do good (beneficence) vs. patient's right to equal access to health care
Billing:	Institution's right to be paid for services vs. patient's right to equal access to health care vs. third party's right to deny coverage
Scheduling:	Patient's right to access to care and fair treatment vs. therapist's right to provide quality care vs. manager's and therapist's obligation to distribute resources fairly

or judgments (Box 10–2).[1(p5)] Ethical acts or judgments can be grounded in rules such as the golden rule (do unto others as you would have them do unto you), ethical principles (beneficence, veracity), or ethical theories (utilitarianism, virtue ethics, deontology). In biomedical ethics, actions and judgments are primarily grounded in ethical principles. By grounding acts and judgments in ethical principles, it is meant that the discussion is anchored in ethical principles.

The specific properties that are embedded in moral principles include (1) importance to society, (2) the potential of reducing conflict, (3) a guide to conduct, (4) prescriptive in form, and (5) supremely authoritative.[2(p11)] Principles that possess the greatest number of these characteristics in a health care organization are *beneficence, nonmaleficence,* and *autonomy* in regard to issues related to patient care and *justice* in issues of governance. There are not many basic codes of conduct for health care facilities. Health care professionals are bound by individual professional codes that stress duty and autonomy, and patient advocates have, in many instances, developed basic codes for patients in the form of a Bills of Rights for patients, which stress justice and liberty. Similar codes for health care managers should stress fairness, rights, and obligations.

MORAL DEBATES

Oftentimes debates that are embedded in values such as the abortion debates result in individuals resorting to a "just because" or "that's the way I was brought up" justification for a point of view. Ethical principles give the individual a rational anchor for actions or judgments. Many ethicists, particularly those in biomedical ethics, take this positivist or rational approach. This justification of actions or judgments in ethical principles or ethical theories is called a discursive argument (Fig 10–1).

There is also a nondiscursive tier of ethical decision making that individuals often use in ethical discussions and debates. This discussion may be grounded in family values, religious tenets, or other aspects of virtue ethics. The individual grounds actions or judgments through storytelling and a moral imagination. It may be that the individual imagines a moral society in which a particular action fits that moral goal. The individual's discussion might sound something like . . . "I think that abortion is wrong because if we let individuals make these decisions based on econom-

BOX 10–2 MORAL PRINCIPLES

Principle	Concepts grounded in principle
Autonomy (self-determination, self-governance)	Informed consent; confidentiality; freedom from coercion; absence from being controlled; refusal of treatment; suicide; abortion; privacy
Nonmaleficence (duty to do no harm)	Killing; letting die; use of extraordinary means; obligation to treat; use of medically indicated treatment; living wills
Beneficence (duty to help others)	Consideration of the greater good; promise-keeping; equal access and opportunity; costs, risks, and benefits; paternalism
Justice (fairness, legitimate claims)	Distribution of benefits and burdens (distributive justice); need, effort, contribution, merit; fair opportunity; classes of individuals; health policy allocations
Veracity (truth-telling, not lying)	Documentation; billing; disclosure

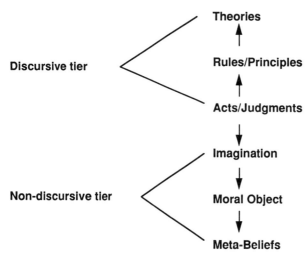

FIG 10–1.
Grounding ethical decisions. (From Nash RJ: *J Thought* 1987; 00: 00.)

ics or sex of the fetus or any other possible set of whims, we will move toward becoming a society which devalues life."

It is important for physical therapy managers to understand that the rational approach to ethical debate is not the only option available to individuals and that the nondiscursive debate has equal validity as an argument for actions and judgments.

RIGHTS

Administrators, personnel, and clients have certain rights by virtue of their responsibilities. "Rights may be rights to act, to exist, to enjoy, to demand."[2(p196)] They are "best understood as justified claims that individuals and groups can make upon others or upon society." [1(p50)] Rights often come into conflict with each other and become the focus of ethical debate. Rights may be absolute rights or prima facie rights. Absolute rights cannot be overridden, whereas prima facie rights may be overridden. Most rights are prima facie rights. Even rights to life are not absolute in our society, or we would not allow capital punishment or excuse mercy killing. Therefore, most rights can be overridden when there is a more compelling right or obligation with which they are in conflict. The rights of the physical therapist and physical therapist assistant through licensing laws are prima facie rights. For example, most laws give therapists the right to perform massage, but not the absolute right, since the state may also license masseuses.

The correlativity thesis states that when one person or group has a right, another person or group may have an obligation to uphold that right. For instance, if a patient has a right to confidentiality, a health care worker has an obligation to keep information related to that patient confidential. Physical therapy personnel should consider not only their own rights and obligations, but also obligations that may be imposed by the rights of patients and other groups.

OBLIGATIONS

Obligations suggest a commitment to acting in a certain way towards those with whom a relationship has been established.[3(p7)] These obligations are often expressed as duties toward others (individuals, groups, or institutions). By virtue of entering into a professional relationship with other people or with an institution, people assume certain obligations. In the organizational environment, administrators, personnel, and clients have certain obligations to each other in that environment, to society, and to the institution.

HEALTH CARE ORGANIZATIONAL RIGHTS AND OBLIGATIONS

The health care institution (represented by the administrative group of the facility) has certain rights and obligations (Box 10–3). The rights of the institution relate to its right to be treated fairly, to bill and collect for services provided by units and employees of the organization, and to pursue its missions without interference from other groups. The organization also has obligations to its clients, the community, the health care system, and employees. These obligations relate to the fair treatment of individuals, the adherence to regulations and laws, and the establishment of systems to assure the delivery of quality services.

The physical therapy manager functions as an agent of the organization and must be responsible for upholding the obligations of the organization as well as advocating for the rights of the organization.

Institutional Review Boards

Of the many obligations that organizations have to clients/patients, one that is mandated by law is the protection of clients/patients when they serve as human subjects in biomedical experiments. Several classic experimental studies conducted in the United States in the early 1920s to 1960s on black subjects, the mentally retarded, and prisoners and the atrocities of the World War II concentration camp experi-

---

BOX 10–3   ORGANIZATIONAL RIGHTS AND OBLIGATIONS

1. Rights
   1.1. To be treated fairly by regulatory agencies
   1.2. To be compensated for services provided
   1.3. To maintain confidentiality (organizational secrets)
   1.4. To pursue organizational missions and goals without interference
   1.5   To establish reasonable expectations of employees (fair day's work for fair day's pay)
2. Obligations
   2.1. Provide a mechanism of quality assurance
   2.2. Provide a safe environment and equipment for personnel and clients
   2.3. Provide adequate staff to support other personnel and accomplish the mission and goals of the organization
   2.4   Develop and maintain personnel policies and procedures
   2.5. Adhere to regulations
   2.6. Adhere to laws
   2.7. Provide mechanisms of information exchange
   2.8. Provide confidential, accurate and timely records
   2.9. To distribute resources fairly
   2.10. To provide fair opportunity
   2.11. To prevent harm
   2.12. To protect clients/patients as human subjects in biomedical research

ments led to federal legislation to protect human beings when they are participants in experiments. In 1972 Congress created the National Commission for the Protection of Human Subjects in Biomedical and Behavioral Research to establish minimal guidelines to regulate experiments in institutions where federal funds were awarded. Basically this legislation identified children and incompetent patients as individuals who must receive maximum protection in the experimental process, it mandated a process of informed consent, and it provided for the establishment of peer review boards that must approve all human experimentation. Most hospitals have institutional review boards that must approve of any experiments in which human or animal subjects are involved. Some private clinics are also beginning to form cooperatives to form ethics committees and review boards.

Clinicians and students may not simply decide to engage in a study and proceed to involve subjects, use medical records, or use patient specimens. All such investigations must be properly reviewed and approved before proceeding to collect any data. It is the responsibility of the physical therapy manager to inform the staff of the procedures to be followed in the institution and to monitor the process to assure that the subjects are protected.

In the 1980s there was a great deal of national debate regarding the rights of parents and physicians to make decisions regarding the starvation of newborn infants who were severely compromised by genetic and medical problems. Following the death of Baby Doe, at the center of this controversy, the federal government intervened by passing the Child Abuse Prevention Amendments of 1984. The regulations that implement this law were revised several times due to the pressure of the American Medical Association and other physician groups. The law restricts the decisions that parents, physicians, and others can make regarding the withholding of treatment for severely involved infants.

The acquired immune deficiency syndrome (AIDS) epidemic and the national debates regarding the treatment and isolation of the AIDS patient or the AIDS population in general renewed the public debates regarding health care. The most recent federal response to these debates has been the creation of a Biomedical Ethics Board and Biomedical Ethics Advisory Board in 1985. These boards report directly to Congress on ethical issues relating to health.

Human experimentation occurs on four basic levels (Box 10–4). Unconscious human experimentation occurs in the normal course of clinical care. It involves the removal of tissues and specimens, the application of treatment processes, and the participation in diagnostic procedures. There is no true attempt to engage in experimentation, but the patient is obviously the center of a clinical "investigation."

Clinical observations go beyond the normal course of treatment. At this level of experimentation, the clinician may collect extra specimens, removed organs may be used in the laboratory, or patient responses to specific exercise routines may be examined against responses of other patient populations. These are intentional obser-

· ·

BOX 10–4 LEVELS OF HUMAN EXPERIMENTATION

1. Unconscious
2. Clinical observation
3. Human experimentation
   a. Therapeutic
   b. Physiological or clinical questions
   c. Physiological observations
4. Genetic engineering

vations in which the patient is not at any risk greater than the risk of engaging in patient care.

Investigators take part in therapeutic research when they design research projects that have as their goal some benefit to the patient within the study. The subjects selected for the research are patients/clients with specific symptoms, diseases, or disabilities.

Research that answers physiological or clinical questions usually offers remote benefit to the subjects of the research. The subjects of this research may be patients/ clients or normal subjects.

When the research focuses on physiological observations, the focus of the research itself is not intended to benefit the patient or subject. The subjects are most often nonpatients, or clients. Drug and equipment studies fall in this category.

The last level of human experimentation is genetic engineering, in which future generations may be manipulated or genes are manipulated to produce disease-free individuals. This is the most controversial level of research.

Informed Consent

The three levels of informed consent are mere consent, informed consent, and educated consent. These levels of consent are defined as follows.

Mere consent. This level of consent is really consent out of ignorance. The individual literally consents to the process without any understanding of the consequences of participation.

Informed consent. The individual is informed of the purpose of the study, the procedures to be employed, the risks and benefits of the procedures, and the medical/psychological services available if any injury occurs during the experiment. The individual is encouraged to ask questions and to have other people present to help make decisions. If the subject is a child, both the child and the parent or guardian are fully informed in language they can understand. The subject and a guardian (if appropriate) then sign a consent form indicating their understanding of the experiment and their willingness to take part.

Educated consent. The individual is given all of the information stated in the informed consent definition. In addition, there is a real attempt to educate the individual regarding the physiological, psychological, physical, or biomedical underpinnings of the study and the risks and benefits without disclosing so much of the study that it biases the subject. The individual is then asked to make a decision from this educated base.

Experimentation challenges the patient's autonomy, principles of justice (fairness), and ethical principles of liberty (freedom) (Box 10–5). The patient's rights to self-determination, privacy, and truth may be overridden by coercion, covert data collection, deception, and breach of confidentiality.

Biomedical investigators have an obligation to inform the subjects, treat them fairly as autonomous agents, and to maximize the benefits of the experiment and minimize the risks. These obligations and the corresponding rights of the subjects are sometimes overridden by biasing of the selection of the subject, unfairly distributing risks and benefits, not informing subjects of risks and benefits, and poor attempts at maximizing benefits and minimizing risks.

The issues of harm to the individual are at the crux of the legislation protecting human subjects. The categories of harm (Box 10–5) clearly state the potential harm to the individual and must be countered with the means by which the professional

. . . .
BOX 10–5 ETHICAL PRINCIPLES CHALLENGED IN EXPERIMENTATION

1. Patient/animal autonomy
   A. Elements:
      (1.) Right of self-determination
      (2.) Right to privacy
      (3.) Right to the truth (veracity)
   B. Violations:
      (1.) Coercion
      (2.) Covert data collection
      (3.) Deception
      (4.) Use of incompetent subjects
      (5.) Breach of confidentiality
2. Justice—fair/equal opportunity
   A. Elements:
      (1.) Informed consent
      (2.) Treating potential subjects as autonomous agents
      (3.) Right to fair treatment
      (4.) Obligation of investigator to maximize benefits and minimize risks
   B. Violations:
      (1.) Social, cultural, racial, and sexual bias in selection of subjects
      (2.) Unfair distribution of risks and benefits based on efforts, needs, and rights
      (3.) Lack of description and delivery of benefits
      (4.) Lack of description of risks
      (5.) Lack of minimizing risks
      (6.) Lack of maximizing benefits
3. Liberty-limiting principles
   A. Elements:
      (1.) Harm, which is often considered in the risks/benefits arguments raised in research
      (2.) Paternalism
   B. Violations :
      (1.) Physiological, emotional, social, or economic harm
         a. Levels of harm
            (i.) No anticipated effects: *usually no risk*
            (ii.) Temporary discomfort (fatigue, headache, tension, anxiety, embarrassment, and stress during study): *minimal risk*
            (iii.) Unusual levels of temporary discomfort (muscle weakness, joint pain, dizziness, fear, and guilt that extends for a period after the study): *risk* (may require follow-up treatment, counseling)
            (iv.) Risk of permanent damage (permanent physical damage, permanent damage to personality, reputation, economic status, and job performance): *high risk*
            (v.) Certainty of permanent damage (organ transplants, early total hip replacements): *usually no risk rating, since risk is 100%*

will minimize the potential of harm, and if harm occurs, the degree of responsibility of the professional or institution to care for the subject after the experiment.

. . . .
EMPLOYEE RIGHTS AND OBLIGATIONS

All physical therapy staff are employees of an organization and may enjoy the rights to be treated fairly, to be provided with equipment and space in which to work, to engage in meaningful work, and to be protected from environmental hazards (Box 10–6). Each employee also has certain obligations to the institution, the client, and the community. These obligations include assuring appropriate education and licensure, performing duties responsibly, understanding and adhering to organizational, state, and regional rules and regulations including practice laws, adhering to the code of the ethics of the appropriate professional bodies recognized by the organization, documenting and billing patients appropriately, protecting the individual and others through liability insurance, and the obligation not to discriminate against any client, patient, or employee.

The American Physical Therapy Association's (APTA's) Code of Ethics imposes a number of obligations on member physical therapists related to the profession and the client. Physical therapists who are members of the association are bound by the code of ethics as are those whose institutions adopt the APTA code of ethics as the professional code of the physical therapy department. A similar document, the Standards of Ethical Conduct for the Physical Therapist Assistant, imposes certain obligations on the physical therapist assistant.

Ethical debate is needed in many areas within physical therapy. Many people feel that there is a need for professions to publicly debate ethical issues and that this debate is healthy for both the professionals involved as well as the consumers of professional services. If mainstream physical therapy does not publicly debate those issues of greatest importance to the profession, the void will be filled by others who will engage in the debate without the appropriate involvement of the profession. For instance, issues such as referral for profit should be openly debated by all parties

. . . .

BOX 10–6   EMPLOYEE RIGHTS AND OBLIGATIONS

1.0 Rights
   1.1   To be treated fairly
   1.2   To have adequate equipment, space, and other resources necessary to perform duties
   1.3   To be protected from environmental hazards
   1.4   To engage in meaningful work
   1.5   To have access to institutional protections (self insurance for liability)
   1.6   To not be discriminated against

2. Obligations
   2.1   Provide evidence of appropriate educational background
   2.2   Provide evidence of licensure in the jurisdiction of practice
   2.3   Provide evidence of specialty certification if representing self as a board-certified specialist
   2.4   Perform duties responsibly and efficiently
   2.5   Be aware of and adhere to institutional rules and regulations
   2.6   Be aware of and adhere to laws governing the practice of physical therapy in the jurisdiction of the practice
   2.7   Adhere to the code of ethics of the American Physical Therapy Association or another appropriate professional code of ethics (business, education)
   2.8   Document all patient care accurately and in a timely fashion
   2.9   Understand fiscal implications of services provided and accurately record all patient charges
   2.10 Understand all contractual responsibilities and discharge all duties as specified in the contract
   2.11 Protect oneself and others through liability insurance
   2.12 Engage in open communications
   2.13 Not to discriminate against any clients/patients

involved, including physical therapists, referral sources, health care facility administrators, and the public. Although the profession of physical therapy is effectively working to eliminate referral for profit, the public remains relatively uninformed of the issues. Public debate in public forums would greatly enhance the public's knowledge of the issues and place the burden on physical therapists to make cogent arguments against these practices.

PATIENT/CLIENT RIGHTS AND OBLIGATIONS

Additional obligations are imposed on the physical therapist and other organizational employees by the rights of the clients or patients. Patients have the right to receive assistance in seeking a second opinion, confidentiality, truthfulness, privacy, competent care, barrier-free access, protection from harm, right to information, full disclosure, freedom of expression, freedom from coercion, and respect (Box 10–7). These rights may be further explained or extended through patient advocacy groups and the development of the patient's Bill of Rights. In defining the rights of the patients, these documents also define the organization's obligations to the patients. Patients also have certain obligations, such as to comply with or refuse treatment, provide information, provide a mechanism to pay bills, follow rules and regulations of the institution, and engage in open communications.

PROFESSIONAL ISSUES

Many of the issues facing the profession of physical therapy have significant ethical components. Referral for profit issues (referral sources—usually physicians—owning a physical therapy practice in which patients are referred by the referral source who then profits from that referral; or referral sources receiving a direct payment

BOX 10–7   PATIENT/CLIENT RIGHTS AND OBLIGATIONS

1.0 Rights
    1.1   Receive assistance in seeking a second opinion
    1.2   Confidentiality
    1.3   Truthfulness
    1.4   Respect of privacy
    1.5   Administration of competent care
    1.6   Barrier-free access to care
    1.7   Protection from harm of person or property
    1.8   Right to information (record)
    1.9   Full disclosure of risks and benefits of treatment (informed consent)
    1.10 Freedom of expression
    1.11 Freedom from coercion
    1.12 Right to have wishes respected (living will)
    1.13 Right to respect for and protection of patient rights
2.0 Obligations
    2.1   Comply with or refuse treatment
    2.2   Provide information including untoward effects of treatment
    2.3   Provide a mechanism to pay bills
    2.4   Follow rules and regulations
    2.5   Communicate openly

from therapists for each referral) are argued on the presumption that there is exploitation or the potential of exploitation of patients and therapists. By exploitation, most physical therapists mean that patient freedom of choice may be denied and that the patient may not be fully informed in such situations. In addition, therapists may be exploited by being coerced to treat patients for longer periods of time than they would under other circumstances.

Direct access (the ability of the therapist to evaluate and treat patients without physician referral) issues are discussed as issues of freedom for the therapist to practice physical therapy without undue influence from physicians who are not grounded in the profession, freedom of the patient to choose practitioners other than physicians as the entry point into the health care system, and fairness to the patient and the insurance companies by reducing unnecessary costs associated with the physician as gatekeeper principle.

One issue that is discussed very little among physical therapists but seems to affect the attitudes of therapists toward each other is the presumed conflict between professional ethics and business ethics.

The profitability of owning a physical therapy business has led to conflict within the profession. Many physical therapists still believe that a profit should not be made from the misfortunes of others. Most physical therapists understand that health care facilities in which the physical therapist traditionally works can impose extraordinary charges for physical therapy services because the facility must support many non–income producing departments, employee benefits, retirement programs, self-insurance programs, buildings, and investments. As these institutions use physical therapy to fund other services over which the physical therapy component of the institution has no decision-making power and reduce the physical therapy manager to employee status, there is great potential for ethical debate in the area of fairness to the profession of physical therapy and physical therapists, the autonomy of professionals and professions, truthtelling in imposing financial burdens on departments in terms of indirect expenses, and the rights of the physical therapists to reasonable benefit from their services.

There seems to be little tolerance within the profession for the fact that the physical therapist owner of a physical therapy practice must also cover significant overhead expenses, plan for an unprotected retirement, develop competitive employee benefit packages, and make investments that will assure the future of the business. The fact that physical therapists are financially successful does not mean that they have been unethical in building their businesses. The questions that must be asked of those therapists might begin with the following.

1. Do other therapists have a fair opportunity to develop similar business ventures? Ethical principle: right to fair opportunity.

2. Is the successful physical therapist being unfair in the manner in which referral relationships are established? Ethical principle: right to choose.

3. Are joint ventures professionally appropriate and fairly established? Ethical principle: fair distribution of resources.

4. Are patients given the freedom of choice in selecting the physical therapy practice setting appropriate for needed services? Ethical principle: right to choose and not inflicting harm by treating problems that are best treated in another setting.

5. Are services or qualifications being misrepresented? Ethical principle: truthtelling.

All physical therapists and physical therapy managers should be challenged to support all aspects of physical therapy regardless of the setting in which the services are provided. Furthermore, physical therapy managers must raise the ethical questions if particular settings or particular therapists are in question, including the issues raised in traditional settings.

Many managers will be frustrated by ethical debates because there usually is no resolution or answer. There is no resultant action to take. The richness of the debate, the posing of concerns, and the grounding of actions and judgments help individuals think about the issues and begin to solidify their personal beliefs. Some physical therapy managers are beginning to facilitate ethical debates among the staff by instituting "lunch and ethics" or "ethics in the afternoon" seminars, in which staff gather voluntarily to discuss real physical therapy cases with chaplains, ethicists, philosophers, psychologists, social workers, psychiatrists, educators, physicians, institutional review board consultants, and other interested individuals.

CASE 10.1

City Hospital Ethics

Cheryl Cooper, P.T., M.S.

The therapists at City Hospital believe that they are facing an ethical dilemma. They are caught in the ever-growing and agonizing realization that the once altruistic health care field, physical therapy included, is making more and more decisions to provide treatment based on the patient's ability to pay for care.

First, it was the health maintenance organization (HMO) subscribers referred for physical therapy. These patients were finding that their insurance plans did not cover the full course of treatment. As the finance and billing departments were physically and operationally separate from the rest of the hospital's patient care functions, it became the job of the physical therapy staff to inform the patients that the rehabilitation benefits of their insurance plans had been exhausted and that they would become responsible for the costs of further treatment. This communication generally resulted in the patient asking for specific costs of treatment procedures. Therapists were uncomfortable with the high charges for the care they delivered. (These charges are set by a state commission and not by the department or the hospital.) The department experienced a drop in productivity as therapists were reluctant to bill for the full extent of services provided to any patient and particularly for those patients who had assumed financial responsibility for their bills.

The public perception of the department and the hospital was that there was an element of discrimination against HMO patients and that the therapists were saying that the patients could no longer be treated. In fact, patients were being told that their benefits no longer covered physical therapy, and should they decide to continue therapy, it would be as a private payer. Staff were unhappy at being the bearers of this news, and the department managers worked with them to intervene with the message, and to determine the best times and ways to discuss the options with the patients. The importance of appropriate and correct billing was discussed often with the staff.

The next critical point in the dilemma came with the state's action in medical assistance (MA) cases. In an effort to reduce spending, the state stopped coverage of all outpatient services provided at the hospital for those patients whose MA was from the state. The problems of the physical therapist staff came with the awareness that there were insufficient community facilities and private practices that accepted MA cases for medical services in general, and physical therapy specifically. In addition, of the clinics and practices providing physical therapy for MA patients, there were only one or two that could deliver the specialized burn rehabilitation care that could be provided at City Hospital. As the private practices that had accepted state MA clients became overwhelmed by the large numbers of patients once seen in hospital clinics, there was a move to cut state medical assistance recipients from the list of patients seen by these practices.

The question of the right to health care and the issue of health care rationing was discussed without resolution. Staff members were clearly uncomfortable with the notion that care was being denied to those in need.

Department managers tried repeatedly to emphasize that treatment was not being denied. Every state MA patient referred to the department for physical therapy would be scheduled for treatment. The critical point, however, was that the patient would be responsible for the cost of the physical therapy services provided. None of these patients could afford to pay for this care. When a patient with state MA was referred to the department, the situation was explained to him or her. The option of treatment at the hospital outpatient department was offered, with the patient being told of his or her responsibility for the cost of treatment. If the patient accepted an appointment, he or she was offered the number of the hospital's financial counselor staff. If the patient declined an appointment, the department staff would provide him or her with a list of private practices and community clinics where physical therapy was available to recipients of state MA. In some cases, the appointments were made for the patient if he or she seemed to need assistance. If patients required specialized services—such as burn rehabilitation—they were seen in the hospital department, regardless of their ability to pay.

Still, the staff had been confronted with an ethical issue for which they could find no completely satisfactory resolution. As more and more community practices turned away state MA clients, the hospital staff felt increasingly uncomfortable with this social situation. The management of the department was at a loss as to how to help the staff feel better about the issue and the role of the hospital in the situation.

Consider the ethical dilemmas of the staff regarding the obligation to do good, the department managers' responsibility to fairly distribute resources and the obligation(s) to the organization, the patients' rights to fair opportunity and fair access to care, the state's responsibility to fairly distribute resources, and the organization's obligations to the community.

. . . .
DEFINITIONS/TERMINOLOGY

Absolute rights: Rights that cannot be overridden.

Beneficence: To do good. Beneficence is generally thought to be more far-reaching than the principle of nonmaleficence because it requires positive steps to help others. Prevention of harm and removal of harmful conditions.

Deontology: Duty-based ethical theory associated with Emanuel Kant. Autonomy of the individual is foremost as is duty for the sake of duty alone. The value of actions lies in the motives. Actions and judgments must satisfy the demands of an overriding principle of duty.

Distributive justice: Justified distribution of benefits and burdens. In management, distributive justice issues refer to the fair distribution of resources within the organization by managers or through institutional policy.

Entering wedge: If an individual allows an action or judgment to occur once, it will continue and escalate. This is much harsher than mere precedent. In ethical terms, it is often the fear that compels people to debate an issue and advocate for laws that prevent the act from occurring.

Equality: A fundamental set of rights. Rights (to make claims to resources) that are not derived from other rights. According to Aristotle, "equals ought to be treated equally and unequals may be treated unequally."[2(p184)] In a physical therapy department, staff ought to have equal rights to resources that are seen as primary goods (needed to do their job).

Goods: When "goods" are referred to in definitions of moral dilemmas, the goods that are in conflict are two or more potentially good outcomes, best decisions, or reasonable approaches.

Justice: When a person has been given what is due or owed, deserved, or legitimately claimed. Fairness.

Law: The ethical minimum. Societally imposed processes to insure compliance with certain basic beliefs.

Liberty-limiting principles: Harm, paternalism. These are principles that restrict an individual's freedom.

Moral dilemma: A situation in which two or more goods are in conflict and when an individual can rely on moral considerations for taking each of two opposing courses of action.

Moral norms: A principle of right action binding upon the members of a group and serving to guide, control, or regulate proper and acceptable behavior.[4] The most basic moral principles governing academic life. These may be expressed in institutional honor codes, tenure rights, and other codes of conduct.

Moral principles: Fundamental rules or codes of conduct. They serve as the foundation for moral rules and a source of justification.

Morality: A social state governed by a specific set of rules and focusing on the relationships of people and how they ought to behave toward one another in the society.

Nonmaleficence: To do no harm. The noninfliction of harm on others. Prevention of harm and removal of harmful conditions.

Paternalism: To take away an individual's freedom to make a decision or choice. To make a decision or choice for another person. To coerce into action because the individual is perceived to be unable to make the "right" decision.

Prima facie rights: Rights that can be overridden.

Slippery slope: The concept that if you act or make a specific judgment around an ethical concept or question, you must act or make the same judgment in all like circumstances.

Utilitarianism: Developed by John Stuart Mill. An ethical theory that is grounded in the concept of the ends justifying the means. The driving force of the theory is that if the end result is beneficial to society or the individual, the acts and judgments that lead to that end are justified.

Virtue ethics: Aristotlian ethics grounded in values of trustworthiness, kindness, faithfulness, and other virtues valued by the society. It is based on people, not behaviors, and stresses the kind of person we ought to be. It is felt by some virtue ethicists that the bonding that may happen in an instant between a patient and a health care professional evolves from the virtues that the therapist displays and therefore gains the patient's immediate trust and confidence.

References

1. Beauchamp TL, Childress JF: *Principles of Biomedical Ethics.* New York, NY, Oxford University Press, 1983.
2. Beauchamp TL: *Philosophical Ethics.* New York, NY, McGraw-Hill Book Co, 1982.
3. Purtilo RB, Cassel CK: *Ethical Dimensions in the Health Professions.* Philadelphia, Pa, W.B. Saunders Co, 1981.
4. *Webster's New Collegiate Dictionary.* Springfield, Mass, GC Merriam, 1976, p. 783.

Suggested Readings

Helmer O: *Looking Forward.* Beverly Hills, Calif, Sage Publications, 1983.

Lasch C: *Culture of Narcissism.* New York, NY, WW Norton Co, 1979.

Lazerson M, et al: *An Education of Value.* Cambridge, England, Cambridge University Press, 1985.

MacIntyre A: *After Virtue.* Notre Dame, Ind, University of Notre Dame Press, 1981.

Nash RJ, Griffin RS: Balancing the private and the public. *Harvard Educ Rev* 1986; 56:20–28.

Nash RJ, Griffin RS: Repairing the public-private split: Excellence, character, and civic virtue. *Teachers College Record* 1987; 88: 549–566.

Nash RJ: Applied ethics and moral imagination: Issues for educators. *J Thought* 1987; 22:68–77.

Purtilo RB: Reading "physical therapy" from an ethics perspective. *Phys Ther* 1975; 55: 361–364.

Purtilo RB: Structure of ethics teaching in physical therapy. *Phys Ther* 1979; 59: 1102–1106.

Purtilo RB: Understanding ethical issues: The physical therapist as ethicist. *Phys Ther* 1974; 54: 239–243.

Purtilo RB: Who should make moral policy decisions in health care? *Phys Ther* 1978; 58: 1076–1081.

Planning and Decision Making in Physical Therapy

INTRODUCTION

Several different strategies are used by physical therapy managers when planning a variety of aspects of the services provided in physical therapy, i.e., managers use planning strategies when they are considering new or enhanced programs, expanding space, building new space, budgeting, and reorganization. Most experienced managers do not use a single planning strategy. The traditional strategies are modified and customized to accommodate the objectives of the system. However, most new managers do follow the tenets of single planning strategies more closely in an attempt to learn the system and reach a predictable end point in the process.

The most basic planning strategy used in organizational planning is the problem-solving process. This process is described by business professionals as well as a number of other professional groups. It utilizes the following steps (Box 11–1).

This basic problem-solving process is employed in many situations involving the management of work and the management of human resources.

IDENTIFY AND DEFINE THE PROBLEM

The first steps in problem solving are to define the problem and write a problem statement containing the following.

1. Future point in time when the problem must be solved (or if not solved, it will result in something).

. . . .
BOX 11–1   PROBLEM-SOLVING PROCESS

1. Identify and define the problem
2. Generate objectives
3. Choose among alternative strategies
4. Decision making
   a. Analyze resources and constraints
   b. Assess adverse consequences
   c. Anticipate potential problems
5. Implement the decision
6. Evaluate the solution

2. Geographic area or parts of the organization that the problem affects.
3. Nature of the problem.
4. Estimate of the size of the problem.
5. Individuals or groups of people affected by the problem.[1(p22)]

The definition of the problem is not only the first step in this process, it is the most important. It is critical to identify the problem, not symptoms of a problem. For instance, morale is a symptom, not the problem. It is the responsibility of the manager to determine why morale might be low if the expectation is that at the end of the problem-solving process morale will be heightened. It is also important for the manager to decide not only what the problem is, but what it is not, so that the limits of the boundaries of the problem can be clarified.

. . . .
GENERATE OBJECTIVES

Once the problem statement has been developed, it must be translated into one or several objectives. Objectives are specific measurable statements of what needs to be accomplished by a given point in time and the degree to which the objective must be met. In assessing the completeness of the objectives, consider the degree to which the objectives *RUMBA*.

Realistic.   Given the resources available and the time frame in which the objective is to be met, is it possible to accomplish it?

Understandable.   Does it make sense? Will it be understood by others?

Measurable.   When considering the measurability of the objective(s), consider the criteria that you will use to assess whether the objective has been met.

Behavioral.   Objectives should not be written as abstract or vague statements. State clearly what will be done.

Achievable.   Does this objective require resources or time periods that are unrealistic? If so, the objective may not be achievable. It is also possible to write the objective so vague or so ambitious that it cannot be achieved within a reasonable timeframe.

· · · · · · · · · · ·
IDENTIFY AND CHOOSE AMONG ALTERNATIVE STRATEGIES

Once the objectives are established, the next step is to identify and choose among alternate strategies. The manager should make an exhaustive list of all ways of reaching the objective. This is one of the most creative aspects of the problem-solving process. Managers should not limit thinking or scope when generating the first list of possible alternatives. All boundaries of the institution, practice, and profession should be eliminated in order to think creatively about the range of possible solutions.

Some alternatives may be eliminated immediately if it is obvious that they will require resources that are not likely to be available for the implementation of the plan or if they break professional or institutional rules which are not malleable. Other alternatives may require more careful analysis. That analysis may begin with a force field analysis, in which both helping and restraining forces are analyzed regarding each strategy. For example, when considering the development of a rehabilitation unit in a small community hospital, the following force field analysis was developed for the alternative of converting unused acute beds to rehabilitation beds (Box 11–2).

Once each of the driving and restraining forces were identified for this one strategy, the manager gathered information that gave relative weighting to each of these forces. From such weightings, the manager can make some preliminary decisions regarding whether this is a viable strategy. The information can be gathered from documents, surveys, observations, or interviews. In the example, both documents and interviews were employed to gather data regarding the forces driving the problem or strategy (Box 11–3).

From this preliminary analysis, the manager can see that the first question which must be answered if this strategy is to be pursued is the question of reimbursement for the rehabilitation beds. It appears that all other restraining forces are manageable if the reimbursement issue is addressed. Furthermore, it appears that the financial loss of unfilled beds is the primary driving force for this particular strategy. A preliminary or rough force field analysis can give the manager a sense of direction in terms of data gathering and incremental problem solving, including whether or not one particular strategy is even worth pursuing.

· ·
BOX 11–2 FORCE FIELD ANALYSIS

Objective: To determine the appropriate size and scope of a bed conversion program at Community Hospital A

Strategy No. 1: Convert "unused" acute beds to rehabilitation beds

Driving Forces	Restraining Forces
Interest of administrators	Reimbursement policies unknown and untested
Interest of physicians	Real need unknown
Interest of community	Commitment of support staff
Ease of conversion	Readiness of support staff
Financial loss if beds continue to be underutilized	Risk of reputation
Perceived need by area health agencies	Time—if pushed too fast, will sacrifice commitment of internal and external groups

BOX 11–3 WEIGHTED FORCE FIELD ANALYSIS*

Driving Forces	Relative Weight		Restraining Forces
Interest of administrators	+++	– – – – – –	Reimbursement policies unknown and untested
Interest of physicians	+++++	– – –	Real need unknown
Interest of community	++	– – –	Commitment of support staff
Ease of conversion	+++++	– –	Readiness of support staff
Financial loss if beds continue to be underutilized	++++++++++	– – – –	Risk of reputation
Perceived need by area health agencies	++	– – – –	Time—if pushed too fast, will sacrifice commitment of internal and external groups

*Minus sign indicates a unit (usually dollars) that restrains the organization from making a decision; plus sign indicates a unit that drives the organization positively toward a decision.

DECISION MAKING

The actual decision-making process is commonly broken into analyzing the resources and constraints, assessing the adverse consequences of the solutions, and anticipating potential problems. There are many strategies available to managers to analyze resources. One strategy is to use a cross-impact analysis. This process involves the use of a grid in which each component of a potential solution is analyzed in terms of people, money, time, and other resources necessary to accomplish the strategy (Fig 11–1).

Another resource analysis strategy is to lay out the plan in terms of the critical incidents that must be accomplished, the time over which the strategy will be implemented, and the resources needed at each critical stage using a program evaluation and review technique (PERT) chart (Fig 11–2). The PERT chart can be used to assess resource needs at each phase of the project. It also aids in scheduling projects by focusing on key steps, sequencing events, and providing a device to monitor and report progress.

To construct a PERT chart the manager must complete the following steps.

1. Identify and define each activity to be performed.
2. Decide the order in which those activities will be performed.

	Professional Staff	Support Staff	Space	Equipment	Supplies
Strategy #1	1	3	0	$10,000	++
Strategy #2	3	4	1600*	45,000	++++
Strategy #3	2	3	3000*	25,000	+++

FIG 11–1.
Resource matrix. Asterisk = square feet of new space; plus sign = approximately an additional $100 a month.

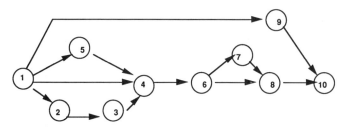

FIG 11–2.
Program evaluation and review technique (PERT) chart. Each circle within the PERT chart represents a milestone. A milestone is a point in terms of time or activity at which a specific activity is accomplished.

3. Determine the time required to complete each activity as well as the entire project.
4. Determine the resources required for each step.
5. Find the critical path.
6. Modify the plan as needed.
7. Monitor and refine the plan.

There are quantitative methods of calculating completion time from milestone to milestone and from beginning to end of the project using three different time estimates for each milestone. If time is the most critical factor, managers should refer to planning texts or consultants to determine specific methods of calculating time within the PERT context.

The critical path method (CPM) is another planning strategy similar to the PERT process. Specific paths and their accompanying time and resource requirements (cost) are considered in planning. The process used is very similar to the PERT process, but the cost of each path is an equally important component (Fig 11–3). When planners focus on this critical path as the planning strategy, it is referred to as the CPM of planning.

For the purposes of this chapter, the PERT and CPM approaches are being used to lay out strategies and to determine resources needed throughout the implementation stage. The time anticipated to complete each phase of the strategy can be explained through use of a Gantt schedule (Fig 11–4).

From the PERT and CPM plans and the Gantt schedule, the physical therapy manager can build a chart of the resources needed to complete the strategy at each phase or milestone. When analyzing staff, the manager must complete job analyses (see Chapter Ten) of each professional and supportive staff position. The job analyses will determine if staff members from existing programs may apply for the positions or if recruitment for the positions will be necessary.

The strategy that is selected must consider the needs of the department and in-

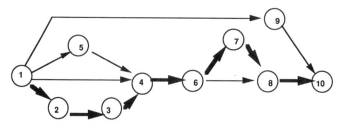

FIG 11–3.
Critical path method of planning.

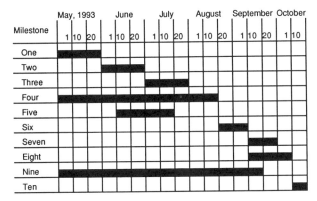

FIG 11–4.
Gantt schedule for completion of the program evaluation and review technique plan.

stitution, noting the characteristics of the various elements of the system and how the strategy will fit with the organization. There are many computer programs in management science and information science that allow the manager to simulate the strategy and analyze the impact on the system. When strategies are expensive and the potential impact on the system is great, it is to the advantage of the organization to develop models or simulations to test the proposed strategy.

· · · · · · · · · · ·
IMPLEMENT DECISIONS

Once the alternatives have been developed and the resources necessary to implement the various strategies analyzed, the physical therapy manager is ready to decide on the strategy to be pursued. If the PERT, CPM, and Gantt tools have been used to develop and analyze each strategy, the manager already has a staged implementation process laid out in these two planning tools.

Most managers make decisions in relative isolation. Decisions may be grounded in intuition, tradition, or management science. The physical therapy manager has many other individuals and groups available to assist in the decision-making process if the manager would like to receive more input (Box 11–4).

Sometimes managers are reluctant to use others in decision making because they feel that they will lose control of the process. The optimal way to use input is to frame the issue or question that is most unclear or variable or less well developed and that would be enhanced by several individuals giving thoughtful consideration to the issue. Using others in the decision-making process does not mean turning

· ·
BOX 11–4 DECISION-MAKING RESOURCES

Individuals involved in making the decision work (the employees)
Administrators above the manager
Peer managers within the institution
Peer managers within the profession (regional or national)
Administration and private practice sections of the American Physical Therapy Association (APTA)
Speciality oriented sections of the APTA
Consultants and experts

over the process to those individuals. It is the manager's responsibility to orchestrate the input that is needed—where it is needed and when.

. . . .

GROUP INPUT TO THE DECISION

When planning the manner in which a strategy will be implemented, it is helpful to ask the employees or individuals who will implement the decision for input. The manager may want to gather the individuals together to give an overview of the strategy and frame the decisions in which the employees will have some input. In order to get the most thoughtful consideration of this input, the employees should then be given an opportunity to ask questions and time to think about the issues and the input that the individual would like to give to the implementation of the strategy. A follow-up meeting in which the employees are asked to brainstorm solutions should then be held.

Brainstorming is an excellent tool to use when the manager wants all of the group's thoughts so that each can be discussed without bias. In order for brainstorming to work, the facilitator of the group process asks each person in the group to present their thoughts. No other member of the group is allowed to offer comments about the value of the comment until everyone has offered input. The facilitator then leads a group discussion on the strengths and weaknesses of each concept until a consensus is reached on the recommendations to go to the manager. If the manager is willing to let the group make final decisions on the recommendations, then the group meeting must result in consensus on the recommendations to be implemented.

The strength of group brainstorming is that it allows each member of the group the opportunity to present and defend concepts and ideas. The weakness is that consensus is difficult to reach. In order for the group to reach true consensus (100% of the group agrees to include certain concepts), an experienced facilitator and a considerable amount of time are required.

If the manager is working with individuals who tend to compete with each other or if some individuals overpower others, the manager may want to use one of two other group consensus methods—the nominal group process or the Delphi process.

The nominal group process also begins with a framing of the decisions to be made. Then small groups (two to three people) are asked to come to consensus on the issues before the next meeting (which may be convened in the next several hours or days). At the next meeting each group presents their consensus without value being placed on the outcomes by the rest of the group. Each group defends the consensus and then the entire group seeks consensus. The strength of this approach is that the consensus in small groups is more likely to be closer to the total group consensus than individual thoughts, since a certain amount of compromise has already had to occur. The weakness is that the small groups have built a stronger connection to the consensus decision and each group member will be highly committed to moving in that direction. The nominal group process usually leads to group consensus faster than brainstorming.

When the manager wants to use groups of experts that are not easily brought together, the Delphi process may be the most appropriate group consensus process. The purpose of the Delphi is to make the best use of a group of experts in obtaining answers to questions from groups of specialists in the area. The Delphi technique was designed to accomplish this with a minimum of interference from the problems of open discussions among panels of experts and to achieve as close a consensus as possible. The process involves a series (usually three) of open-ended surveys. In the first survey, the problem is framed and the experts are asked to brainstorm (individually). The second survey reports the actual individual responses and asks the panel to add additional comments. In the third survey the panel is asked to rate, rank, or eliminate items. The manager then has a document that presents the degree of agreement among experts regarding a particular decision.

With all of this information in hand, the manager is ready to implement the strategy. By the end of the staged implementation process that has been developed in the planning documents, all resources should be in place. As the manager works through the stages of implementation, potential problems will become apparent and contingency plans put in place.

The manager must also consciously determine the control mechanisms that will be a part of the implementation plan. These mechanisms will allow for continuing review of the project and its implementation. The PERT chart, Gantt scheduling chart, and cross-impact analysis of resources are both planning and control documents. The manager is able to monitor progress, time tables, and resource allocation following the planning documents. In addition, the manager must define the communication system within the strategy and how progress and problems will be reported. These communication networks must include those implementing the strategy, the consumers of the services, other managers, and organizational administrative groups.

• • • • • • • • • • •
EVALUATE SOLUTIONS AND REVISE

The evaluation phase of the planning process is critical to the continuing success of the strategy. This evaluation must include an evaluation of the processes within the strategy as well as the outcomes of the strategy. The process evaluation can be based on the control mechanisms put in place to implement the program assessing resource utilization, milestones of accomplishments, and the timeliness of decisions and service delivery. New PERT and Gantt charts will have to be developed to represent the ongoing delivery of services. The outcome assessment must feed back to the original definition of the problem and be tested against that definition to be sure that the problem has been resolved. Evaluation of the system is incomplete without a commitment to make revisions to the process as necessary. A new strategy is unlikely to be perfectly planned or implemented. There will be a need for revisions and fine tuning for a considerable period of time. In addition, the strategy must not only meet the needs it was intended to meet, it must continue to meet the needs of the organization as it grows and changes.

In approaching problem solving, the rational manager takes a logical, sequential approach to each step within the problem-solving process.

The Kepner-Tregoe model of decision making (Fig 11–5) identifies all of the steps that the manager takes in making decisions and solving problems. As this model represents, after the manager recognizes that there is a problem, the causes of the problem must be determined, the best way to solve the problem and implement the plan must be decided, and then again any problems must be determined. Decision-making and program planning are a circular process.

Many managers state that anyone can come up with a solution to a problem, the key is determining the best solution to the problem and then making the solution work (through evaluation and revision). Although the front end of the process, the analytical process of defining the problem and developing a rational plan, is often the most challenging for many managers, the processes of establishing controls and setting up contingency plans are critical to monitoring and adjusting the solutions. There are always nuances to problems, and the likelihood that there is a single best solution that will work without adjustment is minimal. The skillful manager must be prepared to monitor the process and provide thoughtful input and feedback to those implementing the solution.

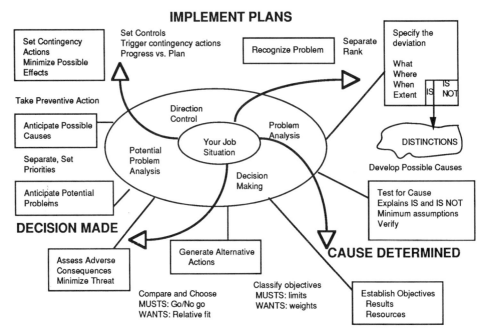

FIG 11–5.
Decision-making model. (From Kepner CH, Tregoe BB: *The Rational Manager.* New York, NY, McGraw-Hill, 1985. Used with permission.)

References

1. Craig DP: *Hip Pocket Guide to Planning and Evaluation.* Austin, Tex, Learning Concepts, 1978.

Suggested Readings

Ackoff RL: *The Art of Problem Solving.* New York, NY, John Wiley and Sons, 1978.

Capelle RG: Changing human systems. Toronto, Canada, International Human Systems Institute, 1979.

Churchman CW: *The Systems Approach.* New York, NY, Dell Publishing Co, 1968.

Drucker PF: *The Practice of Management.* New York, NY, Harper and Row Publishers, 1986.

Friedman LA, et al: A computer simulation model of hospital mergers. *Health Care Manage Rev,* 1983, pp 53–65.

Hampton DR, et al: *Organizational Behavior and the Practice of Management.* Glenview, Ill, Scott, Foresman and Co, 1982.

Hatcher M, Narasinga R: A simulation based decision support system for a health promotion center. *J Med Systems* 1988; 12:11–29.

Hyman HH: *Health Planning: A Systematic Approach.* Germantown, Md, Aspen Publications, 1976.

Johnstone K, et al: Management of Change in a Large PT Department, *Clin Manage* 0000; 5:10–13.

Konrad E: Corporate planning shouldn't be a one-man band. *Innovation* 1970; 00:000.

Lane DS, Mazzola G: The community hospital as a focus of health planning. *Am J Public Health* 1976; 66:000.

Liebler JG, et al: *Management Principles for Health Professionals.* Gaithersburg, Md, Aspen Publications, 1984.

Megginson LC, et al: *Management: Concepts and Applications.* Cambridge, Mass, Harper and Row Publishers, 1989.

Miller JG: *Living Systems.* New York, NY, McGraw Hill, 1978.

CHAPTER 12

Space Designs in Physical Therapy

. . . .

I. Introduction

II. Americans With Disabilities Act Legislation

III. ADA guiding principles: Medical care facilities
    A. Parking
    B. Ramps
    C. Wheelchair maneuverability
    D. Reaching objects from wheelchairs
    E. Bedroom facilities
    F. Toilet facilities
    G. Handrails

IV. Guiding principles: General
    A. Inventory and storage
    B. Flow of traffic
    C. Space flexibility
    D. Equipment placement

. . . .

INTRODUCTION

Given the alternative organizational structures used in physical therapy departments today, it is not possible to predict with a degree of accuracy exactly what the department will physically look like and what the exact equipment needs will be for that department. Therefore, guiding principles will be presented here for the physical therapy manager to consider when adapting or building physical therapy space.

Although many individuals who are physical therapy managers have had a great deal of experience building or renovating commercial and residential space, most physical therapy managers are not space planners, architects, or industrial engineers. It is advisable for the physical therapy manager to consult each of these individuals for their unique professional skills. Likewise, none of these professionals have the unique perspective of the physical therapist regarding the variety of models of delivery of services in physical therapy even in the same facility. Of the professions mentioned, industrial engineers are least consulted by physical therapy managers when designing space. However, it is this professional who is able to provide great insight regarding ergonomically correct work stations and traffic patterns. In considering the guiding principles for building or renovating space, the manager should consider both the ergonomic needs of the staff as well as the space needs of the clients.

The principles that guide the building and renovation of physical therapy space have traditionally come from two domains—regulations (local, state, and federal) regarding new buildings and renovations and elements of architectural design. All managers seeking to build or renovate space must begin with local zoning boards and other governmental agencies to obtain copies of all pertinent ordinances that direct or restrict development. This activity may be completed by an institutional administrator whose primary job is planning and space issues. Increasingly, however, as physical therapy managers either develop their own practices or take on increasing administrative responsibility to develop satellite units, physical therapists will find it important to understand local, state, and federal regulations governing community development.

Many community ordinances are dictated by overriding federal legislation that sets guidelines, such as those that protect wetlands and maintain appropriate transportation networks within the community. Although communities may chose not to follow these guidelines in some instances, failure to do so may deprive the local governing bodies of necessary federal funds to maintain the community. For this reason, it is critical that physical therapy managers seeking to build or renovate space have the guidance of institutional or independent lawyers who are familiar with commercial zoning laws and issues.

In addition, the state has regulations that govern the development of businesses within the state. Again, although others may take responsibility to monitor these regulations, the physical therapist should obtain copies of state guidelines for developing a professional practice within the state and local area. Such regulations can be obtained directly from the Secretary of State in which the practice will be located and from the City or Town Zoning or Planning office for local regulations. Many communities impose business license fees and have strict building ordinances. These fees and ordinances will have different applications if the business is considered for-profit or not-for-profit and should be carefully reviewed with real estate consultants or lawyers. In addition, as a health care facility, especially if the new business is a satellite operation, most states have certificate of need regulations that must be carefully followed before proceeding to build or renovate space.

Many of the regulatory agencies that play a role in the establishment and maintenance of health care agencies have space requirements. For the most part, agencies such as the Joint Commission on the Accreditation of Healthcare Organizations (JCAHO), which are now moving more and more toward outcome assessment, are very general in their space requirements for physical therapy. The guidelines primarily address the adequacy of the space. The Commission on the Accreditation of Rehabilitation Facilities (CARF) is much more prescriptive regarding the amount of space required per rehabilitation bed, recreational units, and rehabilitation activities.

· · · · · · · · · · ·
AMERICANS WITH DISABILITIES ACT LEGISLATION

In 1990 the Americans With Disabilities Act (ADA) was passed by Congress. Accessibility guidelines for buildings and facilities were finalized and became effective in 1992. The law stated that "Title III of the ADA (effective 1/26/92) prohibits discrimination on the basis of disability in places of public accommodation by any person who owns, leases or leases to, or operates a place of public accommodation."[1(p35408)] Public accommodation was defined in the law to include 12 categories of private entities that are presented in (Box 12–1).

··

BOX 12–1 CATEGORIES OF PLACES OF PUBLIC ACCOMMODATION DEFINED IN THE AMERICANS WITH DISABILITIES ACT

1. An inn, hotel, motel, or similar place of lodging
2. A restaurant, bar, or other establishment serving food or drink
3. A motion picture house, theater, concert hall, stadium, or other place of exhibition or entertainment
4. An auditorium, convention center, lecture hall, or other place of public gathering
5. A bakery, grocery store, clothing store, hardware store, shopping center, or other sales or rental establishment
6. A laundromat, dry-cleaner, bank, barber shop, beauty shop, travel service, shoe repair service, funeral parlor, gas station, office of an accountant or lawyer, pharmacy, insurance office, professional office of a health care provider, hospital, or other service establishment

7. A terminal, depot, or other station used for specified public transportation
8. A museum, library, gallery, or other place of public display or collection
9. A park, zoo, amusement park, or other place of recreation
10. A nursery, elementary, secondary, undergraduate, or postgraduate private school, or other place of education
11. A day-care center, senior citizen center, homeless shelter, food bank, adoption agency, or other social service center establishment
12. A gymnasium, health spa, bowling alley, golf course, or other place of exercise or recreation

Item number 6 directs physical therapists, physicians, chiropractors, nurses, hospitals, and ambulatory care centers to make physical accommodations for the handicapped in new or renovated space. Even if this law did not exist, physical therapy clients are likely to be disabled and using wheelchairs or other ambulation aids that make it critical that the facilities in which they receive health care are designed to accommodate for these mobility aides. The *Federal Register* of Friday, July 26, 1991, details the accessibility guidelines for buildings and facilities. The guidelines are extremely specific in terms of building requirements, and the hundreds of pages cannot be duplicated here. However, there are some major guidelines that will determine the overall amount of space needed for specific functions, and those guidelines will be addressed. Some of these guidelines are still open for interpretation as to the extent of the accessibility. For instance, when addressing water fountains, it was determined that only approximately 50% of water fountains had to be accessible. For correct interpretation of these guidelines, it is again critical for the physical therapy manager to seek legal counsel from a lawyer who is familiar with ADA regulations.

The guidelines developed in the ADA legislation incorporate guidelines from traditional health care regulatory agencies (JCAHO, CARF) and then extend those guidelines to incorporate guidelines that have been developed for specific patient populations (arthritis, spinal cord) by advocacy groups. Some of these guidelines had been adopted by individual states and commercial groups prior to ADA. The current legislative guidelines ensure a more uniform degree of accessibility and give the physical therapy manager an exceptional guideline for building and renovating physical therapy space.

· · · · · · · · · · ·

ADA GUIDING PRINCIPLES: MEDICAL CARE FACILITIES*

The minimal requirements for new or renovated space include at least one accessible route from the site of public transportation, accessible parking spaces, passenger loading zones, and public streets or sidewalks to an accessible building entrance[1(35463)]; at least one accessible route connecting accessible buildings; appropriate percentage of accessible parking spaces for the kind of facility; public toilet facilities; appropriate signs designating rooms, directions, and information; designation of accessible facilities by the International Symbol of Accessibility (Fig 12–1); and accessible elevators (new buildings).

Parking

Parking requirements are established by local ordinances as well as state and federal guidelines. Therefore, the physical therapy manager should review all regulations and choose the parking specifications that are most restrictive of the levels of regulations as the guiding principles for development of accessible parking. Most local ordinances are written for commercial establishments and require fewer accessible parking slots than the ADA requirements for health care institutions (Box 12–2). Parking is perhaps the dominant factor in expanding health care institutions today. It is critical to purchase enough land to allow for adequate parking for the present time as well as for planned growth over the next ten years. From a marketing perspective, parking facilities will be one of the first physical aspects of the institution that the client will encounter. Providing accessible and convenient parking for clients will help to ensure their continuing patronage.

Accessible parking can be provided by using the standard accessible parking space that is 96 in. wide with an adjacent 60-in. access aisle. This access aisle will not be large enough for vans with platforms or ramps on the side of the van. An accessible van space would include the 96-in. parking space and an addition 96-in. access aisle. By placing one 96-in. access aisle in the middle of two 96-in. parking spaces, two vans could be accommodated. All health care businesses must provide some van-accessible parking spaces. An alternative is to use the Universal Parking Space

---

*All of the specific measurements and references to sizes in the guiding principles in this chapter were obtained from Americans With Disabilities Act legislation as reported in the *Federal Register,* vol 56, No. 144, Friday, July 26, 1991. Figures in the guiding principles sections of this chapter were also adapted from this same document. The document contains many more specific guidelines for the 12 sites listed in the beginning of this chapter. In addition, there are more specific references to alternatives when the space is being renovated rather than being created in new construction. Readers are encouraged to obtain the full text of the *Federal Register* from: Office of the General Counsel, Architectural and Transportation Board, 1111–18th St, NW, Suite 501, Washington, DC 20036; (202) 653–7834. The document is available in accessible formats (cassette tape, braille, large print, or computer disc) as well as the written format.

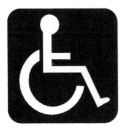

FIG 12–1.
International symbol of accessibility.

BOX 12–2   PARKING GUIDELINES FOR HEALTH CARE FACILITIES

Outpatient	10% of total number of parking spaces must be accessible
Units specializing in treatment of persons with mobility impairment	20% of total number of parking spaces must be accessible

Design (Fig 12–2). This design allows 132 in. for parking space with a 60-in. access aisle between the parking spaces. The advantage of using this design is that no special slots are needed for vans, no additional signs are necessary, there is less variability in the creation and maintenance of the parking area, and greater flexibility is afforded to the disabled driver.

Ramps

Buildings that have stairs to enter the facility must also have a ramp that allows for access from the street level. Most commonly ramps are built with a 1:12 slope projecting for no more than 30 ft. Landings must be as wide as the ramp and will provide at least 60 in. of clear space. If 30 horizontal feet is not available and the ramp is built with a change of direction at the landing, that landing must be 60 × 60-in.

Wheelchair Maneuverability

Within the facility, consideration must be given to accessibility by persons in wheelchairs. The standard wheelchair is approximately 30 in. wide. That means that openings such as doors must be at least 32 inches wide to allow the individual enough clearance for hands to move the wheels of the chair. Corridor or free space must be at least 36 in. wide to allow for operation of the wheelchair over a long space. The depth of the doorway cannot be more than 24 in. to allow the wheelchair user to move through the doorway without being hampered by the closing of the door (Fig 12–3). This will allow the client to move safely through doorways even with a standard 3-sec automatic closer.

If there is a need, as there often is in a physical therapy practice that must accommodate many wheelchair users, for there to be adequate corridor space for wheelchairs moving in opposite directions or passing each other, the minimal clearance width of the space is 60 in. The ADA guidelines also state that if the corridor is less than 60 in. in such a facility, there must be passing spaces of 60 × 60-in. at regular intervals.

When a wheelchair user must navigate around an object 48 in. or more in width,

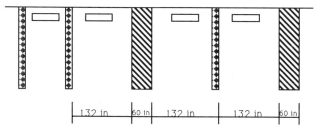

FIG 12–2.
Universal parking space design.

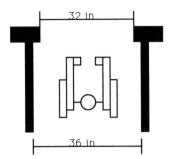

FIG 12–3.
Minimal clearance for single wheelchair.

the space around that object must be arranged in a 36-in. pathway that will allow a 90° turn (Fig 12–4).

When a wheelchair user must maneuver around an object less than 48 inches wide, the pathway space must be at least 42 in. wide, allowing for a 48-in. clearance around the top of the obstacle (Fig 12–5).

Reaching Objects From Wheelchairs

As the individual approaches an object that must be reached from a forward direction (pulleys, weights, balls), the maximum height of the reach should be 48 in. from the floor, and the lowest reach should be 15 in. from the floor. If the individual can approach the object from the side while still in the wheelchair, the reach dimensions are more generous. The maximum side reach height is 54 in. from the floor, and the minimum reach height is 9 in. from the floor.

Counter tops that are intended to be used from a forward approach by a wheelchair user should be approximately 44 in. high and between 20 and 25 in. deep. If counter tops are to be used from a side reach position in a wheelchair, the height of the counter top should be approximately 34 in. from the floor, with no objects placed any higher than 46 in. from the floor (12 in. above the counter top).

Bedroom Facilities

At least 10% of patient bedrooms and toilets are required to be accessible in general hospitals, whereas all bedrooms and toilets in a rehabilitation facility must be accessible and 50% of bedrooms and toilets must be accessible in long-term care facilities. Bedroom accessibility is assured by having wide doors that are easily opened, at

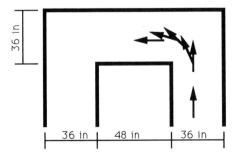

FIG 12–4.
Wheelchair turning around 48-in. object.

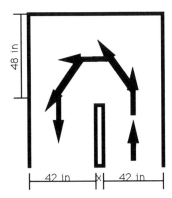

FIG 12–5.
Wheelchair turning around object (x) less than 48 in.

least 36-in. of clear floor space along the side of the bed, and adequate maneuvering space within the room.

Toilet Facilities

Accessible toilet areas in public access areas such as lobbies are often provided within a multiple staff restroom using widened doors, enlarged clear floor space inside the door and around the sinks and stalls, and the enlargement of one toilet stall, which is equipped with appropriate handrails.

Within a physical therapy department it is appropriate to consider individual toileting areas that are designated as universally accessible and used by both men and women. Such facilities should be accessible to each functional area of the department and separate from employee facilities. Commonly, restrooms are located in the waiting or outpatient area, hydrotherapy area, and major treatment area. The restroom in the hydrotherapy area can also serve as a changing area for outpatients and allows patients access without significant climate change.

Toilet seats can be accessed by a wheelchair from a forward, sideward, or diagonal position. For a forward transfer, the patient will need 18 in. access on both sides of the toilet and approximately 20 sq ft of clear floor space. If the toilet is to be approached sideways, it must have at least 42 in. on one side of the toilet and 18 in. on the other side. For a diagonal transfer, the patient will need 18 to 30 in. on one side of the toilet.

The toilet seat should be set at 17 to 19 in. from the floor, with the grab bars at 33 to 36 in. from the floor and extending approximately 42 in. from the wall on which the toilet tank rests to the side of the toilet.

The lavatory should have a 48 × 30-in. clear floor space in front of it to allow a forward approach to the lavatory. The counter surface of the lavatory should be no more than 34 in. from the floor with the bottom of the apron at least 29 in. from the floor and allow at least an 8-in. clearance for the wheelchair user's knees.

The toilet and lavatory are the most common elements of a patient restroom. If the facility also has shower facilities for patients, those facilities must also comply to ADA regulations. A wide variety of shower configurations are possible with and without bathtubs. Again, the major component that will significantly affect construction is the amount of clear floor space necessary for safe accessibility to all toileting facilities. This clear floor space will be dependent on the size of the shower or bathtub. As a general rule, the clear floor space is equal to or somewhat larger than the shower or bathtub space.

Handrails

One of the most common assistive devices used in a physical therapy department is handrails. Handrails can be found in the waiting area, hydrotherapy area, ambulation areas, gyms, and some treatment areas as well as in toileting facilities. The standard handrails have structural strength that allows the application of 250 lb of bending, shear, and tensile stress. The gripping surface is 1¼ to 1½ in. in diameter and 1½ in. from the wall.

· · · · · · · · · ·

GUIDING PRINCIPLES: GENERAL

Inventory and Storage

The modern approach to inventory and storage being used by American business is called just-in-time (JIT) scheduling. Maintaining inventory and the space to store it is a considerable expense to any business. Physical therapy managers should develop relationships with suppliers to provide supplies on a daily to weekly basis. This includes all disposable supplies (supplies that are used up) as well as clean linen and durable supplies that are given or sold to patients. By reducing storage needs, physical therapy space can be planned and used in a more cost-effective way.

The availability of services such as laundry, a durable medical equipment supply company, and a variety of disposable supply distributors is a key factor in being able to use this system. Physical therapy managers in rural settings may have a more difficult time setting up a JIT system, but such systems are very possible by working through purchasing cooperatives, intermediary distributors such as community hospital purchasing departments, and possible local distributors such as pharmacists who can provide supplies but may never have been asked to provide such a service.

Flow of Traffic

The space planners, architects, and industrial engineers consulting on the design of the physical therapy space must know the flow of traffic. The physical therapy manager is the best person to determine the primary diagnostic categories of patients who will use the space and then, working with an industrial engineer, determine the most common flow of traffic for those patient types. When considering the diagnostic categories, the manager may either be asked to consider a single day's traffic flow over a 1- to 2-week period of time or to also consider all levels of disease acuity that will be dealt with within each diagnostic category. For example, a patient in the orthopedic surgery diagnostic category may move by stretcher from the waiting area to the gym for the first 2 days of treatment, by wheelchair from the waiting area to the gym and treatment room for 3 days, and by crutches from the waiting area to the treatment room for the last 2 days of treatment. The most sophisticated analysis of traffic flow will be done by a number of assistants placed at strategic points in the department who collect the traffic flow data. Determinations must be made regarding numbers of wheelchairs, crutchwalkers, and staff moving in a given space for a given period of time. The industrial engineer will then analyze the data and assist in determining the width of high and low traffic pathways, width of doorways, placement of storage areas and supply areas, placement of equipment, location of treatment spaces, and a myriad of other traffic-related decisions.

The space needed for hydrotherapy and the flow of traffic in that space is important knowledge to share with space managers during the space planning process. For instance, the hydrotherapy area (Fig 12–6) must have adequate doors to allow

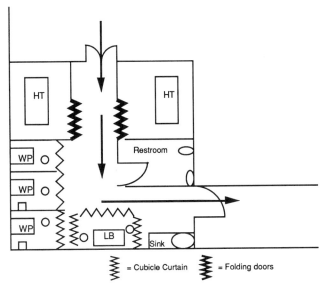

FIG 12−6.
Hydrotherapy *(HI)* area. *WP* = whirlpool; *LB* = low boy; arrow = flow of traffic.

stretchers and wheelchairs to enter the area. Yet, the space planners must realize that the climate in the area will have to be controlled and ideally controlled separately in separate spaces. For instance, if the facility has a regular case load of patients with open wounds or burns, it will be necessary to control the climate in the space where these patients will be treated in order to keep them as comfortable as possible.

In order to maintain as constant a temperature as possible in the space, the hydrotherapy area must be bounded by solid walls, although cubicle curtains can be used within the space for privacy. By strategically placing the cubicle curtains, the space can accommodate several hydrotherapy modalities or provide significant common space for other "wet" activities such as splinting and casting. The cubicle curtains should extend from close to the ceiling to the floor in order to maintain a warm environment for the person who is in any of the hydrotherapy tanks.

Controlling the flow of traffic within this area will also assist in climate control. Ideally there should be automatic doors leading to the area so that an attendant approaching the area can open the doors just prior to reaching them. Automatic doors are doors equipped with power-operated mechanisms that open and close the door automatically upon receipt of a momentary actuator signal. The switch that begins the automatic cycle may be a photoelectric device, floor mat, or manual switch.[1(p35460)] The doors are only open for a minimal amount of time to allow entrance into the area. Without automatic doors, doors have to be propped open while the attendant enters, and then the door is released. This lengthy process makes it more difficult to maintain a constant temperature in the room.

In order to accommodate patient needs and reduce the need for patients to leave the area while they may still be wet, it is advisable to place a patient restroom and dressing or locker area within the hydrotherapy space.

Door opening will also be reduced by placing adequate supply cabinets in the space to store towels, blankets, cleaning supplies, sterile supplies, and debridement equipment.

This will also be a room requiring exceptional lighting for the debridement of wounds and application of dressings. In addition, the installation of heat lamps in the ceiling, especially over hubbard tanks, will allow the therapists to selectively heat the area.

Similarly, the gymnasium area of the physical therapy space must be creatively planned to allow for patients and equipment to be moved easily. This area will house very heavy, cumbersome exercise equipment along with parallel bars and mats that will take up a considerable amount of the floor space available. Space planners must be aware of the most common flow of traffic within the area as patients and staff move between pieces of equipment and other patients are transported in and out of the space.

Just as in hydrotherapy and individual treatment areas, privacy or the option of privacy will enhance the performance of some patients. The placement of solid walls, counter top walls, or solid half walls will separate functions within the gym but still allow accessibility and monitoring of patients. The placement of a counter top wall beside a treadmill allows the patient a measure of privacy that can be increased by pulling a curtain across the top of the counter. At the same time the wall allows equipment to be hung and made accessible for monitoring of the patient. However, these walls may significantly interfere with the flow of traffic in the area. Physical therapy managers may have to work with the space planners to create a "corridor" within the space that will be designated as a traffic area with the appropriate signs and floor covering to direct patients and staff to that area when moving in and out of the space. If the gym is to be covered with low mat carpets to decrease noise and reduce foot-floor impact for ease of working long hours in the space, it may be appropriate to use tile or inlaid wood in the "corridor," which will tend to keep individuals within the corridor as they move in and out of the room.

Most space planners will ask questions about activities in specific areas, but it is the responsibility of the physical therapy manager to creatively think about the space modifications that might significantly enhance the delivery of services in that area.

Space Flexibility

Given the changing nature of patient treatment groups, the growing flexibility of treatment hours, and the probability that space needs will change, it is to the advantage of the manager to plan and use space in the most flexible manner possible. For instance, floor space should be considered to have multiple uses. For that reason, when possible and safe, equipment should be mobile, retractable, and collapsible; platform mats should be mounted on the wall so that they can be raised when not in use in order to use the floor space for other purposes; parallel bars should be collapsible on at least one side even if mounted to the floor on the other side; and treatment tables and small hydrotherapy equipment should be mobile.

Equipment Placement

In addition to the traffic flow issues mentioned above, the manager must also decide where equipment will be placed and the amount of floor space to leave around equipment. Floor space will be determined by the dimensions of the equipment (Box 12–3), the determination of the transportation needs of the patients using the equipment, the point of entry into or onto the equipment, the space the patient needs to safely and effectively use the equipment, and the ADA guidelines for space needs for the transport of patients. For example, the floor space requirement for an upper extremity/lower extremity mobile whirlpool is determined as follows: dimensions of equipment—length, 32 in.; width, 15 in.; patient transport—crutches, wheelchair transfer; ADA guidelines—wheelchair 30 to 42 in. depending on diagonal or sideways transfer; recommended 20 sq ft of clear floor space for transfers (see

· ·

BOX 12-3   FLOOR SPACE DIMENSIONS OF COMMONLY USED PHYSICAL THERAPY EQUIPMENT*

Mobile electrotherapy units	25 in. wide; 14 in. deep
Hydrocollator (12 pack)	30 in. wide; 15 in. deep
Cold pack machine	34 in. wide; 22 in. deep
Diathermy (allow additional 10 in. for arms)	30 in. wide; 15 in. deep
Infrared lamp	20 in. wide; 20 in. deep
Large mobile paraffin bath	10 in. wide; 25 in. deep
Lo boy whirlpool	24 in. wide; 52–66 in. long
Hi boy whirlpool	20 in. wide; 36–48 in. long
UE/LE whirlpool	15 in. wide; 25–32 in. long
Full body tank	24–41 in. wide; 60–95 in. long
Patient lifter (hoyer lift)	22–40 in. wide; 36 in. deep
Electric hi-lo tilt table	28 in. wide; 78 in. long
Electric hi-lo traction table	28 in. wide; 78 in. long
Electric treatment tables	28 in. wide; 78 in. long
Wooden treatment tables	27–30 in. wide; 72 in. long
Parallel bars	17–25 in. wide; 10 ft long
Exercise staircase	Can be custom made
Wall-mounted mat platform	4 ft wide; 7 ft long
Wooden mat platform	4–6 ft wide; 7–8 ft long
Isokinetic system (varies)	Seat unit, 27 in. wide; 27 in. long
Exercise cycle (varies)	18–21 in. wide; 36–44 in. long
Electronic treadmill	16–22 in. wide; 53 in. long
Free-standing pulley weight systems	Varies

*For specialized equipment sizes such as children's rehabilitation equipment, see specialized equipment catalogues.

transfering onto toilet seats for further transfer guidelines); and manager decisions—only the right side of the whirlpool will be accessible; the other side of the whirlpool will have at least 18 in. of space for therapist movement and cleaning; this whirlpool will be placed close to a permanent piece of equipment; as a mobile unit, it can be placed against the wall when more floor space is needed around the permanent equipment.

As more specialized equipment is developed, it will become increasingly difficult for the physical therapy manager to be fully informed regarding the appropriate use of the equipment. Therefore, when making decisions about space, the manager must consult with staff members who will most likely use the equipment regarding space needs around the equipment, benefits and disadvantages of the mobility of the equipment, probable level of usage (staff and patients), and the needs for flexibility of the equipment design.

The early physical therapy departments were add-ons to existing facilities. The space was often in the basement, with little or no design input by the physical therapy manager. The primary role of the manager was to make the space work even if it meant duplication of supplies, unmonitored patients, or unsafe mixing of electrotherapeutic and hydrotherapy equipment. As facilities have grown and physical therapy has become an integral part of the organization, a satellite unit, or an independent entity, the opportunities for physical therapy managers to design creative, efficient, and attractive facilities have grown significantly.

The planning of space is a critical activity that requires expertise in many specialized areas beyond management and physical therapy. The use of space planners, architects, and industrial engineers as consultants will lead to the most efficient and useful space. When physical therapy managers work in large organizations, these consultants are sometimes available through organizational relationships or actual administrative positions. In independent practice situations the physical therapy manager will have to seek those services from independent consultants and professional firms.

References

1. Americans With Disabilities Act. *Federal Register* July 26, 1991, p 56.

Suggested Readings

APTA Resource Guide, P31, Design and Planning of Physical Therapy and Rehabilitation Departments. Alexandria, Va, American Physical Therapy Association, 1990.
Magistro CM: Department planning, design and construction, in Hickok RJ (ed): *Physical Therapy Administration and Management.* Baltimore, Md, Williams and Wilkins, 1982.

CHAPTER 13

Marketing in Physical Therapy

. . . .

. . . .

INTRODUCTION

Peter Drucker, who is credited as the founder of modern management, states that the purpose of a business "must lie outside of the business itself. In fact, it must lie in society since a business enterprise is an organ of society. There is only one valid definition of business purpose: to create a customer . . . Because it is its purpose to create a customer, any business enterprise has two—and only these two—basic functions: marketing and innovation. They are the entrepreneurial functions."[1(p37)]

Marketing has been defined by the American Marketing Association as a "process of planning and executing the conception, pricing, promotion, and distribution of ideas, goods, and services to create exchanges that satisfy individual and organizational objectives."[2(p1)] Unlike the traditional management approach of creating services or products and then looking for markets, the marketing management approach looks at consumer needs, wants, and preferences and develops services and products to match those preferences. This is the key to the marketing management approach.

The traditional approach to management is to develop and offer a product or service. If the product or service is not used by consumers, the manager engages in a process of selling or pushing the product or service harder. If the product or service had been developed based on an analysis of the consumers' needs or preferences, then that service, once appropriately priced, would be promoted through advertising, word of mouth, and a variety of other techniques to the constituents who had indicated a need or want relative to this product or service. This marketing mix—product, place, price, and promotion—characterizes the marketing management approach.

The principles of marketing are the principles of problem solving, planning, budgeting, and decision making applied to consumer and community groups. A separate chapter is devoted to marketing because the marketing approach emphasizes different elements of decision making, paying more attention to the environment and consumer than the institutionally based physical therapist has been exposed to in the past. Physical therapy managers tend to use incremental decision making (decisions are made related to immediate problems, and these decisions lead to other decisions), whereas the marketing approach is a more planned, long-term decision-making process. The concept of promoting as a critical factor in marketing is also relatively new to physical therapy managers.

As recently as 1970, physical therapists were not allowed to advertise, promote, or call special attention to physical therapy services according to the code of ethics of the American Physical Therapy Association. Advertising was seen as selling, and most professionals felt that the selling of services would reduce the profession to the same competitive and capitalistic venturing atmosphere of businesses. Selling has had negative connotations for centuries as merchants have been perceived as taking advantage of buyers. As professions began to understand marketing to include an element of promotion of their services without the concepts of selling or pushing inferior products to uninformed individuals, the profession of physical therapy relaxed its stance in the area of advertising. The majority of physical therapists are still unclear about marketing principles and the differences between marketing management approaches and product- or service-driven approaches. Like many other people, physical therapy managers still confuse marketing with selling.

In the new health care marketplace, services must be marketed with an awareness of competitiveness. The boundaries of communities have broken down in terms of services that consumers seek. As recently as 20 years ago, the consumer would not consider going to a neighboring town or city for health care services. The community hospital, like the local church and school, created a sense of community pride, and members of the community accepted whatever skills and specialties were available through that facility and the other health care organizations within the community.

Today, the consumer who has the ability seeks the best services available and sometimes does not choose the services available in his or her own community. For instance, although superb sports medicine services are available in the Chicago area, an injured athlete from Chicago may choose the highly regarded and aggressively promoted services of sports medicine specialists in Birmingham, Ala.

One of the most telling indicators of the changing marketplace is the name changes of health care facilities. Reflecting on the past focus of the services provided, the name of many health care organizations reflected the community by using the name of the community (Massachusetts General Hospital), a specific organization (Dartmouth-Hitchcock Medical Center) or a renowned member of the community

(Rosalind Russell Arthritis Center). As these organizations have developed distant satellite units, they have attached community specific addenda to the name of the facility (Beaumont Hospital at Troy shortened to Beaumont-Troy). New health care organizations are choosing more generic names such as Rehabilitation Services, Medical Systems, and Medical Professionals.

MARKETING RESEARCH AND PLANNING

The processes used in analyzing the market are problem solving (Chapter 11) and research. The key to marketing is that it is focused on the customer (consumer, patient, client) or potential customer. The goal of marketing research is to find out what the consumer wants and how well competitors are providing services or are poised to provide services. Like other planning approaches, marketing emphasizes the need to base organizational decisions on quantitative and qualitative data. The marketing planning process begins with the problem solving approach.

1. Identify and define the problem.
2. Generate objectives and marketing strategies.
3. Explore the question with internal and external groups (focus groups).
4. Decision making.
    a. Collect and analyze internal and external data.
    b. Analyze resources and constraints.
    c. Assess adverse consequences.
    d. Anticipate potential problems.
5. Implement the program (tactics).
6. Evaluate the program.

Although marketing experts use the problem-solving process, the process is often referred to as strategic market planning; the objectives are referred to as strategies, and the steps in the implementation phase are referred to as tactics. Marketing goes beyond the traditional planning process in that during the implementation phase the manager directs a promotion campaign that will ensure good results of the plan.

The traditional approach to strategic planning focuses on the financial analysis of the organization. Strategic market planning is based on the analysis of both the internal and external market. The external analysis focuses on environmental needs and desires, whereas the internal analysis focuses on the strengths and weaknesses of the organization to meet the needs of the consumers.

DEFINING THE PROBLEM

As in any planning process, defining the true problem to be solved in the planning process or decision-making process is the critical starting point. The problem must be broken into its smallest components to be assured that each component of the problem is solved, therefore solving the whole problem. The problem statement should be as complete as possible and shared with supervisors and subordinates for their input to ensure that the problem is real and that it is set in the appropriate context.

The first step many organizations take in the marketing process is to determine the true needs of its current and prospective users. In large, complex organizations such as hospitals, this will be a long process as each unit engages in an analysis of its constituents. In these kinds of organizations, each unit has a variety of publics (Fig 13–1), while the organization itself has constituents as well.

. . . .
OPPORTUNITIES AND OBJECTIVES

The marketing planning process proceeds from the definition of the problem to the development of the strategic objectives related to this problem and opportunities that may arise from these objectives. The manager's responsibility is to scan the internal and external environment for opportunities. The degree to which these opportunities can be maximized depend on the resources of the organization and environmental factors such as the state of the economy, societal trends, and the political and legal climate.

Case Example

In scanning the environment, a physical therapy manager in a large community hospital decides that there is an opportunity to develop an orthopedic satellite facility in the community. The problem the physical therapy manager is seeking to solve is to find a vehicle to (1) treat outpatient orthopedic patients in an environment that is more conducive to patient motivation than the inpatient unit of the hospital, where outpatient treatment areas are mixed with inpatient treatment areas and to (2) capture more orthopedic outpatient referrals from orthopedic surgeons who are affiliated with the hospital. The organizational resources are available to proceed, but there are two physician-owned orthopedic physical therapy practices in the area and the orthopedic surgeon owners are affiliated with the hospital. It is inappropriate to proceed as long as the other two practices are in the community. Even without an in-depth analysis of the market, the physical therapy manager is certain that the community cannot support a third orthopedic practice, that the exploration of the possibility would create a potential problem with the surgeons who own the other two practices, and that the original goal of capturing more patients from these two surgeons could not be accomplished.

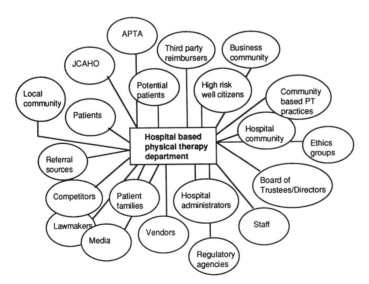

FIG 13–1.
Hospital-based physical therapy department publics. *APTA* = American Physical Therapy Association; *JCAHO* = Joint Commission on the Accreditation of Healthcare Organizations; *PT* = physical therapy.

The physical therapy manager should not abandon the concept, however. Being well informed about professional issues, the physical therapy manager is aware of the Stark legislation limiting physician involvement in business ventures to which the physician makes referrals. Laboratory ownership by physicians is currently restricted if physicians seek medicare reimbursement for laboratory tests, and physical therapy costs in physician-owned clinics are being monitored. The physical therapy manager is sure that the political climate will continue to encourage the restriction of physician ownership, and the orthopedic surgeon owners may want to find an alternative structure in which to meet their practice objectives. The physical therapy manager will begin to discuss the goals of the orthopedic surgeons in relation to physical therapy, scan the political and legal environment, and maintain the organizational resources to make timely decisions regarding this opportunity.

MARKETING RESEARCH

Marketing research includes a combination of quantitative techniques of gathering, analyzing, and interpreting data related to opinions, needs, demands, wants, costs, income, spending, and epidemiological data related to the community of interest.

Qualitative research techniques are also used, especially using focus groups that represent specific marketing targets. Focus groups are usually representative of a specific group of consumers. For instance, if a facility is developing a new program targeted at prenatal and postnatal care, as in the case at the end of this chapter, several focus groups, including pregnant women using the current hospital services, pregnant women not using the hospital services, and women who have given birth within the past 5 years might be interviewed in a focus group environment. The purpose of the focus group is to generate hypotheses, questions, and information to be used in the assessment process, to get impressions on possible strategies, and to facilitate new ideas to improve the service, product, or plans.

The specific qualitative research methods used in marketing research include interviews and observational techniques to assess data related to opinions, attitudes, consumer desires, and changes in community needs.

DEVELOPING A MARKETING PROGRAM

Marketing programs include a plan of action, an implementation phase, and an evaluation strategy. They are based on the aspects of the organization that managers can control. For example, physical therapy managers will develop marketing programs in physical therapy environments. The program is built on an assessment of the external factors (consumer, competitors, environment) and the internal factors (organization).

In marketing arenas, the tools of marketing are referred to as the four Ps—product, price, place, and promotion—or the marketing mix. New research based on surveys of marketing managers and executives has added to this original list of tools, added additional elements, and ranked each element from most to least important (Box 13–1).[3(p10)] Each of these elements will be discussed as they relate to a physical therapy practice.[4(p19)]

MARKETING IN PHYSICAL THERAPY

Customer sensitivity relates to employee attitude, customer treatment, and response to customers. Although physical therapy managers and staff would like to believe

· ·

BOX 13-1 ELEMENTS OF MARKETING*

1. Customer sensitivity	Employee attitude, customer treatment, and response to customers
2. Product	Product quality, reliability, and features
3. Customer convenience	Availability to the customer, customer convenience, and selling
4. Service	Postsale service, presale service, and customer convenience
5. Price	Price charged, pricing terms, and pricing offers
6. Place	Provider accessibility, provider facilities, pricing terms, and availability to customer
7. Promotion	Advertising, publicity, selling, presale services, and pricing offers

that this is not an issue or a problem for physical therapy departments, if the manager asks patients about this issue they are likely to get surprising answers. Marvin Harris, in *America Now,* discusses the concept of why the help don't help. As American society has moved toward a more egocentric society, consumers have sought a greater variety of services to free up more time to take part in activities that are satisfying. Business has tended toward more service orientation, but the employees are still members of society with the same desires to engage in satisfying work and leisure time activities. Many employees (even professionals) see work as an activity that is necessary to provide the resources to engage in more satisfying activities. That means that those individuals are less likely to be helpful, engaging, courteous caregivers.

Assess Employee Attitudes

The first step in marketing management is to assess employee attitudes and response to patients. There are many creative ways to assess these characteristics.

Case example

The problem. The administrative director of the rehabilitation medicine (physiatry, physical therapy, occupational therapy, speech pathology, recreational therapy, cardiac rehabilitation) department of an academic health center was concerned about complaints received from patients about difficulties they were having getting appointments and information from both the clerical and professional staff. The complaints had come from outpatients and three different referral sources.

The evaluation of the problem. The administrator engaged a telephone consultant to conduct a survey of the department. The administrator worked with the consultant to develop a series of simulated telephone inquiries that were commonly posed by patients and referral sources.

Informed consent. The administrator informed the clerical and professional staff of the complaints that had been made and asked the staff to allow a consultant to evaluate telephone behavior over the next 2 months. The administrator explained that simulated telephone calls would be made by a consultant to assess the manner in which inquiries were handled. The consultant would also observe telephone behavior in the department.

Results. Although it might appear that informing the staff in this way would bias their behavior, an interesting result of the project was that the staff behaved on the telephone in ways that they were unaware were not helpful. The consultant made a series of phone calls to therapists, the administrator, the clerical staff, and the support staff over the next 2 months. She also engaged a colleague to make phone calls at specific times while she was sitting in the waiting area to observe the behavior of the clerical staff receiving those calls. At other times, she had permission to sit in the physical therapy office area for the same purpose.

By the end of 2 months the consultant was able to give the staff (and administrator) exact dialogue reflecting discourteous, bored, impatient, and unhelpful responses. In addition, she was able to reflect on the circumstances under which individuals answered the telephone. At times therapists (usually new therapists) would leave patients in the middle of a treatment to take a phone call and then appear to have little patience in answering the caller. Secretaries were observed answering calls while they continued to type or file or even while they continued to try to talk to another party.

This evaluation of telephone behavior was shared with the staff directly by the consultant. The staff, consultant, and administrator then worked together to develop a series of telephone "rules" that greatly improved the telephone communications. Some of those rules can be seen in Box 13–2.

The physical therapy manager must look outside of the department when the physical therapy department is in a complex organization to attend to the sensitivity to customers. The physical therapy consumers will be in many situations in which they must deal with a variety of other departments. This will include physician offices within the facility, billing and insurance offices, the emergency room, the admissions office, nursing service, and the housekeeping, dietary, and maintenance departments. All managers within a complex organization must adopt plans to assess and improve employee sensitivity to the consumers before they can seriously approach new services or products.

· ·
BOX 13–2   TELEPHONE RULES

XYZ Hospital
Rehabilitation Medicine Department

1. Therapists will not be interrupted for telephone calls unless the call is from a referral source or it is an emergency. The suggested response: "I'm sorry, Mr. XXX is with a patient right now." ("This is Dr. YYY, I would like to talk to him about Mrs. AAA.") "I'm sure Mr. XXX would want me to interrupt him, please hold." (This is Ms. KKK, from the APTA) "Mr. XXX could get back to you at 1:00 or 5:00 when he returns his phone calls. Would that be OK?" Then proceed to take the message.
   Note: Do not answer with "Can I tell him who is calling?" as a first response. When you then tell the person that the therapist cannot talk at that time, the person will feel like a second-class citizen. The suggested response above treats every caller the same.
2. Clerical staff will tell all callers who are leaving messages that the calls will be returned at 1:00 PM if a morning call and 5:00 PM if an afternoon call.
3. Therapists will allow 20 minutes at 1:00 and at 5:00 to return phone calls.
4. One clerical staff person will be designated to receive phone calls from 8:00–10:00, another from 10:00—12:00, another from 12:00—2:00, and another from 2:00—5:00. The office manager will determine the rotation system for the staff. While the individual is on telephone duty, the clerical person will be relieved of all other responsibilities and should devote that time to the telephone and the appointment schedule.

Product/Service Quality and Features

Products or services are characterized by styling, features, quality, packaging, and the brand name. In physical therapy, the emphasis is usually on the core service, particular features of the service that are unique to the organization, and the quality of the service and of the outcome of the service. The quality of a physical therapy service within a marketing program must be monitored in the same manner as any physical therapy service and will be discussed in more detail in the next chapter. Of particular concern to the physical therapy manager in implementing a marketing strategy is whether the quality is maintained throughout the implementation phase and ultimately throughout the life of the service. In addition, the manager must be able to monitor quality in a timely fashion so that immediate action can be taken to institute contingency plans, enhance professional performance, or add features to the program targeted at quality improvement.

The styling component of a service includes those aspects of the service that connect it uniquely to the organization/practice. To some degree, the styling depends on the target audience. If the intent of the service is to reach the weekend athlete, then the styling may be much more "low key" than a similar service provided to pre-olympic skating and gymnastics athletes or professional boxers.

The features of the service include aspects of the service that can be added or taken away from the service without affecting the service itself. For instance, in a service targeting a level of cardiovascular fitness for executives, expanding the hours of the service to accommodate their schedules, adding a 10-day outward bound experience to the service, or adding a free 2-month membership in a local health club would be special features of the service.

Although many of the early therapeutic techniques carry names such as PNF (proprioceptive neuromuscular facilitation), NDT (neurodevelopmental techniques), and Brunnstrom stages of recovery, these names are not seen as brand names from a marketing perspective when used as therapeutic techniques. The names were assigned by the experts who developed the techniques. When those individuals (and others) use the names in marketing continuing education programs, videotapes, and publications, the names do serve as brand names. The user is often trading on the reputation of the founders and the techniques to sell a product or service.

Packaging refers to the actual physical wrapping when a product is being described and marketed. In the case of a service, the environment in which the service is produced or delivered serves as the packaging. The reputation of the organization, its visibility, the perceptions of the community toward the organization, and attentiveness to consumers are only a few of the components of the environment that will enhance or detract from the service.

Customer Convenience

The degree to which the service is available to the customer and the degree of inconvenience that the customer must incur to gain access to the service will greatly influence the success of the program. For instance, many physical therapy department managers in complex organizations are moving outpatient functions off site into satellite units. This move away from the crowded medical center environment accomplishes several objectives.

- Parking is enhanced.
- Accessibility of the physical therapy department is enhanced.
- Outpatients are not subjected to the sights, sounds, and smells of a physical therapy department in a short-term care setting.
- The satellite facility can be focused on the target population.

- Other services may be more convenient (drug store, sports shop, durable medical equipment dealer) in a one-stop-shopping environment

In addition, some physical therapy managers are taking services targeted toward the elderly to senior citizen centers and housing developments for senior citizens, pediatric services to the school systems or local youth services building, and prevention programs to health club environments.

The health care industry has always gathered patients together for the convenience of the health care provider. The industry is only beginning to realize that if people are to take part in services, then the services have to be convenient to the individual, not the health care provider.

Service

Service is a component of a product, not usually of a service. It is the follow-up repair and maintenance functions often sold with the product. There are service components to some physical therapy services that must be considered when establishing a new service. For instance, a pain clinic must have an adequate arrangement with a vendor to sell, rent, service, and retrieve transcutaneous electrical neuro stimulator (TENS) units. If a physical therapy manager had established a pain clinic without adequate attention to the servicing of TENS units, the complaints, rental, and sales related to the equipment could totally overwhelm the clerical staff as well as the staff therapists and could lead to considerable financial loss.

Price

The price of a service is determined according to the cost to deliver the service, the demand for the service, or the competition. Physical therapy managers must develop skills in determining pricing of services or find consultants who can develop pricing strategies for the core departmental services, the satellite units, special programs, and new services that grow out of marketing opportunities. The common strategy for many managers is to take the price of services provided in the heavily laden hospital environment and apply the same price to an environment with many fewer overhead expenses. If the satellite unit is to purposefully assume part of the overhead cost of the hospital-based department, that cost should be determined and then added to the base price of the service. This approach to pricing will allow the manager to increase the base service charge when direct costs of delivering the service increase by a known amount and increase the overhead add-on when overhead costs increase.

The breakeven volume of the services provided is determined by subtracting the variable cost from the price of the service and dividing into the fixed cost of providing the service.

$$\text{Break even volume} = \text{fixed cost/price} (-) \text{variable cost}$$
$$\text{Example: } \$300,000/\$110 (-) \$10 = 3,000$$

For example, presume that the fixed cost (including overhead) of delivering a pain clinic service was $300,000. Each patient used approximately $10 of supplies and the usual charge was $110 per treatment. Using the breakeven volume formula, the service would have to treat 3,000 patients per year to break even. This is the most popular form of cost-oriented pricing. The job of the physical therapy manager in this kind of pricing strategy is to determine if it is likely that the program will treat 3,000 individuals in 1 year and if not, when the breakeven point will be reached. If the administration is not willing to take a risk that the breakeven point will not be reached, then the manager must cut the fixed costs. In physical therapy pricing of services is also dependent on governmental regulation, third-party intermediaries, and supplier's costs. Pricing of physical therapy services is covered in more detail in Chapter 15.

The price considerations in a marketing program go beyond the pricing of the service. They also include special promotions, free services, bundling of services in special ways, discounts, payment systems, and credit terms. All of these aspects of cost to the consumer will have an effect on making the consumer aware of and interested in the service.

Place

Place takes into account several of the same factors discussed in consumer convenience when the outcome of the program is a service. The physical therapy manager will have to assure provider accessibility following Americans With Disabilities Act guidelines and zoning laws. In addition, the manner in which the patient is expected to pay for the services is considered in this component of marketing mix. If the billing office is in another facility and there is no mechanism for accepting payment, answering questions, or processing claims on site, then there is likely to be dissatisfaction on the part of the consumer related to these inconveniences.

It is also critical that if the satellite unit is dependent on the larger facility for staff, linen, supplies, and other products that there is a clear mechanism for timely distribution of people and services to the satellite. If the physical therapy manager institutes a just-in-time inventory system in the satellite, there must be assurances that the inventory will be replenished in a timely fashion.

Promotion

Promotion is usually discussed as advertising, publicity, and the selling of products and services. In physical therapy advertising is accomplished through the use of marketing trinkets (key chains, goniometers, sweat bands, mugs), brochures, flyers, direct mailing, and a variety of media opportunities including interviews, features, letters to the editor, and live coverage of special events. Good promotional campaigns give the consumer information about the services and those providing the services, persuade the consumer to try the service, and remind the consumer about the availability of the services. Consumers usually make purchasing decisions about products and services following the traditional steps of awareness-interest-desire-action (AIDA). Physical therapy managers should not underestimate the importance of informing the consumers about the credentials of the physical therapists. The public, claims reviewers, referral sources, and the variety of agencies that physical therapists deal with are not aware of the professional characteristics of physical therapy. Some physicians working in specialties that make a significant number of referrals to physical therapists do not know that physical therapy is an academic discipline with a designated degree. Many other groups and individuals still think that physical therapists are trained on the job. Despite the ongoing efforts of the APTA's promotional campaigns to inform the publics that physical therapy serves or that have an impact on physical therapy the profession is still widely misunderstood.

Promotional campaigns begin with goals related to exposure of the market to the service. High-powered promotional campaigns expose the market to as many as 10 to 12 ads in as short a period of time as 3 months. A physical therapy manager may decide to launch a similarly high-powered promotional campaign to patients and potential patients in exposing the market to the opening of a new satellite general practice facility in a rural area. The following strategies might be used.

1. Flyers placed in all physician and dentist offices.
2. Payroll inserts for all employers of more than ten employees.
3. Newspaper announcements.
4. Yellow pages ad.
5. Radio interview.
6. Speaker at adult education classes.
7. Speaker at major community service organizations (Rotary, Women's Club, Business and Professional Women's Club, Round Table International, Lions, etc).
8. Volunteer at local events (bar-BQ, softball games, muscular dystrophy bowl-a-thon) and sponsor flyers, score cards, T- shirts.

Promotional programs must follow the strategic objectives of the marketing program and cannot be single events. They are made up of multiple advertising opportunities that move from awareness to persuasion to reminders. The persuasion aspect of the promotional campaign must be carefully orchestrated to give the consumer of the service valid statements about the degree of satisfaction that will be obtained if the service is used. This is the phase of the promotional campaign where the physical therapy manager must be aware of the differences between selling and marketing. The goal here is not to sell, it is to persuade. The interviews, advertisements, letters, and speeches must capture the interest of the consumer and help the individual to understand that he or she does have a desire for the service and that taking part in the service will lead to greater wellness, prevention of disability, or less discomfort.

Considerable controversy arose when health care institutions first began advertising to patients and potential patients. One well-known hospital advertised plastic surgery by showing the image of a woman with half of the body showing normal signs of aging and the other half corrected through plastic surgery. Many professionals felt that this kind of advertisement was selling, not informing or persuading. As a full-page ad in the Sunday supplement of a highly circulated newspaper, it was unprofessional because it obviously targeted the general population, depicted aging as an unattractive process. The ad presented the impression that women should appear young through plastic surgery as they grow older.

When physical therapy managers construct promotional campaigns it is important to constantly assess the messages to be assured that they are not sensational or misrepresenting the service or the profession. They should inform, persuade, or remind, but not attempt to sell concepts, performance, or services based on misinformation or the skewing of facts to fit the service. Although many brand name product promotional campaigns use competitive advertising (one product is better than another), most health care organizations do not use competitive advertising. In assessing the market, the physical therapy manager has assessed the competition and knows where the new service's strengths and weaknesses are in comparison to the competition. This information often plays a role in deciding on the promotional message. It is appropriate to point out the strengths of the service or the new aspects for the community.

The audience of the promotional campaign is the target market. That may be a segment of any of the publics of the organization or physical therapy department (Fig 13–1). The market can be patients, clients, third-party reimbursers, governmental agencies, community service organizations, referral sources, employees, peers, and a multitude of other groups. The promotional campaign will be specific to the market being targeted because it will follow the strategic plan of the marketing program and the strategic objectives of the new service.

Marketing is not public relations or another name for selling a product or service. Marketing is a management planning approach to define problems and systematically plan, price, place, and promote strategies that will address the problems. It is an approach that is gaining acceptance in health care and a growing acceptance in physical therapy (see Selected Readings). Marketing management is not used by all businesses, and it will not be used by all health care organizations or physical therapy practices. However, those who use marketing management will focus on the consumer, not the provider. The future success of physical therapy services and the recognition by the public as a professional discipline will depend on greater focus on the consumers of physical therapy services.

CASE 13.1:

New Program/Service

Kathleen Jakubiak Kovacek, P.T.

Eastside General Hospital is a small (150-bed) community hospital located in the suburban Milwaukee area. It offers medical surgical care, ambulatory surgery, psychiatric and rehabilitation services, and a newly built family-oriented childbirth center. This concept revolves around the labor, delivery, recovery, and postpartum (LDRP) focus. The mother labors, delivers, recovers and, along with her newborn, receives postpartum care, all in the same room. These rooms appear comfortable and homelike, but conceal high technological equipment. All necessary equipment can be immediately accessed if the mother or baby need emergency attention.

Even more important in the LDRP concept is how the mother and baby receive care. The same primary nurse attends to both mother and baby. Instead of the common system of one nurse taking care of the mother, with another nurse attending to the infant in a separate nursery setting, this primary nurse provides couplet care. The LDRP focus is complete when the mother works together with her physician, midwife, and primary nurse to make as many decisions as appropriate regarding the care she and her new baby receive.

This concept is becoming increasingly popular. Many hospitals are developing the LDRP concept as a way to attract new patients.

The Physical Therapy Department has been approached to participate in this new program. Specifically, the nurse manager, Jane Smith, is interested in developing prenatal, perinatal, and postnatal exercise programs. She is interested in having sessions three times a week for 6 weeks, with sign up commencing every 6 weeks. Jane is energetic, sincere, and genuinely wants LDRP to succeed. In fact, she applied for this job because she wanted to implement some of the same programs that existed in the Chicago hospital where she used to work.

Kathy Doe is the Director for Physical Therapy. She is also very interested in the LDRP focus from a personal and professional viewpoint. The hospital where she had delivered her second child 2 years ago offered a birthing room, but it was occupied when she was admitted. Therefore, she was systematically moved from a labor room to the delivery room, rested in a separate recovery room, and finally was given a semiprivate room. The obstetrics (OB) staff nurses were separate from the nursery room staff. Questions about her baby couldn't be addressed to the OB nurse assessing her postpartum recovery, since none of the OB staff even read the infants' charts. Likewise, the nursery room staff never assessed the new mothers of their newborn patients.

Since Kathy was a physical therapist, she knew how to plan appropriate exercises that kept her feeling fit throughout her pregnancy. She was also very aware how uncomfortable her roommate, Kim Jones, was with progressive exercises. As a first time mother, Kim had a variety of questions, especially regarding returning to activities, the right exercises to do to shape up quickly, and how to decrease low-back pain. These personal experiences served to boost Kathy's own interest in LDRP.

Kathy and Jane worked closely together on a new proposal to introduce an exercise component to the LDRP service. They enjoyed working together and found the project moving along quickly. They both planned to present the proposal jointly to their respective staffs for input and constructive criticism. Ultimately they would jointly present their ideas to their boss, Elizabeth Anderson, Administrator for Professional Services, to whom they both reported. Elizabeth was a nurse, mother, and had given strong support to developing LDRP in its initial stages.

Kathy proposed that she would be the lead clinician to start up the new program. Along with her personal interest, she had belonged to an OB-GYN Special Interest Group for some time and had participated in the group's inservices. One of her staff physical therapists was also very interested in the new program. She agreed to help with program development, offer backup coverage for her should the need arise, and contribute to the initial stability of the exercise component.

Jane and Kathy were both familiar with a model for prepartum and postpartum exercise classes that met three times per week for 6 weeks. Then the participants were encouraged to continue on a home program or sign up for another session if feasible. The class was to be held in the newly renovated Physical Therapy Department. Part of the department was carpeted. Pillows, blankets, foam supports, floor mats, mat tables, chairs, and plinths were readily available. This saved the inconvenience and expense of moving equipment around three times each week. Along with active participation in the exercise regimes, Kathy planned on educating her patients. She would only need to transport an overhead projector. Topics to be covered included body mechanics, posture, stretching vs. strengthening, aerobic activity, and exercise progression with careful attention given to prenatal and postnatal changes. Since the normal length of stay for an uncomplicated vaginal delivery at Eastside General Hospital was 2.3 days, Kathy decided to incorporate perinatal exercises into the prenatal session. This would give the mothers a chance to ask questions before their babies are born. Jane readily agreed with this modification. It was tough enough teaching new moms how to care for their newborns in the short time that they're in the hospital postpartum, so it made sense to introduce the exercise component before the baby was born.

One last consideration was made. Since the Physical Therapy Department was the chosen site for the classes, Kathy decided that they would be held during the noon lunch hour, so there would be only minimal interruption (if any) of regular patient care.

What would be charged for this new service? The LDRP concept was developed to meet the needs of the obstetrical patient but also to build patient loyalty to Eastside General Hospital. In the United States it is generally the female head of the household who makes the family's health care decisions. To develop loyalty to any one health care facility, a young family may be introduced to that facility via maternity care. If the LDRP experience is positive, the family may return when an emergency room visit is necessary. If the comfort level with that facility remains high, that same family may recommend the facility to friends and their extended family. This, in turn, could become a rehabilitation referral or outpatient surgery choice. In today's competitive health care arena, developing patient loyalty is a top priority. With this in mind, Kathy and Jane decide that they would provide the exercise component free of charge.

Kathy and Jane worked hard to cover every detail. Confident that Elizabeth Anderson would be as enthusiastic about their proposal as they are, they made an appointment to present the "On the Go With Baby and Me" exercise program to their boss.

Elizabeth congratulated them on their enthusiasm, but she had multiple questions after they completed their presentation.

1. Who are the customers of "On the Go With Baby and Me"? Kathy and Jane identified the mothers (patients) as customers (users) of the program. What about physicians, midwives, insurance companies, traditional workout gyms? These groups may be customers as well as potential referral sources.

2. How will high-risk patients be handled? Will every patient need physician clearance to participate? Perhaps only pregnant women will need clearance. Are there special liability concerns if a mother who is 8 weeks postpartum who is no longer technically under an obstetrician's care wants to participate independently?

3. How do Kathy and Jane know there is a market for this service? Will the model they have chosen of three times per week for 6 weeks work? What about working women? How will they participate in the middle of the day? How about mothers with other young children? Will babysitting be provided? Will they be willing to participate in a program that runs for 18 sessions? Can the educational and physiological goals for the program be achieved in any other model?

4. What are the opportunity costs for running this program? In other words, how much revenue could have been generated if regular physical therapy treatments were given during this time period? Stretching it further, why is the Physical Therapy Department shut down completely for an entire hour at noon?

5. If the program is free, will participants value it as much as they would if they had some financial investment in the program? Have insurance companies been approached to consider this as a possible covered benefit? What do other similar programs in the area charge? Should "On the Go With Baby and Me" be priced the same, higher, or lower in relation to the current market?

6. Since LDRP was already on site at Eastside General Hospital, trying out "On the Go With Baby and Me" was a relatively low-risk project. Using the Physical Therapy Department made sense because essentially all the necessary equipment (except the overhead projector) was located there. What will happen if demand increases and it is desirable to have a prepartum and postpartum class running simultaneously? Will there be enough physical space? How will staffing be expanded to cover the exercise classes? Can other members of the health care team competently conduct this program? If so, how can they be trained? Will the charge/coverage be different if some other health professional conducts this program?

7. Kathy and Jane genuinely cared about developing the LDRP focus to include the exercise component. It appears that they let their personal experiences influence their assessment of need for the program. Remember Kathy's roommate who wasn't comfortable with returning to activity after the birth of her child. Kathy never did ask if she would have been willing to participate in any exercise class, especially one that ran three times a week for 6 weeks.

8. What are the demographics of Eastside General Hospital? Are these patients likely to value participating in their own health care decisions? Even if they do wish to participate, how can Kathy and Jane find out what kind of program they would desire most?

. . . .
DEFINITIONS

AIDA: Awareness-interest-desire-action. The traditional steps an individual goes through in making a purchase decision.

Bottom line: Overall profitability measure of performance.

Break even: The number of products or services that must be sold at a specific price to generate sufficient revenue to cover total costs.

Buyer's market: Abundance of goods and services in relation to the level of consumer demand.

Capital equipment: Equipment that is expected to last a long time and must be depreciated over time.

Clayton Act: Federal law passed in 1914 restricting price discrimination.

Cluster sampling: Research sampling technique using geographic areas or clusters.

Competitive bidding: Process in which potential suppliers submit price quotations to a buyer for a proposed purchase or contract.

Consumer rights: Rights to choose freely, to be informed, to be heard, and to be safe.

Demographics: Individual characteristics such as age, sex, socioeconomic status.

Federal Trade Commission Act: Federal legislation passed in 1914 that prohibited unfair methods of competition and established the Federal Trade Commission (FTC) to oversee laws dealing with business.

Focus group: Eight to 12 individuals who meet specific characteristics of a target group and are brought together to provide insight, analysis of products and services, and new ideas.

Inflation: Rising price level that results in reduced purchasing power for the consumer.

Joint venture: An agreement between business partners in two or more businesses in which the partners agree to share risks, costs, and management responsibilities.

Just-in-time inventory system (JIT): Inventory system in which inventory is limited to that inventory needed for a short time span (1 day to 1 week).

Market: Group of people who possess purchasing power and the authority and willingness to purchase.

Marketing: Process of planning and executing the development, pricing, promotion, and distribution of ideas, goods, and services that meet individual and organizational objectives.

Market cost analysis: Evaluation of such items as selling costs, billing, and advertising to determine the profitability of particular customers or products.

Marketing ethics: Standards of conduct in marketing.

Marketing mix: Product, place, price, and promotion.

Marketing planning: Process of determining the course of action designed to achieve marketing objectives.

Marketing research: Systematic approach to gathering, sorting, analyzing, and interpreting data related to marketing problems and opportunities.

Marketing strategy: Program to meet the needs of a group of consumers through marketing techniques.

Nonprofit organization: Organization whose mission and objectives result in something other than the return of a profit.

Penetration pricing: Pricing strategy using a relatively low entry price hoping that this price will result in market acceptance of a service or product.

Positioning: Developing a marketing strategy aimed at a particular market segment and designed to achieve a desired position with the prospective buyer.

Product: Group of physical, service, and symbolic attributes designed to satisfy consumer wants.

Product line: Various related goods offered by an organization.

Profit center: Any part of an organization to which revenue and controllable costs can be assigned.

Public: Distinct group of people who have an interest in and impact on an organization.

Responsive organization: Organization that makes every effort to determine, serve, and satisfy the needs and wants of its clients and publics within the constraints of its budget.

Seller's market: Marketplace characterized by a shortage of goods and services.

Sherman Antitrust Act: Federal legislation passed in 1890. Prohibits restraint of trade and monopolization.

Stagflation: Situation in which an economy has both high unemployment (stagnation) and a rising price level (inflation).

Strategic window: Limited periods during which the fit between the key requirements of a market and the particular competencies of a firm is at an optimum.

SWOT: Strength, weakness, opportunity, threat. The components of an internal evaluation of the organization's ability to meet marketing objectives.

Tactical planning: Implementation of activities specified by the strategic marketing plan that are necessary in the achievement of the organization's objectives.

Trend analysis: Quantitative sales forecasting method in which estimates of future sales are determined through statistical analyses of historical sales patterns.

Unit pricing: Pricing policy under which prices are set in terms of a recognized unit of measurement or a standard numerical count.

References

1. Drucker PF: *The Practice of Management.* New York, NY, Harper and Row, 1982.
2. Staff AMA board approves new marketing definition. *The Marketing News* 1985; 00:000.
3. Berry D: *Marketing News,* December 24, 1990, p 10.

Selected Readings

Adams PM: Marketing a satellite PT clinic. *Phys Ther Today* 1989; 12:000.

Boone LE Kurtz DL: *Contemporary Marketing.* Chicago, Ill, The Dryden Press, 1986.

Boynton PS Fair PA: Becoming a market-driven rehabilitation program: A case study. *Rehab Literature* 1986; 47: 174–178.

Brown G: Changing health care environments—implications for physical therapy research, education, and practice. *Phys Ther* 1986; 66:1242–1245.

Hiam A, Schewe CD: *The Portable MBA in Marketing.* New York, NY, John Wiley and Sons, Inc, 1992.

Cameron J: Making the most of your media opportunities. *Phys Ther Today* 1988; 11:35–37.

Carey RG, Seibert JH: Integrating program evaluation, quality assurance and marketing for inpatient rehabilitation. *Rehabil Nursing* 1988; 13:000.

Connolly J: Customer service in physical therapy. *Phys Ther Today* 1990; 13:10–16.

Crocker KE, Alden J: An investigation of clients' and practitioners' views of the effect of physical therapy advertising and its content. *JHCM* 1986; 3:12–18.

Davidson JP: Becoming your own press agent. *Whirlpool* 1987; 10:000.

Davidson JP: New ways of approaching the marketplace. *Phys Ther Today* 1990; 13:38–44.

Doherty JJ: Marketing your practice through a weekly newspaper column. *Whirlpool* 1986; 9:15–18.

Fremion-Battell B: On the right track . . . wellness programs can bail out hospitals. *Clin Management* 1985; 5:22–25.

Heffernan S: Market research as a tool for the private physical therapy practice. *Whirlpool* 1987; 10:34–38.

Hiam A: *The Vest-Pocket Marketer.* Englewood Cliffs, NJ, Prentice Hall Publishers, 1991.

Hillestad SG, Berkowitz EN: *Health Care Marketing Plans.* Gaithersburg, Md, Aspen Publications, 1991.

Horting M: Marketing strategies: How to enhance reimbursement for PT services. *Clin Management* 1987; 7:36–40.

House SG: Advertising and the individual professional. *Clin Management* 1982; 2:33–35.

Jackson DE, Gazaway JR: Marketing rehabilitation services to home care agencies. *Whirlpool* 1987; 10:38–41.

Kelly KK: Separate yourself from the crowd. *Phys Ther Today* 1989; 12:59–63.

Kotler P: *Marketing for Nonprofit Organizations.* Englewood Cliffs, NJ, Prentice Hall, Inc, 1982.

McCarthy MJ: Marketer zero in on their customers. *The Wall Street Journal* Monday, March 19, 1991.

Momberg WA: A fresh appraisal of your agency's identity. *Whirlpool* 1987; 10:24.

Momberg WA: The 11th commandment: Know thy market. *Phys Ther Today* 1988; 11:34.

Nadoisky JM: The marketing of rehabilitation services. *J Rehabil,* July/Aug/Sept, p 5, 66.

Panos A: Professional advertising. *Clin Management* 1982; 2:36–37.

Rapp S, Collins T: *The Great Marketing Turnaround.* New York, NY, Simon and Schuster, Inc, 1991.

Sabin S: Rehab program's marketing plan was tailored to fit. *Nursing and Health Care,* May 1985, pp 269–271.

Schaefer K, Lewis CB: Marketing geriatric programs. *Clin Management* 1986; 6:14–17.

Schaefer K: Finding your clinic's marketing niche requires a periodic assessment with an objective eye. *Clin Management* 0000; 8:000.

Stevens A: Public relations: A powerful marketing tool for the PT. *Clin Management* 1985; 5:24–25.

Stoline A, Weiner JP: *The New Medical Marketplace.* Baltimore, Md, Johns Hopkins University Press, 1989.

Tanner SE, Klein JB: Market analysis reveals rehab program potential. *Hospitals,* June 1, 1985, pp 65–66.

CHAPTER 14

Quality and Productivity in Physical Therapy

I. **Introduction**

II. **Mandated quality: Institutional regulations and regulatory agencies**

III. **QA**

IV. **TQM**

V. **Productivity**
   A. Measuring productivity

VI. **Utilization**

INTRODUCTION

Since productivity cannot be discussed without also discussing the quality of the services provided, these two concepts are combined in this chapter. Effectiveness and efficiency are critical concepts in managing a physical therapy service. Without documented proof of adequate performance and outcomes, the physical therapy manager will be ineffective in securing accreditation, gaining additional resources, building new programs, marketing new and ongoing services, or securing contracts with other agencies such as health maintenance organizations (HMOs) and preferred provider organizations (PPOs).

In physical therapy, quality care must be a priority of the service for all patients. Health care is in its infancy in terms of quality management just as it is in its infancy in marketing management. These two concepts go hand in hand. The focus on meeting the needs and wants of the consumers is at the core of both approaches. Quality is measured in a number of ways in complex health care organizations, and the physical therapy manager must work closely with other organizational groups to coordinate the evaluation process. Just as physical therapy managers are experimenting with new quality measures and systems, so are a number of other health care managers. Meeting together in work groups or discussion groups will benefit each manager and the organization as a whole. This is an exciting time for health care and for physical therapy administration. It is an opportunity to grow as a manager and make a significant contribution to the organization and the profession of physical therapy by thoughtfully considering the issues of quality management.

The manager has the responsibility to establish and maintain a quality assurance (QA) program for the department, service, or practice. That program must begin with a philosophy statement in which the role of QA in the department is clearly determined and the level of review is determined. That is, if a department's philosophical statement identifies the individual physical therapist as the professional who is responsible for the process of evaluation, treatment, and planning related to the individual patient, then that department must develop a system that assesses the individual's patient-related behaviors and the outcome of the individual's patient care performance. From the mission or philosophical statement of the the department, standards of practice are developed. The standards of practice in physical therapy developed by the American Physical Therapy Association (Appendix 5.4) are often adopted or adapted by physical therapy departments. These standards of practice are broadly stated and are only a beginning point for establishing quality improvement standards.

Quality improvement standards must be collectively established either within a facility or across facilities. The process must involve the input of consumers (referral sources, patients, reimbursement agencies, administration) and professionals. In some instances[1] adequate research has been done to be able to adopt measures of functional performance as the consistent tool to assess treatment outcome. In most situations, however, the lack of reproducibility of measurement procedures chosen by the staff or the lack of consistency of measuring parameters hamper the ability to assess outcome. The evaluation of progress notes based on standards of practice and the mission statement has been the most commonly used quality assurance system in physical therapy. Since these standards are very broadly stated and the assessment is only as good as the standards being used, quality assurance programs in physical therapy have lacked the precision necessary to measure outcome of care.

Quality can only be assured if it is continually assessed and feedback given to the professionals and managers responsible for patient care and professional performance. Total quality management (TQM) focuses on continuous quality improvement with an emphasis on treatment outcomes.

· · · · · · · · · · ·
MANDATED QUALITY ASSURANCE: INSTITUTIONAL REGULATIONS AND REGULATORY AGENCIES

The 1971 amendment to the Social Security Act mandated the development of Professional Standards Review Organizations (PSROs) as a cost savings measure in the funding in medicare patient care. These organizations conducted a number of studies on quality of care and patterns of care within hospitals. In the 1980s the PSROs were replaced by Peer Review Organizations (PROs) whose focus was the quality of medical care of medicare patients. Currently, PROs compete for contracts with the Health Care Financing Administration to monitor medical care of medicare patients and promote cost control mechanisms such as second opinions and retrospective studies of medical care.

The current utilization review processes in hospitals grew out of the federally mandated review processes. Complex organizations (hospitals, HMOs, PPOs) recognized that preadmission review, procedure review, and reviews of levels of care and the medical necessity of admissions and procedures kept costs down and improved the quality of care. Therefore, in organizations that have utilization review systems, physical therapy procedures, duration of physical therapy intervention; frequency of treatments, and timeliness of discharge are all part of the institutional review process. In order to treat patients outside the utilization review guidelines, the therapist must document the potential cost savings as well as the appropriateness of the proposed plan.

Regulatory agencies such as the Joint Commission on the Accreditation of

Healthcare Organizations (JCAHO) also mandate quality assurance systems within the organization and the individual departments providing patient care, whereas the Commission on the Accreditation of Rehabilitation Facilities (CARF) mandates systems of program evaluation. As JCAHO, CARF, and other regulatory bodies move toward more rigorous criteria of measuring program effectiveness and efficiency and outcome assessments, the QA systems in physical therapy are changing to reflect more rigorous systems of quality assessment and a focus on outcome.

A QA program based on outcome assessments focuses less on individual professional practice processes and more on the status of the patient at specific points in time as a reflection of shared philosophies and treatment processes with the patient and other disciplines responsible for the care of the patient. The profession of physical therapy is in the process of moving away from the procedurally oriented QA program to an outcome-oriented QA program. This requires creative involvement of the managers, therapists, patients, employers, and families to assess the outcomes of treatment over time and in a variety of activities and settings.

. . . .
QA

The process of assuring quality services begins with an analysis of the progress note and other forms of documentation of the status of the patient. The most basic QA process is an audit of the clinical record that can be used to assess performance by carefully reviewing the evaluation, treatment, and discharge process or by assessing patient outcomes.

The audit process varies among agencies, institutions, departments, and practices. The common elements of the process are the creation of a QA (audit) committee, the regular audit of medical records, a mechanism for feedback to the individual professional, and a mechanism for the development and monitoring of a process to improve care in areas of deficiencies. Less frequently, physical therapists are beginning to assess outcomes by providing a mechanism for the QA committee to make clinical observations; maintaining contact with patients, family, and other health care providers after discharge; and establishing regular (6-month) follow-up meetings to assess outcomes of physical therapy. This process of assessing outcomes of physical therapy will be the manager's challenge during the next decade.

Prior to engaging in an audit, the department must establish standards of practice that can be reflected in processes and/or outcomes. A performance based audit assesses the physical therapist's performance based on standards of practice and may include the following components.

I. Referral form
   A. Completeness
   B. First treatment within 24 hours of the date of referral (if not within 24 hours, a priority rating is given for the waiting list)

II. Patient assessment
   A. Identifiable data base
   B. Reliability of data
   C. Appropriateness
   D. Entered in the record in timely fashion

III. Problem list
   A. Problem list clearly evolved from patient assessment
   B. Have problems been added appropriately
   C. Psychosocial problems on the problem list

IV. Initial note

A. If the patient assessment is incomplete, is there an explanation for why it has not been completed and is there a plan for completion

B. Initial note entered within an acceptable period of time

C. Is each note in an acceptable format (i.e., SOAP)

D. Initial assessment focuses on the total problem list

E. Goals for each appropriate problem are listed

F. Goals are logical and give date of expected completion

G. A plan is specified for each active problem relating to physical therapy

H. Plans are appropriate

V. Progress notes

A. Progress note on each active problem relating to physical therapy is written regularly

B. Deferred areas from the data base are followed up

C. Each note is dated and signed

D. Each note is in appropriate format (i.e., SOAP)

E. Assessment considers all data and the problem list as indicators of good analytic sense of the problem

F. Problems are added, updated, or resolved as new information is documented in the record

G. There is an indication of a full discussion of the program and progress with the patient and significant others

H. Patient education is documented

I. Plans and goals are clear

J. There is evidence of communication with other team members

K. There is a re-certification form every 30 days (if appropriate)

VI. Discharge summary

A. A discharge summary is complete

B. A discharge note is entered within 24 hours of discharge

C. Discharge note includes a statement on patient education

D. All active problems are addressed

· · · · · · · · · · ·

In reviewing the record, the QA committee looks for completeness of information, the degree to which the treatment is based on the assessment, the logic and efficiency of the treatment approach, and follow-up. If the medical record audit is used to assure quality, it is assumed that the record accurately reflects the quality of care that has been given to that specific patient. It is also assumed that what is not written has not been done. These are huge assumptions. First, it cannot be assumed that any standard of outcome will emerge based on the thoroughness of performing the procedures of evaluation, treatment, and planning as documented in the medical record.

In addition to monitoring the medical record and progress notes, audit committees should monitor performance over time by reviewing notes, flowsheets, follow-up letters, and discharge summaries on a regular basis.

Although physical therapists are improving the documentation of services, that documentation is almost always in the form of progress notes and oftentimes is targeted at the reimbursement agency or other colleagues who may follow-up on the patient. In looking at the medical record in terms of outcomes, the documents that give the most clear view of the quality of services are documents such as surgical reports, postoperative flow sheets, discharge summaries, and physicians' letters to other physicians.

Future efforts in assessing outcomes will have to focus on functional levels of independence, resumption of responsibilities, quality of life measures, and health status measures. Physical therapy managers will have to form alliances with epidemiologists and other health services scientists to appropriately develop the determinants of successful care.

TQM

TQM is discussed briefly in Chapter 7. TQM is not new to American business, but because it focused on the consumer and not the processes of production, this quality improvement system was not adopted when it was first described by W. Edwards Deming in the 1940s. However, Deming found Japanese business leaders to be willing participants in a system that would promise them manufacturing success after World War II. The system thrived in Japan and only now—in the 1990s—is the American manufacturing community recognizing the need to focus on consumer wants and perceptions.

The TQM system fits the marketing management system described in the previous chapter in which the consumer and employee are central to the description of problems, design of strategies, and implementation of plans. The role of management in this system is to coordinate and facilitate the process of work, and the role of the worker is to take responsibility for the output of the system and to generate new ideas about how the process can improve.

Deming's system is capsulated into his 14 points for management. These points were presented in Chapter 7 and are presented here again in Box 14–1 with an indication of those points that directly address quality improvement. Deming stresses that quality assurance cannot be an add-on to the management system. It must not be a process of counting behaviors and processes of observations and inspections. Quality assessment and attention to quality must be a constant or continuous process. Workers must be given the right to take pride in their work, not to feel that the work belongs to the organization and they are simply the mechanics who produce the work.

As Deming has proposed this system for manufacturing, several individuals are bringing this process into nonprofit organizations and health care as well. The challenge for the physical therapy manager is to instill the concepts of continuous quality assessment in the professionals and support staff within the department and then develop mechanisms for getting feedback from the professionals regarding the outcomes of patient care. The manager must also take responsibility to keep all workers well informed of changes in the institution and environment so that the employees can make appropriate adjustments to their expectations. A key to success in the manufacturing community is to fix problems while the system continues to function. The normal route for most managers in the physical therapy environment is to identify the problem as a performance discrepancy with the workers, take the individual out of the system when there is a performance discrepancy or a need for training, and send the person to a program or consultant for remediation. Quality problems do not usually fall on the shoulders of the individual worker. The failure to deliver a quality service is the fault of the system. Managers must therefore work with the workers, consumers, and environment to solve the quality problems. Adequate, up-to-date education is often one of the key elements to providing quality programs. The physical therapy manager should develop relationships with physical therapy

· ·
BOX 14–1 DEMING'S 14 POINTS FOR MANAGEMENT*

1. Create constancy of purpose toward improvement of product and service, with the aim to become competitive and to stay in business, and to provide jobs.
2. Adopt the new philosophy. We are in a new economic age. Western management must awaken to the challenge, must learn its responsibilities, and take on leadership for change.
3. Cease dependence on inspection to achieve quality. Eliminate the need for inspection on a mass basis by building quality into the product in the first place.
4. End the practice of awarding business on the basis of price tag. Instead, minimize total cost. Move toward a single supplier for any one item, on a long-term relationship of loyalty and trust.
5. Improve constantly and forever the system of production and service, to improve quality and productivity, and thus constantly decrease costs.
6. Institute training on the job.
7. Institute leadership. The aim of supervision should be to help people and machines and gadgets to do a better job. Supervision of management is in need of overhaul, as well as supervision of production workers.
8. Drive out fear, so that everyone may work effectively for the company.

9. Break down barriers between departments. People in research, design, sales, and production must work as a team, to forsee problems of production and in use that may be encountered with the product or service.
10. Eliminate slogans, exhortations, and targets for the work force asking for zero defects and new levels of productivity. Such exhortations only create adversarial relationships, as the bulk of the causes of low quality and low productivity belong to the system and thus lie beyond the power of the work force.
11. a. Eliminate work standards (quotas) on the factory floor. Substitute leadership.
    b. Eliminate management by objective. Eliminate management by numbers, numerical goals. Substitute leadership.
12. a. Remove barriers that rob the hourly worker of his right to pride of workmanship. The responsibility of supervisors must be changed from sheer numbers to quality.
    b. Remove barriers that rob people in management and in engineering of their right to pride of workmanship. This means, inter alia, abolishment of the annual or merit rating and of management by objective.
13. Institute a vigorous program of education and self-improvement.
14. Put everybody in the company to work to accomplish the transformation. The transformation is everybody's job.

*From Deming WE: *Out of Crisis.* Cambridge, Mass, Massachusetts Institute of Technology, 1986, pp 23–24.

educational programs to provide team consultation within the facility and to provide real patient care issues and problems in the classroom. Such relationships can improve both the quality of the work and the quality of the education.

This system cannot be instituted; it must be developed with shared goals and shared meaning among patients and other consumers, professionals, support staff, and management. Deming feels that if the system is to work, it must be the only system in place within the institution. Physical therapy managers will be challenged to abandon old systems and develop a new one based on TQM and to be able to develop the system within the work environment with employees, consumers, and managers working cooperatively. Once developed, the job is only beginning. This is a continuous quality improvement system. The process is a constant one and the goal is continual review, revision, refinement.

Individuals interested in more in-depth reading in TQM, cases and further description of methods should begin with the reference list at the end of this chapter.

· · · · · · · · · · ·
PRODUCTIVITY

Productivity is not a simple counting of service units per unit of time. "Because much of healthcare is labor intense, productivity systems have emphasized FTEs per discharge, or man hours, divided into a specified product descriptor such as x-ray procedures, physical therapy procedures, surgical cases, etc."[2(p5)] Productivity must be measured along with quality and related to the many personal and interpersonal factors related to personnel management discussed in earlier chapters. Employee morale may play a significant role in productivity and morale is affected by several factors. Among the top reasons for physical therapists leaving jobs, lack of a sense of accomplishment has been given as a major reason.[3] A national survey of retention and recruitment of physical therapists in hospitals demonstrated that 62% of therapists were frustrated because they could not deliver quality care and 88% felt that the demand was high and there were not enough therapists.[4] Given the human resource shortages in physical therapy discussed earlier in this book and the fact that physical therapy services in complex organizations are particularly challenged to find ways to retain and recruit experienced physical therapists, it is not surprising that the demand on the individual therapist has increased.

Measuring Productivity

Both hospital-based and private practice physical therapy managers are using a variety of charge systems. These include charge systems based on the following:

- Modalities
- Time
- Procedures
- Relative value units

The most common productivity standard is between 85% and 90%, and the most common productivity measure is the procedure, although the trend is toward the adoption of the relative value unit as a productivity measure. This shift is consistent with the shift away from charging by the procedure to charging by the visit. The relative value unit is the standard unit of measurement or value of the volume of physical therapy activities associated with a patient visit.

There are several methods of monitoring productivity. The most objective of these systems begins with an actual time study to determine the amount of time those staff who treat patients spend in the treatment processes. The majority of complex organizations do not base their relative value units on time studies. Some simply assume the national standard, others negotiate with the administration for the productivity standard. One of the important reasons to determine the productivity standard of the department is to staff each component of the department appropriately.

The relative value unit is also forming the foundation for some third parties to determine the costs of delivering services (especially in the outpatient, private practice setting) and therefore the rate at which the service will be reimbursed. It is critical for the physical therapy manager to be as objective as possible in determining the productivity quotient of the department.

Several methods of determining productivity have been identified in the literature and by individual therapists. Two commonly used systems are represented in the following text and Box 14–2 . These methods were developed by Natalie Finegold Lapin, P.T., Director of Rehabilitation at Southfield (Michigan) Rehabilitation Hospital and Peter R. Kovacek, M.S.A., P.T., Owner of Kovacek Physical Therapy Services, Harper Woods, Mich.

. . . .
BOX 14–2 PRODUCTIVITY MONITORING: METHOD 2 WORKSHEET

Date: _____ Day: _____
Staff Hours Total

PT 1: _____ Aide 1: _____
PT 2: _____ Aide 2: _____
PT 3: _____ Aide 3: _____
PT 4: _____ Aide 4: _____
PT 5: _____ Sec: _____
PT 6: _____
PT 7: _____
A. Staffed minutes (Staff×480 minutes): _____
   Staff comments: _____

Workload Indicators:

1. Evaluate new patients(39+41)	(45): _____	2. #1 Total: _____
3. Gait training	(25): _____	4. #3 Total: _____
5. Ultrasound	(20): _____	6. #5 Total: _____
7. Small whirlpool	(35): _____	8. #7 Total: _____
9. Medium whirlpool	(45): _____	10. #9 Total: _____
11. Large whirlpool	(60): _____	12. #11 Total: _____
13. Transcutaneous electrical neurostimulator units	(20): _____	14. #13 Total: _____
15. Therapeutic exercise	(25): _____	16. #15 Total: _____
17. Traction	(25): _____	18. #17 Total: _____
19. Discharge plan	(60): _____	20. #19 Total: _____
21. Paraffin	(10): _____	22. #21 Total: _____
23. Hot pack	(19): _____	24. #23 Total: _____
25. Cold pack	(17): _____	26. #25 Total: _____
27. Ice massage	(10): _____	28. #27 Total: _____
29. Electric stimulation	(24): _____	30. #29 Total: _____
31. Massage	(15): _____	32. #31 Total: _____
33. Diathermy	(25): _____	34. #33 Total: _____
35. Special dressing	(30): _____	36. #35 Total: _____
37. Patients transported	(24): _____	38. #37 Total: _____
39. New inpatients	(35): _____	40. #39 Total: _____
41. New outpatients	(35): _____	42. #41 Total: _____
43. Delays	(10): _____	44. #43 Total: _____

45. Total workload units (Add 2 through 44)=   _____
46. Total staffed minutes ("A" above)   =   _____
47. Fixed minutes   =   (1322)
48. Workload units + total fixed minutes
    (45 + 47)   =   _____
49. Variance (48 − 46)   =   _____
50. Productivity quotient (46 ÷ 48)   =   _____
51. No shows, inpatient _____ 52. 51 Total: _____
53. No shows, outpatient _____ 54. 53 Total: _____

Productivity monitoring: Method 1

1. Output:
   A. Use number of generated (i.e., billed) relative value units or timed treatment units.
2. Input:
   A. Determine those personnel involved in only direct patient care. This would generally be physical therapists (PTs), physical therapist assistants (PTAs), and treating aides.
      (1.) Count the regular payroll hours worked over a month
      (2.) Sick, vacation, holiday, and conference (seminar) hours do not count.
   B. Identify those personnel who are partially involved in direct patient care. This will usually include supervisors, secretary/aide (if both functions are performed).
      (1.) Identify what average percentage of time the above are involved in patient care.
      (2.) Use that percentage of the hours for productivity calculation. Example: A supervisor who is considered to be 0.5 full-time equivalent (FTE) for supervisory time and 0.5 FTE for treatment would have only half the payroll hours counted in the month's productivity.
   C. Add together the total hours of direct patient treatment time.
3. Productivity:
   A. Total units generated
      (1.) Total number of direct patient treatment hours. Example:

Person	Position	Payroll (hr)	Productivity (hr)
A	Staff PT	100	100
B	Staff PTA	100	100
C	Treating aide	100	100
D	PT Supervisor	100	75
E	PT Director	100	50
F	Secretary	100	0
G	Transport aide	100	50
	Total		475

   (2.) Conclusion: If the department generated 1400 units of 15 minutes each:

$$1400 \text{ units}/475 \text{ hours} = 2.95 \text{ units/hour}$$
$$2.95 \text{ units/hour}/4.0 \text{ units/hour} = 73.7\% \text{ productivity}$$

Productivity monitoring: Method 2

1. Variable time monitors
   A. Treatment Related Variables: therapeutic exercise, ultrasound, hot pack, transcutaneous electrical neuro stimulator units, electric stimulation, cold pack, whirlpool (by size), wound care, gait training, evaluation
   B. Nontreatment Related: Nonroutine cleaning, cancellations, no shows, delays, new patient scheduling, discharge planning, charting, nonbillable instruction
2. Fixed time monitors

    A. Administrative time, supervisory time, education, orientation, meetings, supply/inventory, clerical time
3. The formula:

$$\frac{(\text{Fixed inputs} + \text{variable inputs})}{\text{Actual staff time}} = \text{productivity quotient}$$

4. Ideal productivity quotient (Pq) = 100%
5. Pq formula accounts for nonbillable but valuable activities in the department.
6. The process
    A. Define goals
    B. Describe to staff
    C. Describe to administration
    D. Set start time table
    E. Staff involvement in scoring
    F. Define formula
    G. Commitment from staff and administration
    H. Trial data collection period
    I. Staffing contract
    J. Implementation
    K. Review and revise

Method 2 relies on accurate time study data collected by the staff and then analyzed by the physical therapy manager. The data are analyzed using the worksheet in Box 14–2.

These productivity analyses are important in preparing and monitoring the physical therapy budget and are discussed further in Chapter 15. Once the productivity quotient for the core physical therapy service has been determined, the physical therapy manager cannot simply apply that quotient to all other services. Physical therapy managers know intuitively that the quotient will be different for satellite units on the intensive care floor, in the sports outpatient facility, and in outpatient areas. Productivity analyses must be completed for each service area.

UTILIZATION

The weakness of the approach to productivity described above is that it assumes that there is either a natural end point to the treatment of individual patients or that there is no end point and that treatment is necessary. In addition to the productivity quotient, the physical therapy manager must also begin to determine, with the staff and through clinical research, what the normal end point of treatment is for the myriad of diagnoses treated in a physical therapy department.

The Health Care Financing Administration (HCFA) has already proposed screens (edits) (Box 14–3) for medicare patients that limit the number of visits by category of patient. As with many screens, the Health Care Financing Administration edits do not account for the severity of illness or injury.

Before the bureaucratic agencies impose utilization screens on the physical therapy manager, it would be appropriate to establish physical therapy utilization screens that reflect the national practice data available as well as the professional judgment that must be applied when data are not available.

In a national study of patterns of practice in outpatient physical therapy, Alan Jette presented data on a stratified sample of outpatient physical therapy patients

· ·

BOX 14–3 PARTIAL LISTING OF MEDICARE EDITS*

Edit ID No. (mo)	Diagnosis	ICD-9-CM	No. of Visits	Duration
1	Cancer	162.0–163.9	7	1
		165.0–165.9	24	2
2	Parkinson's disease	332.0–332.1	13	1
3	Meningitis	320.0–323.9	16	2
	Huntington's chorea	333.4–333.7	16	2
	Multiple sclerosis	340	16	2
4	Cerebrovascular accident, acute	436.0	32	3
	Concussion	850.4	32	3
5	Transient ischemic attack	435.0	7	1
6	Paralytic syndromes	344.0–344.9	39	4
	Spinal cord injury	952.0–952.9	39	4
7	Late effects, polio	138	19	2
	Peripheral nerve injury	953.0–957.9	19	2
8	Diabetes	250.7	13	1
	Lymphedema	457.0–457.9	13	1
9	Diabetes with ulcer	250.8	29	2
	Hansen's disease	030.0–030.9	29	2
	Cellulitis	681.0–682.9	29	2

*From Medicare Medical Review Manual. There are 26 categories of medicare edits and hundreds of diseases and symptoms covered in these categories. This representation covers only nine of the categories and does not depict all of the diseases or symptoms covered.

ICD-9-CM is the International Classification of Diseases (ICD)-9-Clinical Manifestations codification system. Unlike the older ICD system, the ICD-9 system classifies symptoms such as weakness, swelling, and contractures as well as traditional disease entities. This classification system is traditionally used in billing by physical therapists and other disciplines and is also used to collect and report clinical outcome data in individual departments as well as publications.

from both hospital-based and private practice settings. The results of this study indicate that short-term care (up to 60 days) accounted for 80.2% of outpatients in hospital-based practices and 66.8% of outpatients in private practices. The majority of patients seeking outpatient physical therapy presented with back injury and upper and lower extremity muscle tears. These data are consistent with other data in the literature.

The Oregon Physical Therapy Association has developed a document that identifies the criteria for care for outpatient physical therapy services for specific diagnosis. An example of the criteria for temporomandibular joint dysfunction is shown in Box 14–4.

From this information and information gathered within the individual department, physical therapy managers must begin to understand the utilization patterns of the department or practice. It is going to be increasingly important to be able to demonstrate to reimbursement agencies how decisions are made to treat and to terminate treatment. The only approach to cost containment that has worked has been prospective payment. Reimbursement agencies will continue to look for ways of predicting costs before the patient begins the process and to set limits beyond which payment will not be continued. The American Physical Therapy Association (APTA) is engaged in numerous activities to collect data related to utilization. Physical therapy managers may want to contact the APTA for assistance in looking at patterns of practice or form a partnership with a physical therapy educational program to design the appropriate clinical studies to develop practice pattern data.

· ·

BOX 14–4   CRITERIA FOR TEMPOROMANDIBULAR JOINT DYSFUNCTION*

Sample Criteria for Care for Outpatient Physical Therapy Services
Oregon Physical Therapy Association
Title: Temporomandibular Joint (TMJ) Dysfunction and Associated Symptoms (i.e., headache, neck pain, tinnitus, dizziness)

I. Justification for service: Physical therapy is indicated for one of the following reasons:
   A. Traumatic onset
   B. Loss of opening/closing range of motion
   C. Headache associated with TMJ dysfunction
   D. Muscle guarding/spasm
   E. Improper posture or body mechanics
   F. Clenching, grinding, or bruxing
   G. After surgery

II. Number or length of service (frequency)
   A. Up to twice daily while hospitalized
   B. Outpatient treatment:
      a. Daily up to 3 weeks
      b. 3 times/week up to 15 weeks
      c. Care beyond 15 weeks depends on outcomes

III. Exceptions: Complications that would alter expected outcome, length of service, or specific treatment
   A. Re-injury
   B. Impaired ability to retain information or follow instructions
   C. Additional undiagnosed pathology
   D. Degenerative condition

IV. Critical aspects of care
   A. Upon physician referral, evaluation by physical therapist to determine present status and services necessary to achieve expected outcomes
   B. Treatment program should include at least one of the following:
      a. Modalities and manual techniques to decrease pain, muscle tension, and muscle guarding
      b. Manual techniques and exercise to improve ROM on opening/closing and to improve symmetry and sequence of motion
      c. Exercise to improve ROM, strength, posture, and body mechanics as related to head, neck, and jaw function.
      d. Biofeedback techniques to increase awareness of clench, brux, and proper posture.
      e. Training in proper body mechanics, posture, and movement for prevention of re-injury and aggravation.

V. Status at completion of service episode (outcome)
   A. Improved symmetry and range of motion of open/close
   B. Demonstration of understanding of self-care as related to body mechanics, posture, and position of tongue/jaw
   C. Diminished headache, jaw and facial pain, tension and guarding.
   D. Demonstrates independence in home exercises

*From Burles B: Criteria for care for outpatient physical therapy services. *Orthop Practice* 3:91. Used with permission.

References

1. Carey RG, Seibert JH: Integrating program evaluation, quality assurance, and marketing for inpatient rehabilitation. *Rehabil Nursing* 1988; 13:66–70.
2. Rich JM: Physical therapy productivity systems: Fact or myth? *Phys Ther Forum,* April 1, 1992; pp 4–8.
3. Harkson DG, Unterreiner AS, Shepard KF: Factors related to job turnover in physical therapy. *Phys Ther* 1982; 62:1465–1470.
4. Staff: *Recruitment and Retention of Physical Therapists in Hospitals.* Report of the 1989 House of Delegates, Alexandria, Va, American Physical Therapy Association, 1989.
5. Burles B: Criteria for care for outpatient physical therapy services. *Orthop Practice* 1991; 3:8–11.

Selected Readings

Bohannon RW: Productivity among physical therapists: An evaluation of one department. *Phys Ther* 1984; 64:1242–1244.

Bohannon RW: Statistical analysis of productivity in one physical therapy department. *Phys Ther* 1987; 67:1553–1557.

Buller B: Consolidation raises staff productivity. *Hospitals* 1984; 58:49–50.

Deming WE: *Out of the Crisis.* Cambridge, Mass, Massachusetts Institute of Technology Center for Advanced Engineering Study, 1982.

Gabor A: *The Man Who Discovered Quality.* New York, NY, Times Books, 1991.

Gay P: Get it in writing. *Nursing Manage* 1983; 14:32–35.

Hancock WM, et al: A model to determine staff levels, cost, and productivity of hospital units. *J Med Syst* 1987; 11:319–330.

Hays P: A change of pace: Alternate work schedule options. *Clin Manage Phys Ther* 1989; 9:26–28.

McLaughlin MA: Monitoring the quality of contracted therapy services provided by a vendor: A model for home health services. *QRB,* 1988, pp 40–44.

Rase CW: Reliability of the auditing process at the University of Montana's physical therapy department. *Phys Ther* 1984; 64:1088–1090.

Schackenberg LA, et al: Quality assurance: A team approach. *Caring,* Sept 1983, pp023–24.

Scherkenbach WW: *The Deming Route to Quality and Productivity.* Washington, DC, Ceep Press, 1991.

Staff: *Productivity in Physical Therapy.* Alexandria, Va, American Physical Therapy Association. APTA Department of Practice Monograph.

Staff: *Progress Notes for Physical Therapy.* Alexandria, Va, American Physical Therapy Association. APTA Department of Practice Monograph.

Stocks K: *Total Quality Management, Management Memos, Section on Administration.* American Physical Therapy Association, Alexandria, Va, May 1991.

Walton M: *The Deming Management Method.* New York, NY, Perigee Press, 1986.

CHAPTER 15

Fiscal Management of Physical Therapy Services

INTRODUCTION

There was a time in the history of physical therapy when the physical therapy manager's fiscal responsibility was limited to the development of an annual budget based on the budget of the previous year plus an inflationary factor and the monitoring of that budget throughout the year. Although budgeting and budget accountability remain an important management function, the scope of fiscal responsibility of the physical therapy manager has changed significantly.

Most physical therapy managers are now responsible for budget planning, budget projections, meeting the fiscal goals of market management, assuring payment for services, estimating reimbursement levels of the patient population being served, and appealing reimbursement decisions to third-party reimbursers.

. . . .
BUDGETARY CONTROL

Budgets are not a simple projection of revenues and expenditures. They are a mechanism of assessing the success and progress of the organization or department, programs, and projects in terms of budget projections. Budget projections are determined from the facts that are known related to the previous budget period plus assumptions that the physical therapy manager and the administration believe will be true of the environment, institution, markets, and consumers.

When used on a regular basis by the physical therapy manager, budgets are a mechanism of controlling the implementation of programs or services and assessing the incremental progress or failure to progress of the program or service to meet projected fiscal targets. Budgets express the anticipated income and expenditures of the programs and components within a unit and are set in the context of organizational and departmental plans. Revenues and expenditures arc planned and spread over specific budget units of time and focus on personnel, buildings and space, equipment, and supplies. Budget periods can vary. For example, the budget period for personnel and supplies is usually 1 year, whereas the budget period for capital expense may be 5 to 10 years depending on the anticipated life of the equipment.

Planning-Programming-Budgeting Systems

Budgets are an integral part of the planning process. The plan for a new program or service is developed from the mission and objectives of the organization and the budget builds upon the plan. Planning-programming-budgeting systems (PPBS) were developed to assist managers in reducing duplication of costs associated with activities within an organization. This system of budgeting focuses on planning, analyzing the anticipated costs and benefits of each program within an organization, and then allocating resources to those programs that are accepted by the organization for the next fiscal period. The resources needed for each increment of a planned program are determined using planning strategies such as Program Evaluation and Review Techniques (PERT), critical path method (CPM), and cross-matrix analyses. Organizational fiscal administrative staff must be able to predict incremental revenues and expenditures in order to assess the progress of the organization, unit, or department. The PPBS approach demands that the manager develop a process for evaluation of costs and revenues at critical points in the implementation of the program and a mechanism to transmit that information as a mechanism of control.

When plans are developed, as discussed in previous chapters on planning and marketing, the physical therapy manager must assess the need for specific resources at given points in time (milestones) to implement organizational plans. Some physical therapy managers use milestone budgeting for new programs. As each major phase of the project is completed, the actual costs are determined and new budget projections are made for the next phase of the project. It may be necessary to continue to approach a new service with this kind of budgeting for a prolonged period until the service is well developed.

Zero-Base Budgeting

Zero-base budgeting (ZBB) takes a fresh look at the organization's goals, activities, and resources associated with activities at the beginning of each budget period. The cost of running a program is then computed from a zero base as if the program never existed.

Some administrators will use a variation of ZBB in which the physical therapy manager is asked to submit three budgets—one with no change from the previous year, one with a 30% (will vary among institutions and with the economy) increase, and one with a 30% decrease. The purpose of developing this kind of budget is to see which programs will fall out or be put in place with a substantial decrease or increase in the budget. The administrator can then more appropriately assist in the decision making regarding programs to keep and discard based on the intensity of resources needed for the program and the decisions of the physical therapy manager regarding program changes.

Break-Even Budgeting

The traditional approach to budgeting within a physical therapy service is incremental budgeting with a focus on breaking even at the end of the fiscal period. Organizations usually base departmental or unit budgets on certain increases (or decreases) from the amounts granted for the previous fiscal period.

Productivity-Based Budgeting

Many physical therapy managers adopt budgeting systems that are based on productivity and break-even budgeting. These systems rely on the manager's decisions regarding staffing levels needed to provide services to projected volumes of patients, as discussed in Chapter 14. The manager then projects gross revenues using the unit cost system adopted by the department and the corresponding charge system in order to cover costs of providing services.

. . . .
PREPARING BUDGETS AND REPORTS

When the budget within a complex organization is prepared, the institution will already have guidelines, forms, formats, codes, and other basic budget tools to use during the budgeting process. Many institutions ask for a budget for the next fiscal year with comparison budgets for the current and past year. In addition, many administrators find it helpful to have projections for the remainder of the current year to discuss performance and projections.

The complete budget for a specific department in a complex organization is multifaceted. It contains yearly fiscal performance and projections, capital equipment costs spread over a 5- to 10-year period, new projects with projections of costs on a monthly basis for the start-up phase of the project and indications of impact on the total budget, and a discussion of marketing opportunities and potential ventures for the department over a 5-year period. By providing a complete picture of the budget, the physical therapy manager is helping the administration understand how the current and projected budget fit into a larger picture of planned growth or reconfiguration of the physical therapy services.

The specific reports that the physical therapy manager will be asked to produce include income and expense statements. Physical therapy managers in independent practice will also want to produce a balance sheet that balances the assets of the business against liabilities and the equity (capital, equipment, building, investments) the owner has in the business.

The mechanics of developing income and expense statements are the mechanics of fiscal accounting. The physical therapy manager in a complex organization has a great many resources available to assist in the mechanics of developing a budget. These resources are available through the facility's chief financial officer, marketing and personnel professionals, and the administration. In an independent practice, the physical therapy manager usually employs accountants to develop balance sheets and income and expense statements. Although these skills are important to the manager, they are skills that other professionals possess and use and refine every day. It is to the advantage of the physical therapy manager to use professional accountants to assist in the preparation of fiscal reports. The key skills for physical therapy managers are a very clear understanding of the charge system used in the department and the development and monitoring of a successful reimbursement system.

· · · · · · · · · · ·
CHARGE/COST SYSTEMS

Since the profession of physical therapy first began billing for services, the most common unit cost system utilized by physical therapy managers has focused on either modalities of care or units of time. In many instances these charge systems were based on the volume of modalities of care provided and the resultant costs to be assigned to those units of care in order for the department to break even. The formulas used within departments have focused on the cost of maintaining the department plus indirect costs (Box 15–1) offset by the unit costs associated with a specific volume of patients. For example, if the cost of personnel, supplies, and equipment of a small physical therapy department is $300,000 and the institution assesses the department an indirect overhead rate of 60%, the total cost of maintaining the department for the budget period (1 year) is $480,000 (Box 15–2). If the physical therapy manager projects a volume of 4,800 units of care for the year, then the unit cost for that year will be set at $10 a unit.

The unit may be described as actual modalities of care (hot pack, ultrasound, electrotherapy, therapeutic exercise) or as units of time. There has been a considerable move away from cost systems based on modalities of care because this system does not reflect the actual level of services provided for the individual patient. For example, in a system in which the minimal unit carries the same value, a patient who receives a hot pack is charged the same as a patient who receives therapeutic exercise. One modality may be primarily delivered by an aide, whereas the other is delivered by a physical therapist. Although this system results in a break-even point for the department, individual patients are not equitably charged according to the level of services received.

The time unit charge more appropriately bills the patient for services rendered but again does not in itself distinguish the level of care provided. Many physical therapy managers have adopted per-visit charge systems that take into account aide, assistant, and physical therapist time and the degree of complexity of the services provided. A first-visit charge will assume a large evaluation time component, whereas a

· ·
BOX 15–1 EXAMPLES OF COSTS ASSUMED IN INDIRECT COST RATES WITHIN AN ORGANIZATION

1. Maintenance department costs
2. Administration (administrative services that can be related to the oversight of the department/service)
3. Electricity
4. Rent/space costs
5. Water
6. Laundry services
7. Housekeeping
8. Housekeeping supplies (i.e., lightbulbs)
9. Percentage of non–revenue producing services and departments assigned to the department

BOX 15–2 TOTAL COSTS OF A SMALL PHYSICAL THERAPY DEPARTMENT

Physical Therapy Department
Annual Budget
Direct Costs

Department manager	$ 60,000
Senior physical therapist	$ 40,000
Staff physical therapists at $30,000	$ 90,000
Physical therapist assistant	$ 20,000
Physical therapist aide	$ 14,000
Secretary	$ 15,000
Receptionist	$ 12,000
Transporter	$ 12,000
Equipment	$ 10,000
Supplies, telephone, mail	$ 27,000
Total direct cost	$300,000
Indirect Cost Rate = 60%	$180,000
Total cost	$480,000

recheck visit will assume a small evaluation time component and a treatment visit may assume no or minimal evaluation time components.

As the variety of charge systems have grown in physical therapy, there has been an increasing need of third-party reimbursement agencies to understand the charge systems and work toward a more uniform charge system. The resource-based relative value system (RBRVS) is such a system and is discussed further later in this chapter.

REIMBURSEMENT

Reimbursement levels for physical therapy services within a hospital are included in the negotiation process of the institution with third-party reimbursers. Although the systems may be complex, the reimbursement levels of physical therapy services are oftentimes directly connected to other reimbursement formulas for the institution.

One of the frustrations for physical therapy managers within a complex organization is that physical therapy reimbursement is a relatively small component of the reimbursement system of the organization. Most physical therapy managers will not be aware that the majority of denied claims for physical therapy in a complex organization are not questioned by the billing clerks and financial officers of the institution. When institutions are dealing with charges for surgery, intensive care, radiographs, laboratory tests, and daily inpatient stays, denial of 25% of physical therapy bills may be considered insignificant. It is the responsibility of the physical therapy manager to make these individuals aware of the significant impact that uncollected fees have on the overall cost and budget of the department. It may also be of benefit to the institution for the individual physical therapy manager to employ a billing clerk whose sole responsibility is to follow up on denials of physical therapy bills. In many instances simply adding a code number, changing a procedural code, or interpreting a progress note will result in a successful resubmission of a claim.

Understanding physical therapy reimbursement for physical therapists working in an independent practice situation is important to understanding both current reimbursement issues for physical therapy as a separate entity as well as the future of physical therapy reimbursement. The charges for a specific service or set of services are subjected to medicare edit standards, coding standards, and RBRVS standards, and then the reimbursement level is determined for those charges (Fig 15–1)

Medicare Edits

As discussed previously, the Health Care Financing Administration (HCFA) recently developed a set of Medicare Edits to be used for Level II medical review for outpatient physical therapy reimbursement. The edits provide information regarding the number and frequency of reimbursable physical therapy treatments within the medicare program (Chapter 5, Table 5–1). These edits are used to initially determine the necessity of a service. When a claim is reviewed, the edits provide a screen to determine if physical therapy is appropriate for the particular diagnosis. Furthermore, they give an indication of the duration and frequency of treatments for the specific diagnosis. If a claim is submitted to Blue Cross/Blue Shield specifying four physical therapy treatments over a 2-week period for balance training for a patient with Parkinson's disease, the claim reviewer will check the edits (Table 5–1) and note that physical therapy is appropriate for Parkinson's disease (332.0–332.1) for up to 13 treatments over a 1-month period.

In addition to the edits, medicare also imposes other restrictions on physical therapy, including a 30-day recertification process, in which the physician must review the patient's progress and recertify the need for physical therapy. A $750 limit is on the medicare patient receiving care from an independent practitioner of physical therapy.

Coding Systems

Coding systems have been established by physician groups and insurers "to maximize uniformity in defining services for record keeping and payment purposes."[1(p20)] The coding systems that are particularly important to physical therapists are the Current Procedure Terminology (CPT) developed by the American Medical Association and adopted by most third-party reimbursement agencies for the billing of procedures in a physician's office or by independent practitioners of physical therapy; the Health Care Financing Administration (HCFA) Common Procedure Coding System (HCPCS); the International Classification of Diseases, Clinical

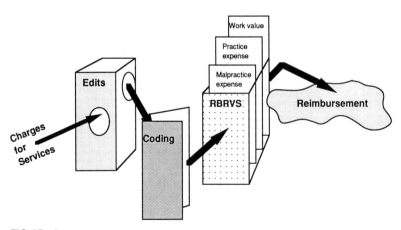

FIG 15–1.
Reimbursement for charges by an independent physical therapist. *RBRVS* = resource-based relative value system.

Manifestations (ICDA-9-CM); local codes that may be designated by individual insurance carriers; and modifiers that are used to indicate special circumstances (e.g., CPT code for therapeutic exercise is 97110, and 97110-52 indicates therapeutic exercise in a group setting). Modifiers and local codes are not universally accepted by all third-party reimbursers and should be carefully discussed with each carrier.

It is important for the physical therapy manager to understand the insurance coverage of the individual patient. "Billing problems apparently due to coding may actually be due to coverage. It is important to distinguish among the causes for these problems in order to remedy them. For instance you may find it difficult to get reimbursed for evaluation. There is a series of CPT codes that are appropriate for evaluation: the CPT's 90000-series codes for office and home visits. However sometimes insurers simply exclude those types of services from coverage for physical therapists."[1(p21)]

Some insurers may link coding systems. The most common link is ICD-9-CM as the diagnostic code with CPT as the procedural code. This link can be seen in the commonly used HCFA 1500 billing form. This form asks for ICD diagnostic codes and then asks for a link between the CPT procedure delivered and the specific diagnostic code for which it was delivered (Box 15–3). If appropriate reimbursement is to be obtained, it is important to use these coding systems properly.

RBRVS

Relative value units are the standard unit of measurement of the value or worth of physical therapy activities associated with a patient visit. The HCFA requires independent physical therapy practitioners or physical therapists working in a physician-owned clinic to use the RBRVS when billing for services.

When the worth of a service is determined, RBRVS takes into account the work value indicated by the degree of stress, judgment, and labor associated with the activity, the practice expense reflected in overhead and the cost of support staff, and the cost of malpractice insurance. The process that HCFA uses in determining the reimbursement rate in a relative value system is to determine the basic value of the service (e.g., muscle testing with exercise=1.08, therapeutic exercise=0.54, extended physical therapy=0.27). This value is then multiplied by a national conversion factor in dollars. For 1992 the national conversion factor was $31. So, muscle testing with exercise would be

BOX 15–3 EXCERPT FROM HEALTH CARE FINANCING ADMINISTRATION (HCFA) 1500 BILLING FORM

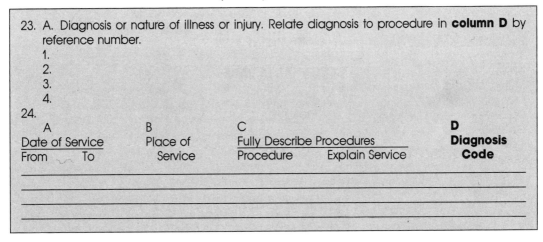

reimbursed at a rate of \$33.48 (1.08×\$31). RBRVS is very attractive to reimbursement agencies at the present system. The basic flaw of the system that now exists is that the system has been built on medicare data, not on actual physical therapy assessments of the work value of the units assigned to each category. The American Physical Therapy Association (APTA) and the Private Practice Section will continue to work with HCFA to refine this process so that a system can be developed which fairly reflects the work of the physical therapy staff in delivering services.

Reimbursement Issues Related to Direct Access

In 1992, there were 42 states that allowed evaluation of patients without referral and 27 states that allowed both evaluation and treatment of patients without physician referral. Attaining passage of laws that permit practice without referral have not automatically assured reimbursement without physician referral. The physical therapy community is actively seeking practice without referral legislation in all states within the United States, and insurers are increasingly paying for those services (Boxes 15–4 and 15–5).

Obtaining reimbursement within individual states has varied widely. In some states it was only necessary for the physical therapy community to point out to the insurance commissioner that direct access was now law in that state and reimbursement followed relatively quickly. In other states, the physical therapy community has had to lobby widely and engage in legal debates in order for reimbursement to be considered. Many physical therapists are still unable to seek reimbursement for direct access services within their state, and HCFA continues to require a physician's review of the case every 30 days in order for continuing reimbursement of medicare patients.

· · · · · · · · · · ·
CLAIMS REVIEW

Claims review at the level of the insurer is most commonly performed by non–physical therapists. It is important for the physical therapy manager to understand the review process and to make contact with responsible parties at the insur-

· ·
BOX 15–4 INSURERS PAYING FOR PHYSICAL THERAPY EVALUATION WITHOUT PHYSICIAN REFERRAL

Aetna	CT, IL, IA, KY, MD, NY, NC, TX*
Blue Cross	AK, CO, ID, IL, KY*, MD, MA, MN, MT, NC, SD, VT
Cigna	AK, CT, IA, LA, NC, TX
Equitable	IL, IA, MD, MN, NY, NC, TX
John Hancock	IL, MD
Metropolitan	CO, CT, KY*, MD, NY
Mutual of Omaha	KY*, MT
New York Life	MD, MT
Prudential	CT, KY*, MD*, MT, NY
State Farm	KY
Travelers	IL, KY*, MD, NY
Great West	MD*
Susquehana	MD*
SAMBA	MD*

*Under certain conditions/coverages. The Department of Reimbursement of the American Physical Therapy Association (APTA) maintains an up-to-date list of all insurers that pay for physical therapy services. For the most current information, contact the Department of Reimbursement, APTA, 1111 N Fairfax St, Alexandria, VA 22314. Used by permission from APTA.

BOX 15–5 INSURERS PAYING FOR PHYSICAL THERAPY TREATMENT WITHOUT PHYSICIAN REFERRAL

Aetna	IA, KY, NC
Blue Cross	AK, CO, ID, IA, KY, MD, MA, MT, NC, SD, VT
Cigna	AK, ID, IA, NC
Equitable	IA, MD, MN, NC
John Hancock	MD
Metropolitan	KY
Mutual of Omaha	ID, MT
New York Life	MD, MT
Prudential	KY
State Farm	KY
Transamerica	AZ
Travelers	AZ, MD, MT
Virgina Mason Health Plan	WA*

*Under certain conditions/coverages. The Department of Reimbursement of the American Physical Therapy Association (APTA) maintains an up-to-date list of all insurers that pay for physical therapy services. For the most current information, contact the Department of Reimbursement, APTA, 1111 N Fairfax St, Alexandria, VA 22314. Used by permission from APTA.

er's claims review office or department to ascertain guidelines for review that the insurer is willing to share. Some insurers will not pay for three modalities delivered within one treatment session. There may be no particular rationale to such a guideline other than the insurer's attempt to identify patterns of abuses and to develop guidelines to reduce those abuses. It is very helpful to give insurers information that will help them develop reasonable guidelines to reduce abuse.

The APTA is beginning to develop guidelines for the insurers to identify patterns of potential abuse (Box 15–6). Physical therapy managers may want to take this contact with insurers one step further and volunteer to provide a series of educational sessions for claims reviewers in the practice of physical therapy.

In addition to not knowing the practice of physical therapy, many reviewers are not familiar with physical therapy terminology. In addition to actual terminology, physical therapy shorthand can often cause a reviewer to deny a claim simply because they cannot read the progress notes or claims forms. Commonly used shorthand can be found in Appendix 15.1 following this chapter. The entire profession of physical therapy must develop a common nomenclature not only to standardize the collection of data and to ease internal communication, but also in order to assure that other parties, such as third-party reimbursers, understand the work that the physical therapist has done. Documentation problems are the key problems facing physical therapy and managers of physical therapy services. Poor documentation make quality assessment activities more difficult and may seriously jeopardize reimbursement. It is the responsibility of the physical therapy manager to monitor documentation and provide continuing incentives to improve documentation. Novice physical therapists must realize that progress notes have multiple consumers, with the major consumer being the reimbursement agency. Notes must be written in clear, concise language focusing on patient behaviors as they reflect the outcomes of physical therapy services.

ACCURATE FISCAL REPORTING

Perhaps the greatest challenge for the manager of a physical therapy service is the tendency of physical therapists to give away services by inaccurate reporting of time

. . . .

BOX 15–6 PATTERNS OF POTENTIAL ABUSES IN PHYSICAL THERAPY

The most common physical therapy treatments that may appropriately be done either simultaneously or consecutively:
Hot packs (97010) and traction, mechanical (97012)
Ultrasound (97128) and electrical stimulation (manual) (97118)
Therapeutic exercise (97110)49electrical stimulation (unattended) (97014) or (manual) (97118)
The following are virtually synonymous or likey* to be inappropriate if billed together in the same session:
Microwave (97020) and diathermy (97024)
Whirlpool (97022) and hubbard tank (97220)
Iontophoresis (97120) and electrical stimulation (unattended) (97014)
Microwave (97020) and infrared (97026)
Infrared (97026) and ultraviolet (97028)
Functional activities (97114) and activities of daily living (97540)
Orthotics training (97500) and prosthetic training (97520)
The following are considered controversial techniques:
Alexander technique
Hot clay/mud
Hellerwork
Inversion therapy
Myotherapy
Rolfing

*In rare clinical circumstances, both services in each pair may be appropriate. Used by permission from the American Physical Therapy Association.

spent with the patient or procedures completed. Physical therapy managers have found that this problem usually stems from two primary problems. The first is inadequate recording of time or procedures at the time of treatment so that when the therapist produces the daily charges (usually at the end of the day), that therapist may have to rely on memory. This problem is fairly easily corrected by monitoring the therapists and developing fiscal recordkeeping forms and formats such as daily log forms that the therapist can carry during the day.

The more difficult problem faced by the manager of the physical therapy service is the therapist's attitude that the service provided may not be worth the charge. That therapist then manipulates the charge system to reflect fewer charges for the services provided. The physical therapy manager must recognize this problem early and not let it continue to disrupt the charge/reimbursement system. Careful orientation of the new employee with attention to the manner in which the charge system has been developed, the reimbursement levels of the charges, and the impact on the department if services are not adequately billed is critical. In addition, managers must recognize that this is not just an issue for the novice or new employee. As the cost of delivering care continues to increase, physical therapy charges rise as well. The physical therapist who once delivered care for $50 may feel that the level of care has not changed but that the same service is now being charged at a $75 rate. Remarkably, most professionals do not tie their increasing salary and personal benefits into charge systems, and they do not necessarily stay well informed regarding the cost of health care. Regular inservices by the physical therapy manager, personnel department professionals, financial officers, marketing professionals, and hospital administrators will give the professional and support staff opportunities to ask questions related to costs of service delivery and to understand the changing environment of health care systems.

In order to assure accuracy of billing data, many physical therapy managers are training billing clerks to check billing data, make changes as appropriate, maintain regular contact with insurers, attend reimbursement workshops, and follow up on denied claims. This investment has proven to significantly improve reimbursement.

· · · · · · · · · · ·
DEFINITIONS

Bundled services: When several procedures may be grouped into a single designation such as "office visit."

COB: Coordination of benefits. An example of coordination of benefits is family coverage through a spouse.

CPT codes: Current procedural terminology codes are designed and maintained by the AMA for use by physicians. For example, 90000 = brief level of service, new patient.

Deliverables: Items or services that you must provide at the end or within a budget period.

Direct expenses: Expenses specifically incurred by a department or service.

HCPCS codes: HCFA's (Health Care Financing Administration's) common procedure coding system. Designed and maintained by HCFA, these codes include CPT and additional nationally uniform codes. For example, M000X = physical therapy office visit.

ICD codes: International classification of diseases. For example, 847.0 = sprain, cervical.

ICD-9-CM codes: International classification of diseases, Ninth Revision, clinical modification.

Indirect expenses: Expenses incurred by the organization as a whole.

Line-item budgets: The budget is presented as a long list of items to be evaluated one by one.

Local codes: Designed and maintained by individual insurers. Specific services and codes will vary.

Modifiers: Alphanumerics used to indicate special circumstances, e.g., in CPT, 97110 is therapeutic exercise, but 97110-52 is therapeutic exercise in a group setting.

Sales budgets: Budgets that are based on sales. The sales may be reflected in historical form, by consumer group, or a number of other ways.

SOC: Start of care. The date when services began. Often listed on insurance forms as SOC date: _____.

UB82: Uniform Bill for facility services.

Unbundled services: Procedures or services are reported as specific separate services or procedures.

Variable budgets: Expense budgets that are expressed as a percentage of sales instead of absolute dollars.

Zero-base budgets: Used to budget staff and overhead. It assumes a starting point of zero in planning the next budget period and all programs must be justified from that base rather than automatically considering the program to continue at some increment above or below the previous level of funding.

References

1. Rasmussen B: Billing codes: Problems, options. *Clin Management* 1991; 11:20–23.

Suggested Readings

Brown SR: Selling your practice. *Phys Ther Today* 1990; 13:60–61.

Campbell TL, et al: *Principles of Accounting,* San Diego, Calif, Harcourt Brace Jovanovich, 1989.

Deaton WC: Establishing or expanding your practice: Forecasting your initial cash needs. *Phys Ther Today* 1989; 12:19–24.

Deaton WC: Obtaining financing for the private practice. *Phys Ther Today* 1989; 12:48–53.

DePaoli TL: Medicare reimbursement in home care. *Am J Occup Ther* 1984; 38:739–742.

Domenech MA, et al: Utilization of physical therapy personnel in one hospital. *Phys Ther* 1983; 63:1108–1112.

Ferguson C: Balancing the budget. *Rehab Management* 1990; 3:73–84.

Front J: A consideration for reimbursement. *Whirlpool* 1986; 9:22–26.

Harvard Business Review: *Getting Numbers You Can Trust: The New Accounting.* Boston, Mass, Harvard University Press, 1991.

Hill CJ: Never Say "Die" (or "Deny"). *Phys Ther Today* 1989; 12:63–66.

Magary JL: The fundamental elements of medicare documentation. *Phys Ther Today* 1988; 11:23–30.

Milakovich ME: Creating a total quality health care environment. *Health Care Manage Rev* 1991; 16:40–45.

Nolan MF: Documenting patient care with TENS suggestions for reducing reimbursement denials. *Clin Management* 1988; 8:16–19.

Nold EG: Developing reports. *Am J Hosp Pharm* 1983; 40:1968–1975.

Rodriguez D: Strategic financial planning for rehabilitation companies. *Phys Ther Today* 1988; 11:32–34.

Schorr B: Health care business deals: Kickbacks or capitalism? *Phys Ther Today* 1989; 12:35–42.

Zuidema GD, et al: Documentation of care and prospective payment. *Ann Surg* 1984; 199:515–521.

APPENDIX 15.1:

Common Physical Therapy Shorthand

A–B

AA	Active assistive
Abd	Abduction
AC joint	Acromioclavicular joint
ACL	Anterior cruciate ligament
ADD	Administration of development disabilities
Add	Adduction
ADL	Activities of daily living
AE	Above elbow
AFO	Ankle foot orthosis
AK	Above knee
AKA	Above-knee amputation
Ant	Anterior
ASIS	Anterior superior iliac spine
AWP	Arm whirlpool
B	Bilateral
BE	Below elbow
Bil	Bilateral
BKA	Below-knee amputation

· · · · · · · · · · ·
B—H

BME	Brief maximal effort
BP	Blood pressure
CB	Contrast baths
CCS	Crippled children's service
CHI	Closed head injury
CMV	Cytomegalovirus
COTA	Certified occupational therapy assistant
CP	Cerebral palsy
CPM	Continuous passive motion
CPT	Chest physical therapy
CTLSO	Cervicothoracolumbosacral orthosis (scoliosis brace with neck ring)
CW	Continuous wave
D (prefix)	Direct
D1,2	Diagonal 1, 2 (PNF patterns)
DC	Discontinue
DD	Developmental disabilities
DIP joint	Distal interphalangeal joint
DS	Down's syndrome
DTR	Deep tendon reflexes
DVC	Direct voltage current
Dx	Diagnosis
EDX	Electrodiagnostic examination
EM	Electromagnetic radiation
EMF	Electromotive force
EMG	Electromyogram
EMR	Educable mental retardation
EMS	Electrical muscle stimulation
ERA	Effective radiating area
ES	Electrical stimulation
EX	Exercise
Ext	Extension
Ext rot	External rotation
FE	Free exercise
FES	Functional electrical stimulation
Flex	Flexion
FO	Foot orthosis (shoe inserts)
FW	Free weights
FWB	Full weight bearing
GaAs	Gallium arsenide laser
GFI/GFCI	Ground fault circuit interrupter
GT	Gait training
GTO	Golgi tendon organ
H & C	Heat and cold
H/O	History of
HBO	Hyperbaric oxygen
HCP	Hemicorporectomy
HD	Hip disarticulation
HeNe	Helium neon laser
HFC	Hip flexion contracture
HKAFO	Hip knee ankle foot orthosis (long leg brace)

. . . .
H–P

HP	Hot pack
HPV	Hemipelvectomy
HT	Hubbard tank
Hx	History
Hz	Hertz
I (prefix)	Indirect
IEP	Individual educational plan
Int rot	Internal rotation
IPSF	Immediate postsurgical fitting
IR	Infrared
J cane	Single-tipped cane
KAFO	Knee ankle foot orthsis
KD	Knee disarticulation
KFC	Knee flexion contracture
Lat	Lateral
LBQC	Large based quad cane
LBWP	Low boy whirlpool
LCL	Lateral collateral ligament
LE	Lower extremity
LEA	Local educational administrator
LOM	Limitation of motion
LPTA	Licensed physical therapist assistant
LSO	Lumbosacral orthosis (corset)
LWP	Leg whirlpool
MCH	Maternal and child health
MCL	Medical collateral ligament
MCP joint	Metacarpalphalangeal joint
MD	Muscular dystrophy
MED	Minimal erythemal dose
Med	Medial
MH	Moist heat
MHz	Megahertz
MMT	Manual muscle test
MPQ	McGill Pain Questionnaire
MR	Mental retardation
MS	Multiple sclerosis
MSK	Musculoskeletal
MTP joint	Metatarsalphalangeal joint
MVA	Moving vehicle accident
MW	Microwave
NCV	Nerve conduction velocity
neg	Negative
NK Table	Table for exercising lower extremities
nl	Normal
NWB	Nonweight bearing
OPD	Outpatient department
ORIF	Open reduction internal fixation
OT	Occupational therapist
P-bars	Parallel bars
Para	Paraplegia, paraplegic
PB	Powder board
PCL	Posterior cruciate ligament

. . . .
P–T

PD	Postural drainage
PE	Physical exams
PH	Past history
Phono	Phonophoresis
PIP joint	Proximal interphalangeal joint
PMR	Physical medicine and rehabilitation
PMR	Profound mental retardation
PNF	Proprioceptive neuromuscular facilitation
POMR	Problem-oriented medical record
pos	Positive
Post	Posterior
PPOC	Patient plan of care
PRE	Progressive resistance exercise
PSIS	Posterior superior iliac spine
PT	Physical therapist
pt	Patient
PTA	Physical therapist assistant
PTA	Prior to admission
PTB	Patellar tendon bearing (prosthesis or orthosis)
PUW	Pick up walker
PW	Pulsed wave
PWB	Partial weight bearing
Quad	Quadriceps, quadriplegia, quadriplegic
R/O	Rule out
RL	Residual limb (substitution for stump)
RM	Repitition maximum
Rmin	Repitition minimum
ROM	Range of motion
Rx	Treatment
s/p	Status post
SA	Standby assistance
SACH	Solid ankle cushion heel (prosthetic foot)
SAQ	Short arc quads
SAR	Specific absorption rate
SB	Sandbag
SBQC	Short based quad cane
SC joint	Sternoclavicular joint
SCI	Spinal cord injury
SCM	Sternocleidomastoid muscle
SCSP	Supracondylar suprapatellar
SEA	State educational administrator
SI joint	Sacroiliac joint
SOAP	Subjective, objective, assessment, plan
SOB	Shortness of breath
SW (SWD)	Short wave diathermy
SWID	Shortwave induction drum
SWP	Sterile whirlpool
Sx	Symptom
T strap	Shoe correction
TBI	Traumatic brain injury
TDWB	Touch down weight bearing
TE	Therapeutic exercise

T–Z

TENS	Transcutaneous electrical nerve stimulation
THA	Total hip arthroplasty
THR	Total hip replacement
TKE	Terminal knee extension (short arc quads)
TKR	Total knee replacement
TLSO	Thoracolumbosacral orthosis (hyperextension brace)
TMJ	Temporomandibular joint
TMR	Trainable mental retardation
TPR	Temperature, pulse, respiration
TT	Tilt table
TTWB	Toe touch weight bearing
Tx	Traction
UCB	Univ of CA at Berkeley shoe insert
UE	Upper extremity
US	Ultrasound
UV	Ultraviolet
VC	Vital capacity
VO	Verbal order
VR	Vocational rehabilitation
WB	Weight bearing
WBAT	Weight bearing as tolerated
WBTT	Weight bearing to tolerance
WC	Wheelchair
WCE	Work capacity evaluation
WL	Weight loading
WNL	Within normal limits
WP	Whirlpool
xs	excess

SYMBOLS

≈	approximately	↑	increase, up
↓	decrease, down	Ⓛ	left
°	degree	<	less than
=	equal	♂	male
/	extension	‖	parallel bars
♀	female	1°	primary
✓	flexion	Ⓡ	right
'	foot, feet	2°	secondary
>	greater than		
"	inch, inches		

CHAPTER 16

The Future of Physical Therapy Management

. . . .

    I. The health care system in the United States

   II. Cost containment

 III. Health care organizations

  IV. Recruitment and retention

   V. Career paths for physical therapy managers

. . . .

THE HEALTH CARE SYSTEM IN THE UNITED STATES

In a survey conducted by the Gallup Organization in late 1990, ninety-one percent of 387 chief executives from the Fortune 500 service and industrial lists felt that fundamental changes or complete rebuilding of the [health care] system is needed.[1] In 1992 there were over 20 bills submitted to Congress proposing some form of national health insurance. The common trend among these bills was cost containment. Health care costs have grown steadily over the past 40 years as have the number of underinsured individuals in the United States. Although there were many attempts to control health care costs (certificate of need [CON], professional services review organization [PSRO], managed health care, peer review organizations [PRO]) in the 1980s, very little resulted from these attempts.

The cost of health care as an employment benefit drives the cost of goods and services up in those industries where health care benefits are provided. A little over half of all Americans rely on employer-sponsored health insurance programs. Employers spent $176.8 billion dollars in 1989 for health benefits. Some major manufacturing companies in the United States spend in excess of $1 billion dollars per year to provide health care benefits to employees. For most smaller companies, the costs of providing health care benefits are prohibitive, leaving millions of individuals without insurance or with inadequate insurance.

Whatever national health system or piecemeal health legislation is adopted over the next decade, it is certain to focus on cost containment. Many of the bills in Congress suggest incentive programs for individuals to take care of themselves by not smoking and engaging in stress and weight-reduction programs. There is also a focus on quality assessment and a closer monitoring of the effectiveness of treatment. At some point health care professions and professionals will have to re-establish their ability to police themselves as tort (malpractice) reform places caps on awards to patients and their families. Perhaps the hardest of all jobs and one that will involve all health care managers is the rationing of health care or the determination of minimal health services needed for varying age groups and disability groups. The careful development and testing of triage systems in physical therapy now will lay the groundwork for these systems in the future.

COST CONTAINMENT

Currently the profession of physical therapy is more reactive than proactive when it comes to cost containment and reimbursement issues. There is little nationally available epidemiological data in physical therapy upon which to build effective cost-containment systems. However, the local clinical practice abounds with data. Physical therapy managers must form partnerships or engage epidemiologists and health service researchers to develop recording systems and train individuals to appropriately collect and analyze the data. Local reimbursement agencies are anxious to receive well-grounded data, but without it, they will develop systems of reimbursement based on their experience with the discipline. This kind of approach could be disastrous to the fiscal base of the service delivery in physical therapy.

In addition to the task of collecting data, physical therapy managers can begin building a relationship with major insurers to provide expert opinions and input when these agencies move ahead with decisions related to physical therapy. Many disciplines have as little national data available as physical therapy, but they are recognized as experts when decisions are made that may affect the discipline.

HEALTH CARE ORGANIZATIONS

As health care becomes more complex, health care management at all levels also becomes more complex. Physical therapy managers in large complex organizations or in independent practice settings must possess management skills that reach beyond the intuitive skills that propelled many physical therapists into these positions in the past. Physical therapy managers must be able to plan, assess the market, develop innovative management approaches to problems, maximize reimbursement for services, and creatively manage scarce resources of people, time, money, space, and equipment.

Many physical therapy departments are faced with the dilemma of being managed by non–physical therapists who have acquired the advanced management skills necessary to function in the complex environment. Some physical therapy departments are experimentally engaging in alternative organizational structures such as service line management in order to deliver services most effectively and efficiently with less duplication of programs and services. In some cases these systems are working, but in many organizations physical therapy managers are either not chosen for these management positions, are not able to manage these multidisciplinary units, or are not interested in moving into this aspect of management. Many physical therapist managers state that alternative organizational structures work for physical therapy if a physical therapist is in charge, but they don't work when other disciplines are in charge. Why? Physical therapy managers must move away from traditional modes of management and reconsider organizational structures and departmental boundaries in order to compete in the evolving health care system.

Health care systems will continue to move toward multihospital and multiservice centers where costs can be centralized, referral systems enhanced, services streamlined, and costs controlled. It will be a challenge to the physical therapy manager to keep pace with the changing systems, plan innovative programs and services, and provide state-of-the-art services in new environments.

Competition will also continue to drive both complex and simple organizations. The physical therapy manager will be obligated to gain skills in marketing management in order to understand the competition and to recognize and create marketing opportunities.

The Japanese management system and its emphasis on continuing quality assessment will continue to have an influence on American industry. Although the success of this approach was greatly enhanced by the Japanese culture, American business (including the health care industry) is becoming convinced that continuous quality improvement is a key to turning out better products and keeping employees more satisfied in their work environment. The Deming principles are already being applied to physical therapy practice settings with emphasis on the ongoing assessment of quality, correction of performance discrepancies within the worksite, and a shift away from assessment of quality that is based on the end product which "blames" or "rewards" the individual worker. Physical therapy managers are learning that success or failure of a service is a dynamic process that must be dynamically analyzed and corrected.

RECRUITMENT AND RETENTION

As the profession of physical therapy continues to grow and diversify, it will become increasingly difficult to attract and keep physical therapists in complex organizational structures where autonomy is limited. The physical therapy manager must consider the physical therapist and physical therapist assistant as a target market and develop strategies to recruit and retain these individuals within the system. Creative benefit packages, day care, public transportation, enhanced parking, sabbaticals, leaves of absence, rotation to a variety of services and facilities, the opportunity to advance clinically, continuing education, and consulting experts on the premises are just a few of the considerations that will have to be explored to attract the limited number of physical therapists.

Physical therapy managers will also have to lead the way for partnerships with educational institutions to increase physical therapy class sizes to meet the growing demand for physical therapists. Higher education develops curricula that produce quality graduates. The class size is determined primarily by the resources available at the university. In order to increase class sizes, physical therapy educational program directors are considering partnerships with the health care industry to develop creative programs to retrain physical therapists who have been out of the field for some time, to provide second career tracks for individuals already in the health care system or related systems, and to provide quality education to a larger number of traditional applicants. At the same time, physical therapy managers must be open to new clinical education models such as student-run clinics that allow a greater number of students to engage in the clinical education component of the educational program.

CAREER PATHS FOR PHYSICAL THERAPY MANAGERS

The majority of physical therapy managers find themselves in management positions because of longevity, interest, perceptions of advancement, networking, or coercion. Many physical therapy managers are promoted to managerial positions because they are exceptional physical therapists with outstanding communication skills. After agreeing to take on the job of managing the department, the manager discovers the myriad of skills needed to be an effective manager and is then faced with the dilemma of letting go of some of the practice skills that propelled the individual to the management position in order to pursue continuing and formal education in management. This is the traditional path. Although this path continues to work, it will not prepare the physical therapy manager in management theory and advanced management skills and will not necessarily give the manager skills that are easily marketed to other environments.

Health care management is complex, and it is an academic discipline. Continuing education courses in management usually provide or enhance skills, but these courses do not advance the management novice in a predictable manner to apply management theory to increasingly complex situations with a special emphasis on health care. Although many fine administrators come from traditional management academic backgrounds, the majority have had extensive coursework in health care management. For those managers who are not inclined to pursue formal education, they may have to consider non–physical therapy managers as partners or colleagues within the management level of the department. If these individuals are in systems with changing administrative structures, they may also face extinction as new administrators set new goals and administrative challenges for the physical therapy manager.

The administrator can play a key role in career development. The physical therapist who is considering management as a career can often volunteer to work on special projects with managers, administrators, and staff from a variety of disciplines. In addition to making these opportunities available, the administrator can provide feedback concerning skills in planning, marketing, developing innovative concepts, and a variety of other skills that demonstrate the individual's acumen for a career in management. Most physical therapists have the intelligence to pursue a formal education in management. In addition, the individual should seek counsel regarding analytical interests and personal characteristics as they apply to careers in management. Career counselors or career centers can provide batteries of tests to determine the individual's likelihood of success in this career path.

Within the department, career ladders focusing on management skills are usually available to physical therapists. These ladders include the opportunity to engage in projects, senior physical therapist positions, and a variety of jobs at the Assistant Director level. Once a therapist has indicated a desire to move in this direction and the manager and administrator agree that the individual is likely to succeed, then in-house training may be available as well as job rotations, special projects, tuition assistance, and job enrichment opportunities.

A time of change is also a time of opportunity. The health care system and the physical therapy profession are changing drastically. Managers are faced with challenges that were not imagined 10 years ago. With change comes the opportunity for innovative planning and implementation. Managing in a time of scarcity forces new thinking and planning activities. A career as a physical therapy manager should not be a case of moving into a position with a relative degree of incompetence. It should be a conscious choice in which the individual is academically prepared, understands the job of the manager as well as those of superiors and subordinates; is able to assess the environment; and is equipped with management tools that are necessary to facilitate the delivery of the highest possible level of services with the highest possible return to the institution.

Reference

1. 1990 national executive poll on health care cost and benefits. *Business Health,* 1990, pp:25–38.

Index

· ·